The Diabetes
Problem
Solver

The Diabetes Problem Solver

Nancy Touchette, PhD

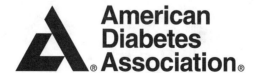
American Diabetes Association

Book Acquisitions, Robert J. Anthony; *Editor,* Laurie Guffey; *Production Director,* Carolyn R. Segree; *Production Coordinator,* Peggy M. Rote; *Composition,* Harlowe Typography, Inc.; *Text and Cover Design,* Wickham & Associates, Inc.; *Printer,* Port City Press, Inc.

Printed in the United States of America
1 3 5 7 9 10 8 6 4 2

The suggestions and information contained in this publication are generally consistent with the *Clinical Practice Recommendations* and other policies of the American Diabetes Association, but they do not represent the policy or position of the Association or any of its boards or committees. Reasonable steps have been taken to ensure the accuracy of the information presented. However, the American Diabetes Association cannot ensure the safety or efficacy of any product or service described in this publication. Individuals are advised to consult a physician or other appropriate health care professional before undertaking any diet or exercise program or taking any medication referred to in this publication. Professionals must use and apply their own professional judgment, experience, and training and should not rely solely on the information contained in this publication before prescribing any diet, exercise, or medication. The American Diabetes Association—its officers, directors, employees, volunteers, and members—assumes no responsibility or liability for personal or other injury, loss, or damage that may result from the suggestions or information in this publication.

ADA titles may be purchased for business or promotional use or for special sales. For information, please write to Lee M. Romano, Special Sales & Promotions, at the address below.

American Diabetes Association
1660 Duke Street
Alexandria, Virginia 22314

Library of Congress Cataloging-in-Publication Data
Touchette, Nancy.
    The diabetes problem solver / by Nancy Touchette.
       p.   cm.
    Includes index.
    ISBN 1-57040-009-1 (pbk)
    1. Diabetes Popular works.   I. Title.
RC660.4.T68   1999
616.4'62—dc21   99-28366
                                        CIP

To the memory of my father, Hermes F. Touchette,
who showed me what living with diabetes is all about.

Table of Contents

Preface

If you or someone close to you has diabetes, you probably already realize the importance of healthy living. Living well with diabetes simply means living well. Eating the right foods and getting enough exercise isn't just good advice for people with diabetes—it's good advice for anyone. If you have diabetes, you have learned—or perhaps are still learning—how to balance your food intake and physical activity with your insulin or oral medication in order to keep your blood glucose levels where you want them. This is the cornerstone of diabetes care and will go a long way in preventing the complications of diabetes and helping you live a long and healthy life.

Even if you practice healthy habits and have mastered the art of good blood glucose control, problems are bound to come up every now and then. Your blood glucose level falls too low, you develop an infection, or you are having problems coping. Sometimes it is clear what is happening and you know how to handle the situation. But there may be times when you experience symptoms you aren't used to and you don't know what to do. That's where *The Diabetes Problem Solver* comes in.

This book can help you recognize the signs and symptoms of some of the conditions you may encounter as a person with diabetes. It is not intended to substitute for a doctor's care or advice, but simply to point you in the right direction so you can start asking questions. If you are in doubt about something you are feeling, *The Diabetes Problem Solver* can help you identify symptoms you are experiencing and help you decide whether you need to wait out the problem, call your doctor, or get treatment at once. Of course, if you are ever in doubt about any kind of health problem or medical condition, are experiencing unusual symp toms, or are in great pain or discomfort, call your doctor or a member of your health care team right away.

The Diabetes Problem Solver is divided into two major sections. The first section, "Guide to Symptoms of Diabetes," consists of a series of flowcharts to help you decide what you need to do about a particular condition or symptom. The second section, "Problems of Diabetes," provides more detailed information about many of the problems people with diabetes face, from controlling blood glucose levels or dealing with the complications of diabetes to facing discrimination in the schools or enjoying a fulfilling sex life.

You can use *The Diabetes Problem Solver* in two ways. If you already know you have a particular condition, or want more information on a particular condition, you can go straight to the second section and look up the condition directly. The chapter contents are listed in the Table of Contents or you can look up subjects in the index. Once you find the particular condition you are interested in, you can read about it in more detail. Each section is organized to provide you with the following information:

- SYMPTOMS tell you what to look for
- RISKS provide information about who is at risk for the condition and what risk the particular condition poses for you
- WHAT TO DO tells you what your immediate course of action should be
- TREATMENT tells you how your condition may be treated in a medical setting
- PREVENTION provides information about how to prevent the condition from developing

You can also use *The Diabetes Problem Solver* to guide you to possible conditions that may be causing your symptoms by turning to the flowcharts on page 1. For example, if you are experiencing nausea, you can go to chart 1, Nausea. You will be asked a series of yes and no questions. As you answer the questions, you will be guided through a path that will provide you with a possible condition that may be causing your symptoms. Bear in mind that this is not an accurate diagnosis, and should not substitute for a call to your health care team. The charts can, however, provide you with information to help you decide whether your situation is an emergency and whether it requires prompt attention. Once you have an idea of what might be causing your problem, you can go to the second section for further information about a particular condition.

As you work your way through any particular chart, make sure to also look at alternative paths through the chart. The chart is designed to guide you to a particular condition based on the symptoms that most people experience. However, you may not always experience all those symptoms, or you may experience one or two symptoms differently than anyone else. Also, you may have more than one complicating condition, which could further confound your attempts to determine the source of your problem. Look at each chart as an overview, then try to narrow down your search for your particular problem. Don't necessarily exclude one pathway because you are missing one of the symptoms.

At the end of each pathway, you will be told where in this book you can find further information. You will also be given advice about what to do. If you are told to call your doctor or seek emergency help immediately or without delay, it means to take action **within minutes**. This could be a life-threatening situation in which every minute counts. If you are told to call your doctor right away, it means to take action **within a few hours**. The condition may not be an emergency, but it could be serious and needs prompt attention. If you are told to call your doctor as soon as possible, it means to call your doctor **within a few days**. Of course, any time you are in great discomfort, experiencing pain, or simply feel that something is not quite right, call your doctor right away. This book is in no way intended to substitute for good medical care. Rather, it is my hope that it will point you in the right direction as you look for the information you need.

No one cares about your health as much as you do. I hope that *The Diabetes Problem Solver* will serve as a useful tool in helping you take charge of your diabetes care. The more you know about diabetes, the better equipped you are to work with the members of your health care team to ensure you get the very best care and live a long and healthy life.

Nancy Touchette, PhD

Acknowledgments

I would like to thank Peter Banks for suggesting this book and serving as a guiding light throughout the writing process, Laurie Guffey for patience beyond the call of duty, and Laura James for guidance and support. Most of all, thanks to my family, Caroline, Julie, Katy, and Randy Bryant, for pitching in and putting up with my erratic schedule as the eleventh hour closed in.

Guide to
Symptoms of Diabetes

Below is a list of flowcharts (and the page numbers where you'll find them) that give you information on some of the common problems you may be experiencing. Please read the Preface, pages xiii–xv, to learn how to use these flowcharts and what some of the directions you'll find there mean.

1. Nausea
Feelings of nausea, upset stomach, and stomach discomfort

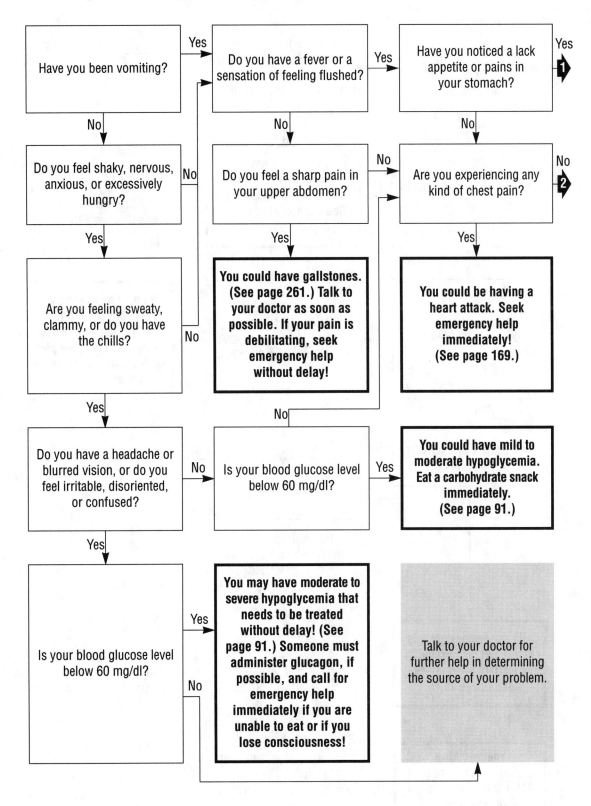

Have you been vomiting?

→ Yes → Do you have a fever or a sensation of feeling flushed?

→ Yes → Have you noticed a lack appetite or pains in your stomach?

→ Yes → **1**

No ↓

Do you feel shaky, nervous, anxious, or excessively hungry?

No → Do you feel a sharp pain in your upper abdomen?

No → Are you experiencing any kind of chest pain?

→ No → **2**

No ↓ (from fever box)

Yes ↓

Are you feeling sweaty, clammy, or do you have the chills?

No →

Yes ↓ (sharp pain) →

You could have gallstones. (See page 261.) Talk to your doctor as soon as possible. If your pain is debilitating, seek emergency help without delay!

Yes ↓ (chest pain) →

You could be having a heart attack. Seek emergency help immediately! (See page 169.)

Yes ↓

Do you have a headache or blurred vision, or do you feel irritable, disoriented, or confused?

No → Is your blood glucose level below 60 mg/dl?

→ Yes → **You could have mild to moderate hypoglycemia. Eat a carbohydrate snack immediately. (See page 91.)**

No (from abdomen/chest) →

Yes ↓

Is your blood glucose level below 60 mg/dl?

→ Yes → **You may have moderate to severe hypoglycemia that needs to be treated without delay! (See page 91.) Someone must administer glucagon, if possible, and call for emergency help immediately if you are unable to eat or if you lose consciousness!**

No →

Talk to your doctor for further help in determining the source of your problem.

1. Nausea
Feelings of nausea, upset stomach, and stomach discomfort *(Continued)*

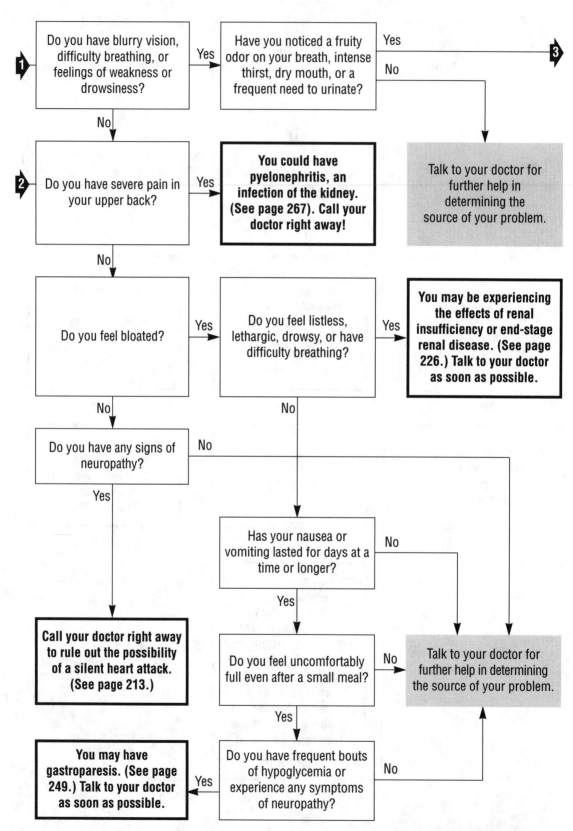

1. Do you have blurry vision, difficulty breathing, or feelings of weakness or drowsiness? — Yes → Have you noticed a fruity odor on your breath, intense thirst, dry mouth, or a frequent need to urinate? — Yes → **3.** / No → Talk to your doctor for further help in determining the source of your problem.

No ↓

2. Do you have severe pain in your upper back? — Yes → **You could have pyelonephritis, an infection of the kidney. (See page 267). Call your doctor right away!**

No ↓

Do you feel bloated? — Yes → Do you feel listless, lethargic, drowsy, or have difficulty breathing? — Yes → **You may be experiencing the effects of renal insufficiency or end-stage renal disease. (See page 226.) Talk to your doctor as soon as possible.**

No ↓

Do you have any signs of neuropathy? — No →

Yes ↓

Call your doctor right away to rule out the possibility of a silent heart attack. (See page 213.)

Has your nausea or vomiting lasted for days at a time or longer? — No → Talk to your doctor for further help in determining the source of your problem.

Yes ↓

Do you feel uncomfortably full even after a small meal? — No → Talk to your doctor for further help in determining the source of your problem.

Yes ↓

Do you have frequent bouts of hypoglycemia or experience any symptoms of neuropathy? — No → Talk to your doctor for further help in determining the source of your problem.

Yes → **You may have gastroparesis. (See page 249.) Talk to your doctor as soon as possible.**

1. Nausea
Feelings of nausea, upset stomach, and stomach discomfort *(Continued)*

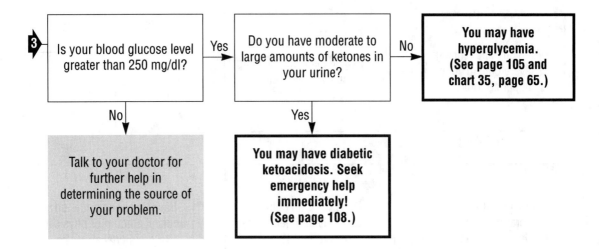

3 Is your blood glucose level greater than 250 mg/dl?

Yes → Do you have moderate to large amounts of ketones in your urine?

No → **You may have hyperglycemia. (See page 105 and chart 35, page 65.)**

No ↓ Talk to your doctor for further help in determining the source of your problem.

Yes ↓ **You may have diabetic ketoacidosis. Seek emergency help immediately! (See page 108.)**

2. Stomach Pain
Feeling any kind of pain or cramping in the stomach or abdomen

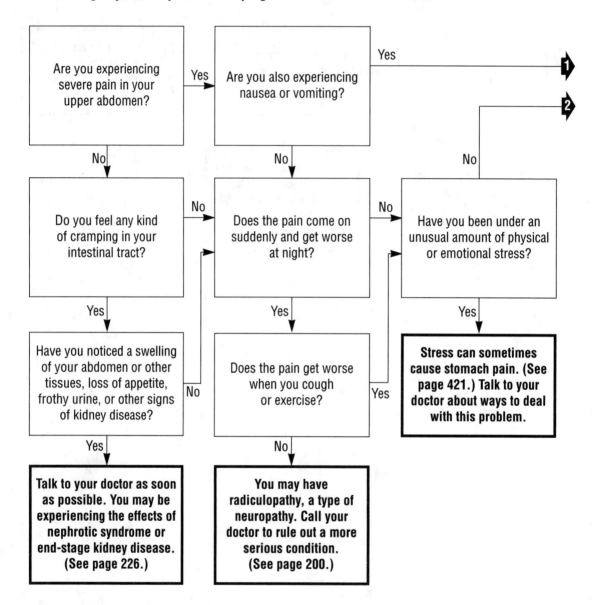

2. Stomach Pain
Feeling any kind of pain or cramping in the stomach or abdomen *(Continued)*

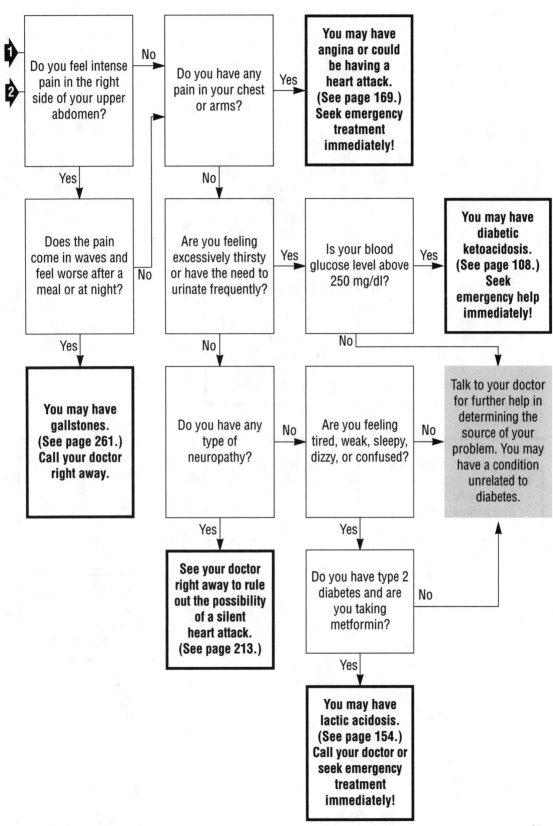

3. Difficulty Breathing
Feeling breathless, short of breath, or tightness in the chest

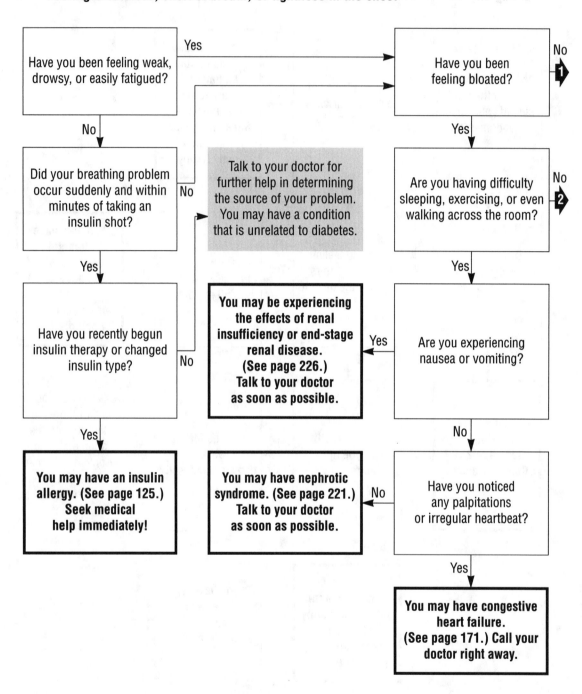

Have you been feeling weak, drowsy, or easily fatigued?

Yes →

Have you been feeling bloated? — No → ❶

No ↓

Yes ↓

Did your breathing problem occur suddenly and within minutes of taking an insulin shot?

No → Talk to your doctor for further help in determining the source of your problem. You may have a condition that is unrelated to diabetes.

Are you having difficulty sleeping, exercising, or even walking across the room? — No → ❷

Yes ↓

Yes ↓

Have you recently begun insulin therapy or changed insulin type?

No → **You may be experiencing the effects of renal insufficiency or end-stage renal disease. (See page 226.) Talk to your doctor as soon as possible.**

Are you experiencing nausea or vomiting?

Yes → (to renal box)

No ↓

Yes ↓

You may have an insulin allergy. (See page 125.) Seek medical help immediately!

You may have nephrotic syndrome. (See page 221.) Talk to your doctor as soon as possible.

No → **Have you noticed any palpitations or irregular heartbeat?**

Yes ↓

You may have congestive heart failure. (See page 171.) Call your doctor right away.

3. Difficulty Breathing

Feeling breathless, short of breath, or tightness in the chest *(Continued)*

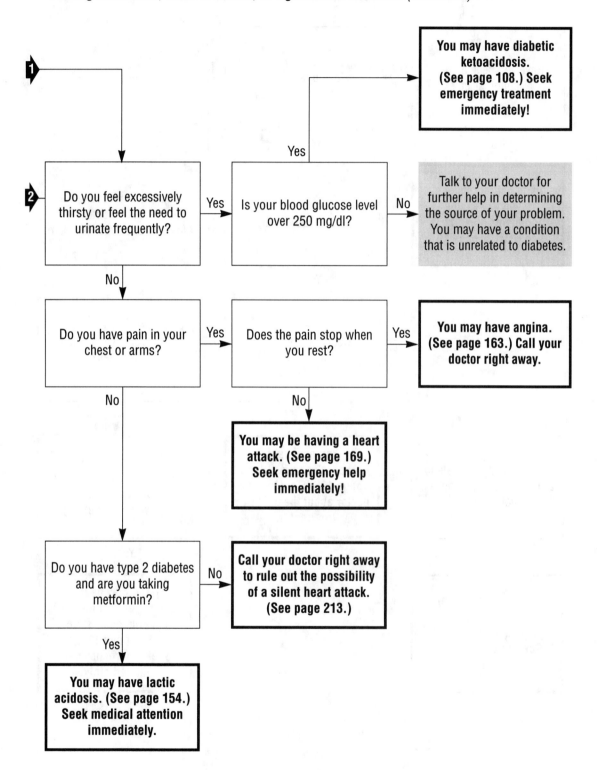

1

You may have diabetic ketoacidosis. (See page 108.) Seek emergency treatment immediately!

Yes

2 Do you feel excessively thirsty or feel the need to urinate frequently? → Yes → Is your blood glucose level over 250 mg/dl? → No → Talk to your doctor for further help in determining the source of your problem. You may have a condition that is unrelated to diabetes.

No

Do you have pain in your chest or arms? → Yes → Does the pain stop when you rest? → Yes → **You may have angina. (See page 163.) Call your doctor right away.**

No — No

You may be having a heart attack. (See page 169.) Seek emergency help immediately!

Do you have type 2 diabetes and are you taking metformin? → No → **Call your doctor right away to rule out the possibility of a silent heart attack. (See page 213.)**

Yes

You may have lactic acidosis. (See page 154.) Seek medical attention immediately.

4. Feeling Tired
Feeling tired, unusually sleepy, weak, or lacking energy

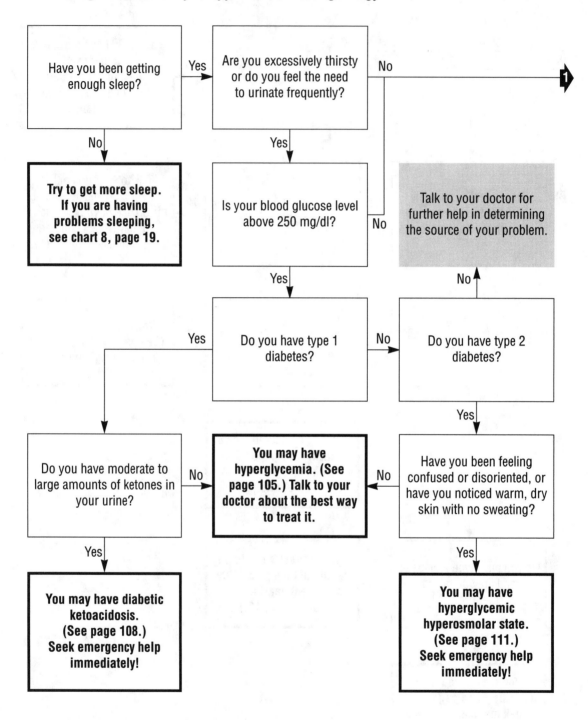

Have you been getting enough sleep?

— Yes → Are you excessively thirsty or do you feel the need to urinate frequently?

— No → **1**

Have you been getting enough sleep? — No → **Try to get more sleep. If you are having problems sleeping, see chart 8, page 19.**

Are you excessively thirsty or do you feel the need to urinate frequently? — Yes → Is your blood glucose level above 250 mg/dl?

Is your blood glucose level above 250 mg/dl? — No → Talk to your doctor for further help in determining the source of your problem.

Is your blood glucose level above 250 mg/dl? — Yes → Do you have type 1 diabetes?

Do you have type 1 diabetes? — No → Do you have type 2 diabetes?

Do you have type 2 diabetes? — No → Talk to your doctor for further help in determining the source of your problem.

Do you have type 1 diabetes? — Yes → Do you have moderate to large amounts of ketones in your urine?

Do you have moderate to large amounts of ketones in your urine? — No → **You may have hyperglycemia. (See page 105.) Talk to your doctor about the best way to treat it.**

Do you have moderate to large amounts of ketones in your urine? — Yes → **You may have diabetic ketoacidosis. (See page 108.) Seek emergency help immediately!**

Do you have type 2 diabetes? — Yes → Have you been feeling confused or disoriented, or have you noticed warm, dry skin with no sweating?

Have you been feeling confused or disoriented, or have you noticed warm, dry skin with no sweating? — No → **You may have hyperglycemia. (See page 105.) Talk to your doctor about the best way to treat it.**

Have you been feeling confused or disoriented, or have you noticed warm, dry skin with no sweating? — Yes → **You may have hyperglycemic hyperosmolar state. (See page 111.) Seek emergency help immediately!**

4. Feeling Tired
Feeling tired, unusually sleepy, weak, or lacking energy *(Continued)*

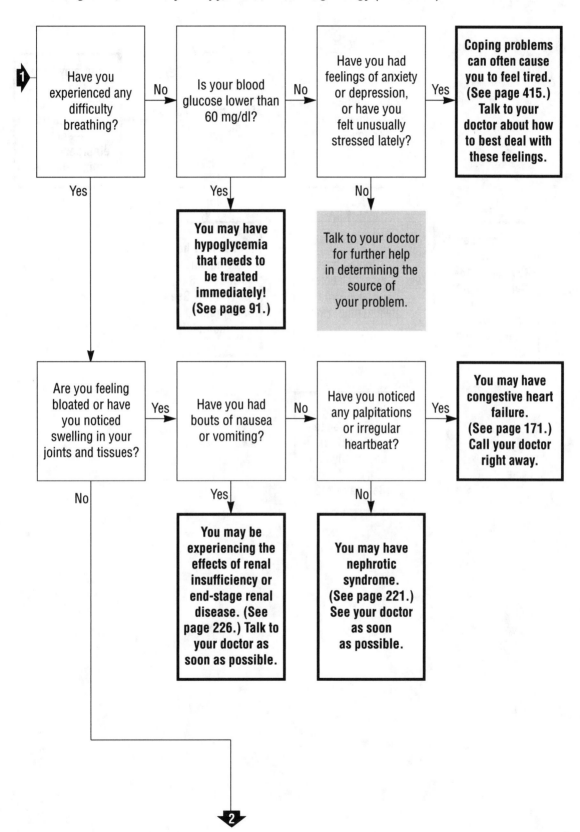

1 Have you experienced any difficulty breathing?

— No → Is your blood glucose lower than 60 mg/dl?

— No → Have you had feelings of anxiety or depression, or have you felt unusually stressed lately?

— Yes → **Coping problems can often cause you to feel tired. (See page 415.) Talk to your doctor about how to best deal with these feelings.**

Yes (from blood glucose) ↓
You may have hypoglycemia that needs to be treated immediately! (See page 91.)

No (from anxiety) ↓
Talk to your doctor for further help in determining the source of your problem.

Yes (from difficulty breathing) ↓

Are you feeling bloated or have you noticed swelling in your joints and tissues?

— Yes → Have you had bouts of nausea or vomiting?

— No → Have you noticed any palpitations or irregular heartbeat?

— Yes → **You may have congestive heart failure. (See page 171.) Call your doctor right away.**

Yes (from nausea) ↓
You may be experiencing the effects of renal insufficiency or end-stage renal disease. (See page 226.) Talk to your doctor as soon as possible.

No (from palpitations) ↓
You may have nephrotic syndrome. (See page 221.) See your doctor as soon as possible.

No (from bloated) ↓ **2**

4. Feeling Tired
Feeling tired, unusually sleepy, weak, or lacking energy *(Continued)*

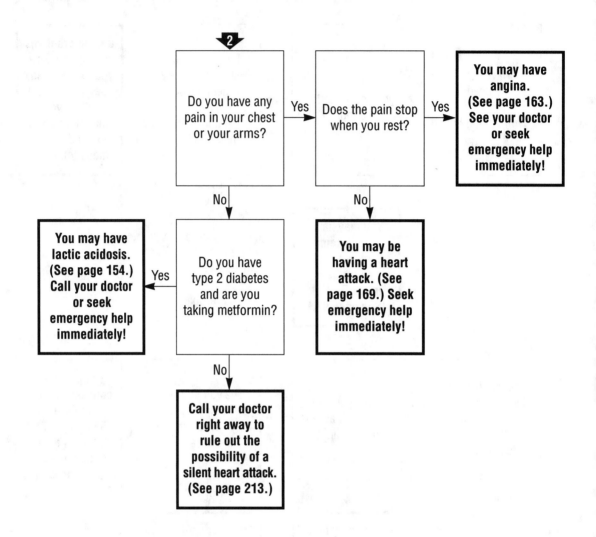

2

Do you have any pain in your chest or your arms?

— Yes → Does the pain stop when you rest?

— Yes → **You may have angina. (See page 163.) See your doctor or seek emergency help immediately!**

— No ↓

Do you have type 2 diabetes and are you taking metformin?

— No (from chest pain) ↓

— No (from pain stop when you rest) → **You may be having a heart attack. (See page 169.) Seek emergency help immediately!**

— Yes → **You may have lactic acidosis. (See page 154.) Call your doctor or seek emergency help immediately!**

— No ↓

Call your doctor right away to rule out the possibility of a silent heart attack. (See page 213.)

5. Vomiting
Throwing up of stomach contents, without nausea or stomach pain

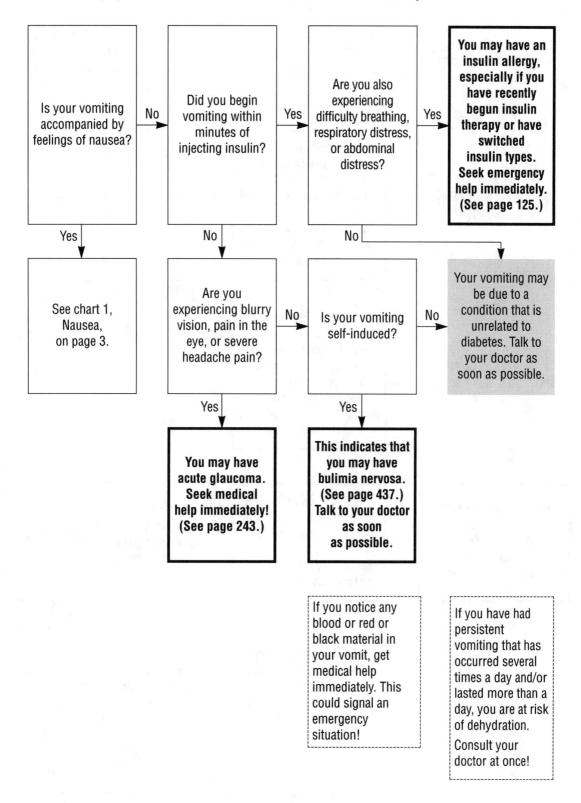

Is your vomiting accompanied by feelings of nausea?

No →

Did you begin vomiting within minutes of injecting insulin?

Yes →

Are you also experiencing difficulty breathing, respiratory distress, or abdominal distress?

Yes →

You may have an insulin allergy, especially if you have recently begun insulin therapy or have switched insulin types. Seek emergency help immediately. (See page 125.)

Yes ↓

See chart 1, Nausea, on page 3.

No ↓

Are you experiencing blurry vision, pain in the eye, or severe headache pain?

No →

Is your vomiting self-induced?

No →

Your vomiting may be due to a condition that is unrelated to diabetes. Talk to your doctor as soon as possible.

Yes ↓

You may have acute glaucoma. Seek medical help immediately! (See page 243.)

Yes ↓

This indicates that you may have bulimia nervosa. (See page 437.) Talk to your doctor as soon as possible.

If you notice any blood or red or black material in your vomit, get medical help immediately. This could signal an emergency situation!

If you have had persistent vomiting that has occurred several times a day and/or lasted more than a day, you are at risk of dehydration.

Consult your doctor at once!

6. Blurry Vision
Having vision that is blurred, out of focus, or hazy

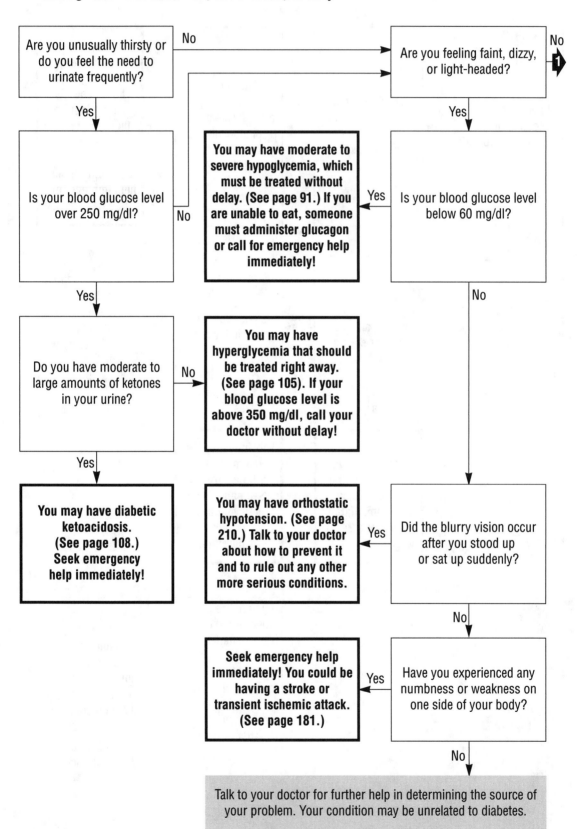

Are you unusually thirsty or do you feel the need to urinate frequently? **No** → Are you feeling faint, dizzy, or light-headed? **No** ➊

Yes ↓

Is your blood glucose level over 250 mg/dl?

No → You may have moderate to severe hypoglycemia, which must be treated without delay. (See page 91.) If you are unable to eat, someone must administer glucagon or call for emergency help immediately!

Yes ← Is your blood glucose level below 60 mg/dl?

Yes ↓

Do you have moderate to large amounts of ketones in your urine? **No** → You may have hyperglycemia that should be treated right away. (See page 105). If your blood glucose level is above 350 mg/dl, call your doctor without delay!

Yes ↓

You may have diabetic ketoacidosis. (See page 108.) Seek emergency help immediately!

You may have orthostatic hypotension. (See page 210.) Talk to your doctor about how to prevent it and to rule out any other more serious conditions. ← **Yes** Did the blurry vision occur after you stood up or sat up suddenly?

No ↓

Seek emergency help immediately! You could be having a stroke or transient ischemic attack. (See page 181.) ← **Yes** Have you experienced any numbness or weakness on one side of your body?

No ↓

Talk to your doctor for further help in determining the source of your problem. Your condition may be unrelated to diabetes.

6. Blurry Vision
Having vision that is blurred, out of focus, or hazy *(Continued)*

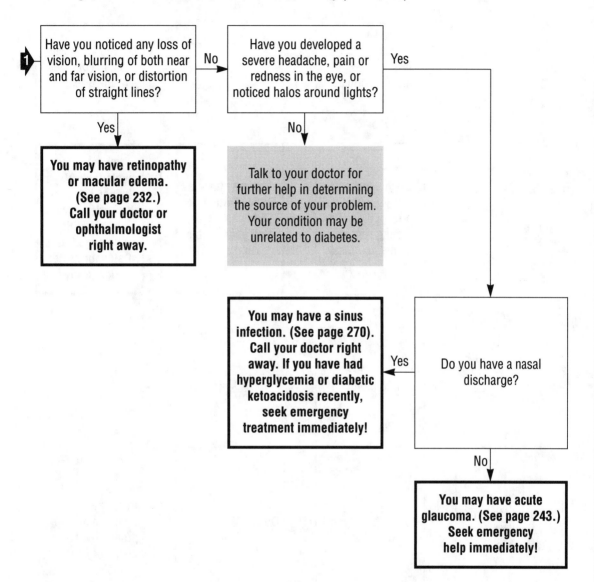

1 Have you noticed any loss of vision, blurring of both near and far vision, or distortion of straight lines?

No →

Have you developed a severe headache, pain or redness in the eye, or noticed halos around lights?

Yes →

↓ Yes

You may have retinopathy or macular edema. (See page 232.) Call your doctor or ophthalmologist right away.

↓ No

Talk to your doctor for further help in determining the source of your problem. Your condition may be unrelated to diabetes.

You may have a sinus infection. (See page 270). Call your doctor right away. If you have had hyperglycemia or diabetic ketoacidosis recently, seek emergency treatment immediately!

← Yes

Do you have a nasal discharge?

↓ No

You may have acute glaucoma. (See page 243.) Seek emergency help immediately!

7. Fever
A body temperature of 100°F or above or skin that is warm to the touch

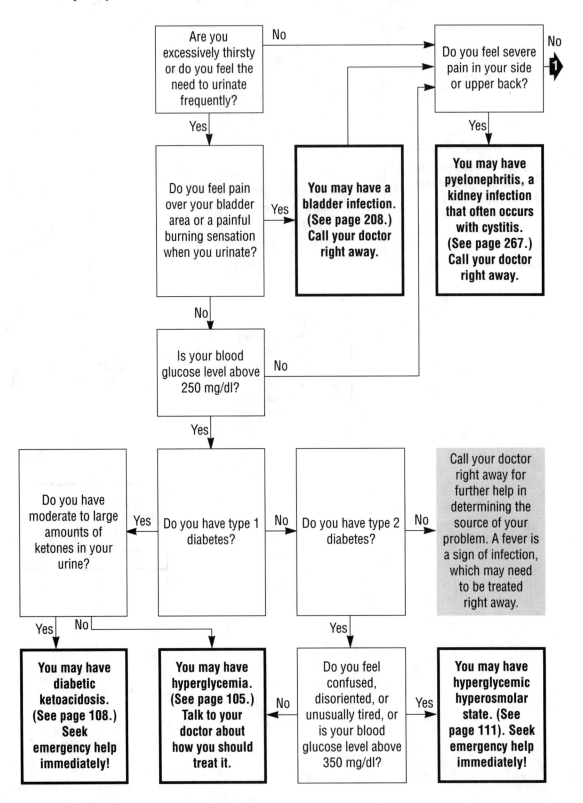

Are you excessively thirsty or do you feel the need to urinate frequently?

No → Do you feel severe pain in your side or upper back? **No** → ❶

Yes ↓

Do you feel pain over your bladder area or a painful burning sensation when you urinate?

Yes → **You may have a bladder infection. (See page 208.) Call your doctor right away.**

Do you feel severe pain in your side or upper back? **Yes** → **You may have pyelonephritis, a kidney infection that often occurs with cystitis. (See page 267.) Call your doctor right away.**

No ↓

Is your blood glucose level above 250 mg/dl? **No** →

Yes ↓

Do you have moderate to large amounts of ketones in your urine? ← **Yes** — Do you have type 1 diabetes? **No** → Do you have type 2 diabetes? **No** → Call your doctor right away for further help in determining the source of your problem. A fever is a sign of infection, which may need to be treated right away.

Yes ↓ / **No** ↓

You may have diabetic ketoacidosis. (See page 108.) Seek emergency help immediately!

You may have hyperglycemia. (See page 105.) Talk to your doctor about how you should treat it.

Do you feel confused, disoriented, or unusually tired, or is your blood glucose level above 350 mg/dl? **No** ← / **Yes** → **You may have hyperglycemic hyperosmolar state. (See page 111). Seek emergency help immediately!**

7. Fever

A body temperature of 100°F or above or skin that is warm to the touch *(Continued)*

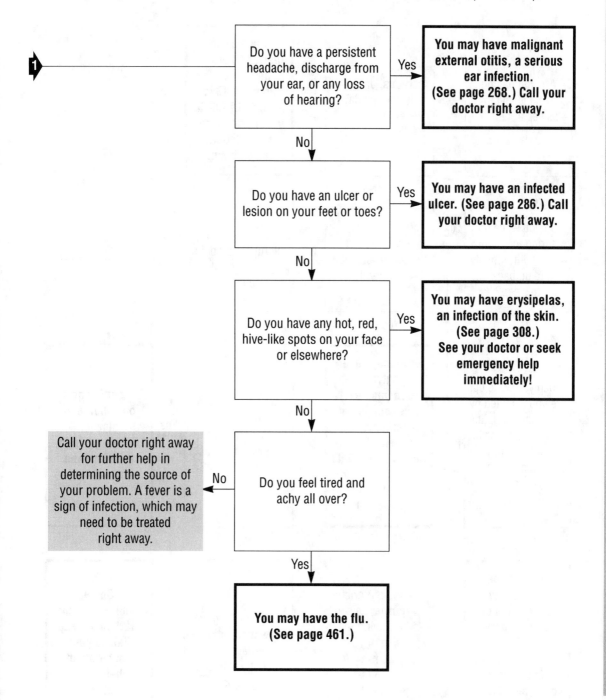

1

Do you have a persistent headache, discharge from your ear, or any loss of hearing?

Yes → **You may have malignant external otitis, a serious ear infection. (See page 268.) Call your doctor right away.**

No ↓

Do you have an ulcer or lesion on your feet or toes?

Yes → **You may have an infected ulcer. (See page 286.) Call your doctor right away.**

No ↓

Do you have any hot, red, hive-like spots on your face or elsewhere?

Yes → **You may have erysipelas, an infection of the skin. (See page 308.) See your doctor or seek emergency help immediately!**

No ↓

Call your doctor right away for further help in determining the source of your problem. A fever is a sign of infection, which may need to be treated right away.

No ← Do you feel tired and achy all over?

Yes ↓

You may have the flu. (See page 461.)

8. Trouble Sleeping
Having problems falling asleep or staying asleep during the night

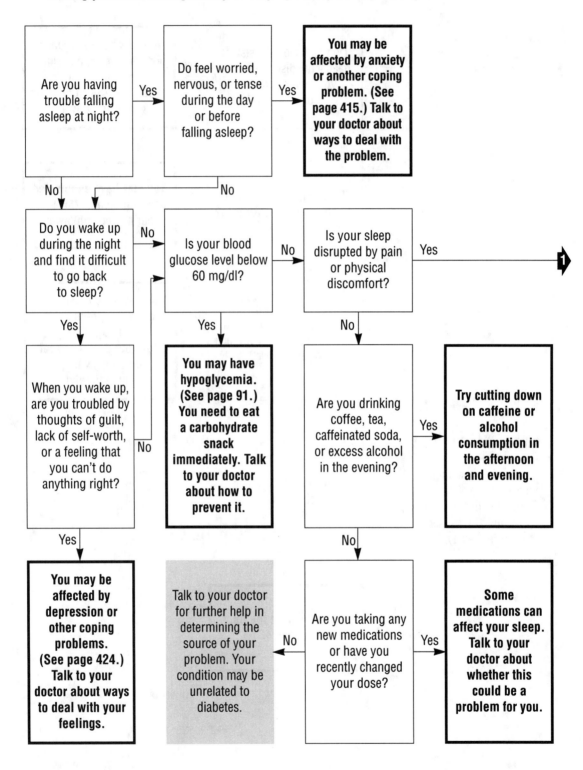

Are you having trouble falling asleep at night?

Yes → **Do feel worried, nervous, or tense during the day or before falling asleep?**

Yes → **You may be affected by anxiety or another coping problem. (See page 415.) Talk to your doctor about ways to deal with the problem.**

No ↓ / No ↓

Do you wake up during the night and find it difficult to go back to sleep?

No → **Is your blood glucose level below 60 mg/dl?**

No → **Is your sleep disrupted by pain or physical discomfort?**

Yes → **1**

Yes ↓ **When you wake up, are you troubled by thoughts of guilt, lack of self-worth, or a feeling that you can't do anything right?**

Yes ↓ **You may have hypoglycemia. (See page 91.) You need to eat a carbohydrate snack immediately. Talk to your doctor about how to prevent it.**

No ↓ **Are you drinking coffee, tea, caffeinated soda, or excess alcohol in the evening?**

Yes → **Try cutting down on caffeine or alcohol consumption in the afternoon and evening.**

No ↓

Yes ↓ **You may be affected by depression or other coping problems. (See page 424.) Talk to your doctor about ways to deal with your feelings.**

Talk to your doctor for further help in determining the source of your problem. Your condition may be unrelated to diabetes.

No ← **Are you taking any new medications or have you recently changed your dose?**

Yes → **Some medications can affect your sleep. Talk to your doctor about whether this could be a problem for you.**

8. Trouble Sleeping
Having problems falling asleep or staying asleep during the night *(Continued)*

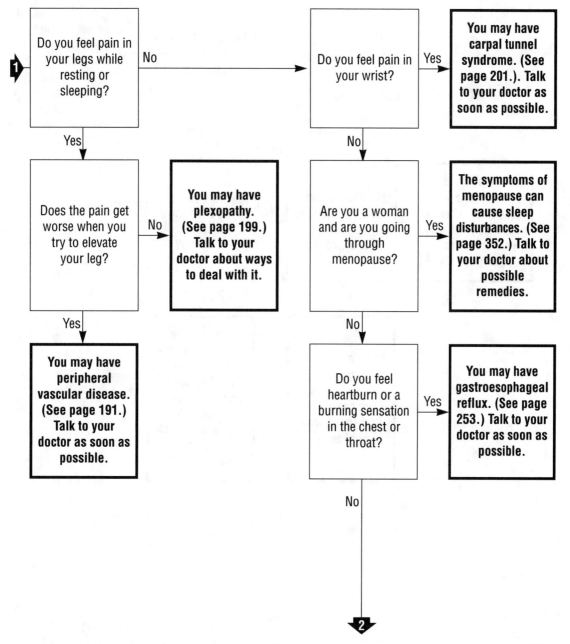

1

Do you feel pain in your legs while resting or sleeping? — No → Do you feel pain in your wrist? — Yes → **You may have carpal tunnel syndrome. (See page 201.). Talk to your doctor as soon as possible.**

Yes ↓

Does the pain get worse when you try to elevate your leg? — No → **You may have plexopathy. (See page 199.) Talk to your doctor about ways to deal with it.**

No ↓ (from wrist)

Are you a woman and are you going through menopause? — Yes → **The symptoms of menopause can cause sleep disturbances. (See page 352.) Talk to your doctor about possible remedies.**

Yes ↓ (from elevate)

You may have peripheral vascular disease. (See page 191.) Talk to your doctor as soon as possible.

No ↓ (from menopause)

Do you feel heartburn or a burning sensation in the chest or throat? — Yes → **You may have gastroesophageal reflux. (See page 253.) Talk to your doctor as soon as possible.**

No ↓

2

8. Trouble Sleeping
Having problems falling asleep or staying asleep during the night *(Continued)*

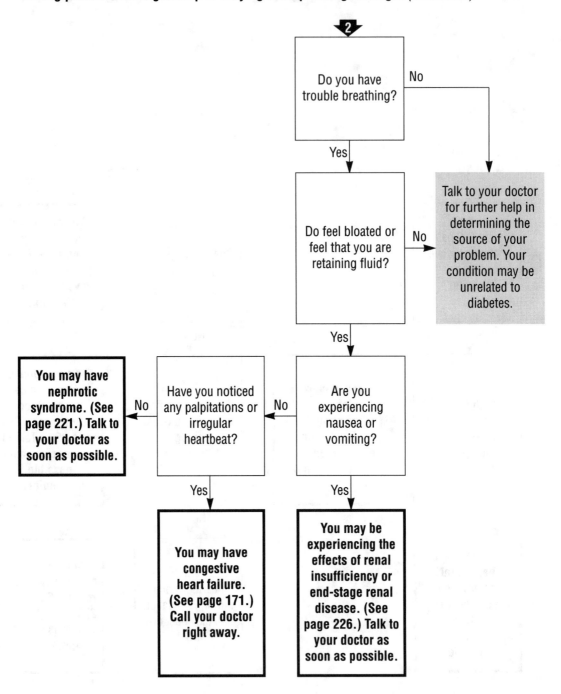

2

Do you have trouble breathing?

No → Talk to your doctor for further help in determining the source of your problem. Your condition may be unrelated to diabetes.

Yes ↓

Do feel bloated or feel that you are retaining fluid?

No →

Yes ↓

Are you experiencing nausea or vomiting?

No →

Have you noticed any palpitations or irregular heartbeat?

No →

You may have nephrotic syndrome. (See page 221.) Talk to your doctor as soon as possible.

Yes ↓ (palpitations)

You may have congestive heart failure. (See page 171.) Call your doctor right away.

Yes ↓ (nausea)

You may be experiencing the effects of renal insufficiency or end-stage renal disease. (See page 226.) Talk to your doctor as soon as possible.

9. Convulsions or Seizures
A violent, involuntary series of muscle spasms, with or without loss of consciousness

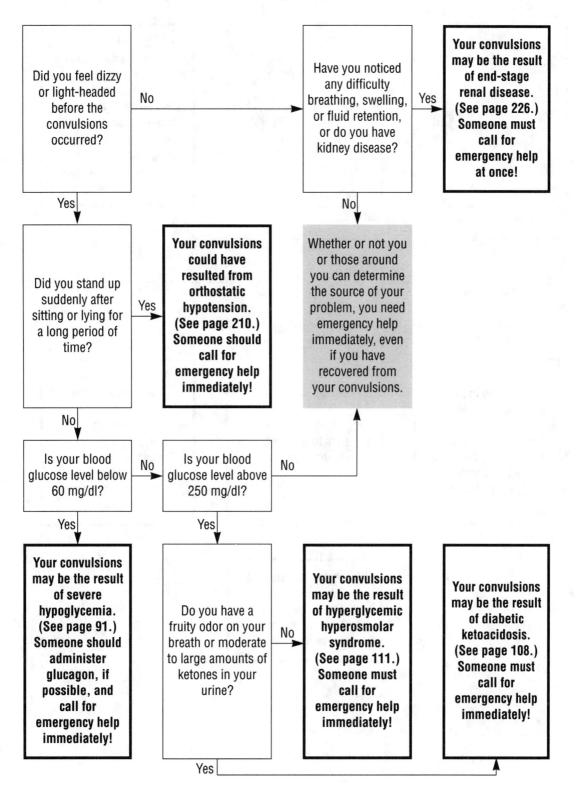

Did you feel dizzy or light-headed before the convulsions occurred?

No →

Have you noticed any difficulty breathing, swelling, or fluid retention, or do you have kidney disease?

Yes →

Your convulsions may be the result of end-stage renal disease. (See page 226.) Someone must call for emergency help at once!

Yes ↓

Did you stand up suddenly after sitting or lying for a long period of time?

Yes →

Your convulsions could have resulted from orthostatic hypotension. (See page 210.) Someone should call for emergency help immediately!

No ↓ (from kidney disease)

Whether or not you or those around you can determine the source of your problem, you need emergency help immediately, even if you have recovered from your convulsions.

No ↓

Is your blood glucose level below 60 mg/dl?

No →

Is your blood glucose level above 250 mg/dl?

No →

Yes ↓ (below 60)

Your convulsions may be the result of severe hypoglycemia. (See page 91.) Someone should administer glucagon, if possible, and call for emergency help immediately!

Yes ↓ (above 250)

Do you have a fruity odor on your breath or moderate to large amounts of ketones in your urine?

No →

Your convulsions may be the result of hyperglycemic hyperosmolar syndrome. (See page 111.) Someone must call for emergency help immediately!

Your convulsions may be the result of diabetic ketoacidosis. (See page 108.) Someone must call for emergency help immediately!

Yes →

10. Confusion
Feeling disoriented, losing a sense of reality, or experiencing loss of memory

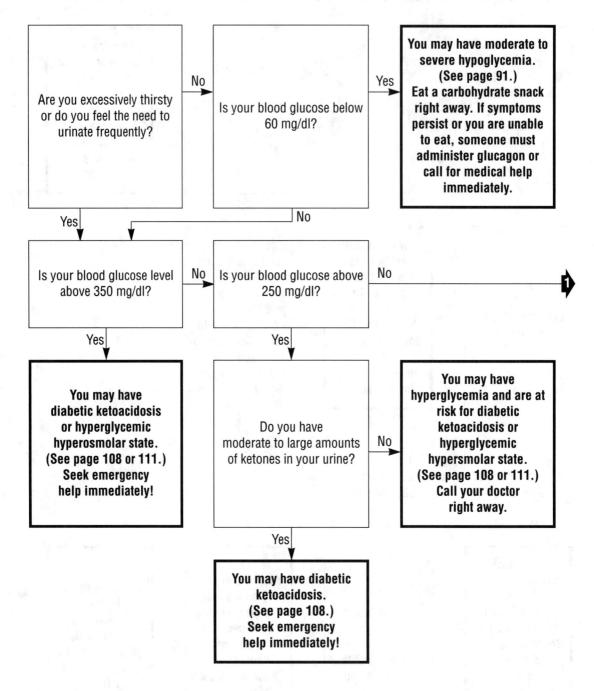

Are you excessively thirsty or do you feel the need to urinate frequently?

No →

Is your blood glucose below 60 mg/dl?

Yes →

You may have moderate to severe hypoglycemia. (See page 91.) Eat a carbohydrate snack right away. If symptoms persist or you are unable to eat, someone must administer glucagon or call for medical help immediately.

Yes ↓   **No** ↓

Is your blood glucose level above 350 mg/dl?

No →

Is your blood glucose above 250 mg/dl?

No → **1**

Yes ↓

You may have diabetic ketoacidosis or hyperglycemic hyperosmolar state. (See page 108 or 111.) Seek emergency help immediately!

Yes ↓

Do you have moderate to large amounts of ketones in your urine?

No →

You may have hyperglycemia and are at risk for diabetic ketoacidosis or hyperglycemic hypersmolar state. (See page 108 or 111.) Call your doctor right away.

Yes ↓

You may have diabetic ketoacidosis. (See page 108.) Seek emergency help immediately!

10. Confusion
Feeling disoriented, losing a sense of reality, or experiencing loss of memory
(Continued)

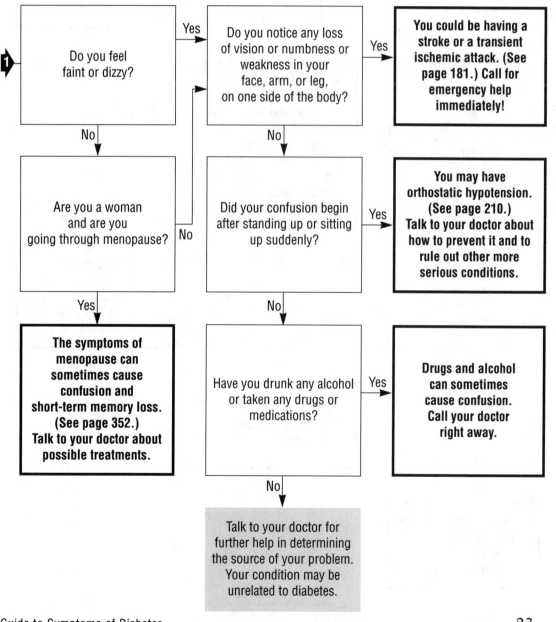

1

Do you feel faint or dizzy?

— **Yes** → Do you notice any loss of vision or numbness or weakness in your face, arm, or leg, on one side of the body?

— **Yes** → **You could be having a stroke or a transient ischemic attack. (See page 181.) Call for emergency help immediately!**

No ↓

Are you a woman and are you going through menopause?

No → (to confusion question)

No ↓ (from vision/numbness box)

Did your confusion begin after standing up or sitting up suddenly?

— **Yes** → **You may have orthostatic hypotension. (See page 210.) Talk to your doctor about how to prevent it and to rule out other more serious conditions.**

Yes ↓ (from menopause box)

The symptoms of menopause can sometimes cause confusion and short-term memory loss. (See page 352.) Talk to your doctor about possible treatments.

No ↓ (from standing up box)

Have you drunk any alcohol or taken any drugs or medications?

— **Yes** → **Drugs and alcohol can sometimes cause confusion. Call your doctor right away.**

No ↓

Talk to your doctor for further help in determining the source of your problem. Your condition may be unrelated to diabetes.

11. Sweating
Excessive or abnormal patterns of sweating

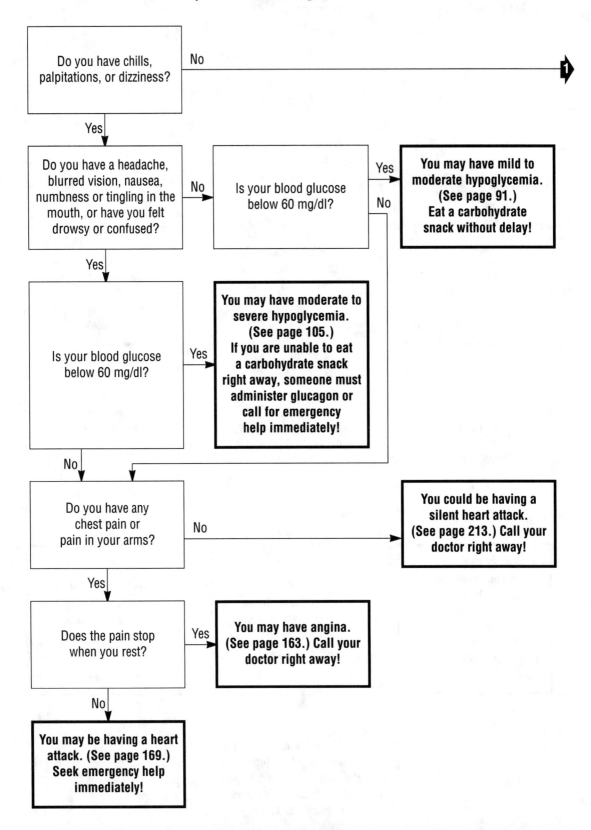

Do you have chills, palpitations, or dizziness? — No → **1**

Yes ↓

Do you have a headache, blurred vision, nausea, numbness or tingling in the mouth, or have you felt drowsy or confused? — No → Is your blood glucose below 60 mg/dl? — Yes → **You may have mild to moderate hypoglycemia. (See page 91.) Eat a carbohydrate snack without delay!**

No →

Yes ↓

Is your blood glucose below 60 mg/dl? — Yes → **You may have moderate to severe hypoglycemia. (See page 105.) If you are unable to eat a carbohydrate snack right away, someone must administer glucagon or call for emergency help immediately!**

No ↓

Do you have any chest pain or pain in your arms? — No → **You could be having a silent heart attack. (See page 213.) Call your doctor right away!**

Yes ↓

Does the pain stop when you rest? — Yes → **You may have angina. (See page 163.) Call your doctor right away!**

No ↓

You may be having a heart attack. (See page 169.) Seek emergency help immediately!

11. Sweating
Excessive or abnormal patterns of sweating *(Continued)*

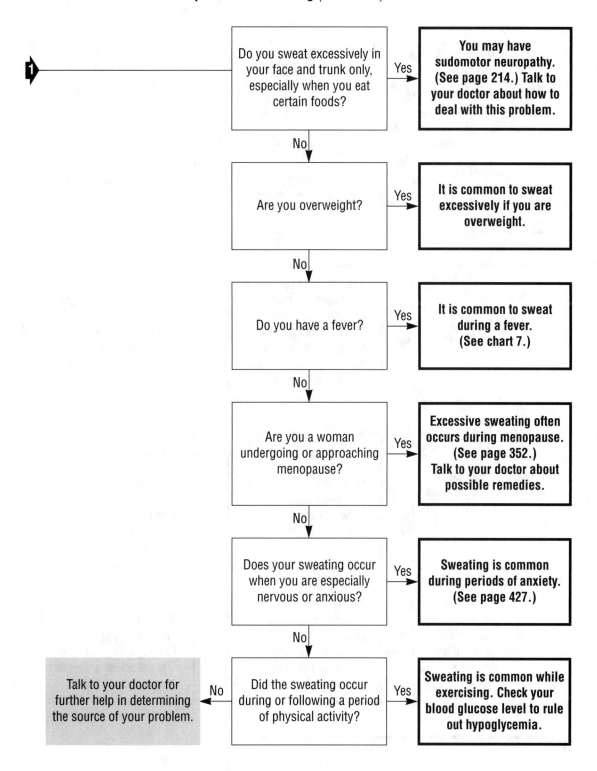

1 ──────────────────→ Do you sweat excessively in your face and trunk only, especially when you eat certain foods? ──**Yes**→ **You may have sudomotor neuropathy. (See page 214.) Talk to your doctor about how to deal with this problem.**

↓ **No**

Are you overweight? ──**Yes**→ **It is common to sweat excessively if you are overweight.**

↓ **No**

Do you have a fever? ──**Yes**→ **It is common to sweat during a fever. (See chart 7.)**

↓ **No**

Are you a woman undergoing or approaching menopause? ──**Yes**→ **Excessive sweating often occurs during menopause. (See page 352.) Talk to your doctor about possible remedies.**

↓ **No**

Does your sweating occur when you are especially nervous or anxious? ──**Yes**→ **Sweating is common during periods of anxiety. (See page 427.)**

↓ **No**

Talk to your doctor for further help in determining the source of your problem. ←**No**── Did the sweating occur during or following a period of physical activity? ──**Yes**→ **Sweating is common while exercising. Check your blood glucose level to rule out hypoglycemia.**

12. Chills and Cold
Experiencing chills or feeling unusually cold

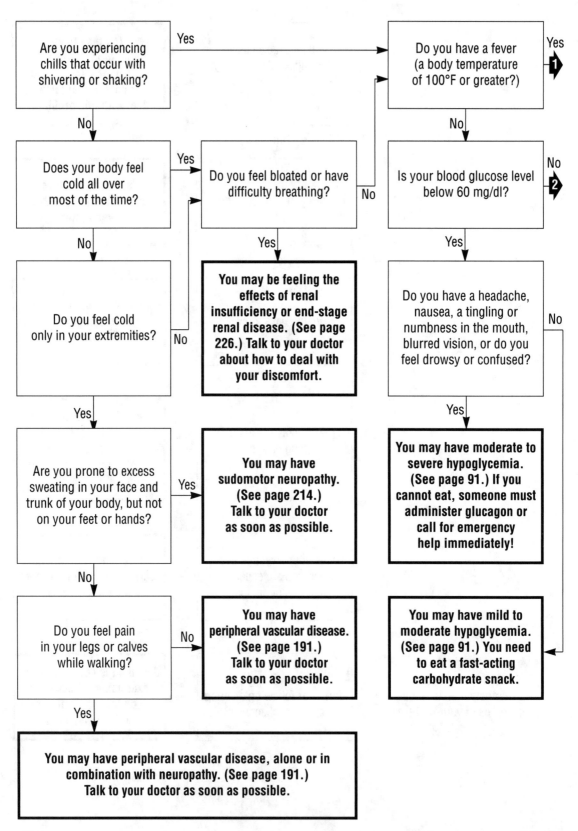

Are you experiencing chills that occur with shivering or shaking? — Yes → **Do you have a fever (a body temperature of 100°F or greater?)** — Yes ① / No ↓

No ↓

Does your body feel cold all over most of the time? — Yes → **Do you feel bloated or have difficulty breathing?** — No → (to fever box)

Is your blood glucose level below 60 mg/dl? — No ② / Yes ↓

No ↓

Do you feel cold only in your extremities? — No → (to bloated/breathing box)

Do you feel bloated or have difficulty breathing? — Yes ↓

You may be feeling the effects of renal insufficiency or end-stage renal disease. (See page 226.) Talk to your doctor about how to deal with your discomfort.

Do you have a headache, nausea, a tingling or numbness in the mouth, blurred vision, or do you feel drowsy or confused? — No → / Yes ↓

Yes ↓

Are you prone to excess sweating in your face and trunk of your body, but not on your feet or hands? — Yes → **You may have sudomotor neuropathy. (See page 214.) Talk to your doctor as soon as possible.**

You may have moderate to severe hypoglycemia. (See page 91.) If you cannot eat, someone must administer glucagon or call for emergency help immediately!

No ↓

Do you feel pain in your legs or calves while walking? — No → **You may have peripheral vascular disease. (See page 191.) Talk to your doctor as soon as possible.**

You may have mild to moderate hypoglycemia. (See page 91.) You need to eat a fast-acting carbohydrate snack.

Yes ↓

You may have peripheral vascular disease, alone or in combination with neuropathy. (See page 191.) Talk to your doctor as soon as possible.

12. Chills and Cold
Experiencing chills or feeling unusually cold *(Continued)*

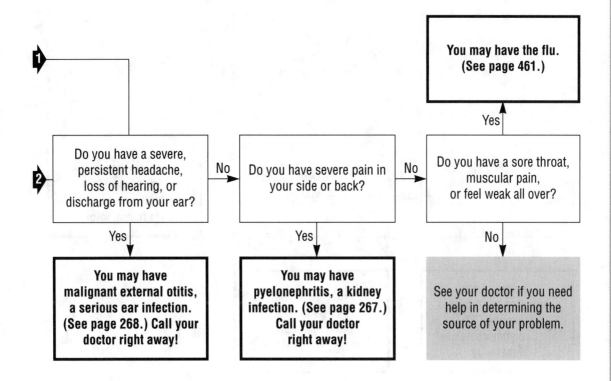

You may have the flu. (See page 461.)

Yes

① ②

Do you have a severe, persistent headache, loss of hearing, or discharge from your ear? → No → Do you have severe pain in your side or back? → No → Do you have a sore throat, muscular pain, or feel weak all over?

Yes

You may have malignant external otitis, a serious ear infection. (See page 268.) Call your doctor right away!

Yes

You may have pyelonephritis, a kidney infection. (See page 267.) Call your doctor right away!

No

See your doctor if you need help in determining the source of your problem.

13. Palpitations
Having a sensation of a more rapid, stronger, or more irregular heartbeat than normal

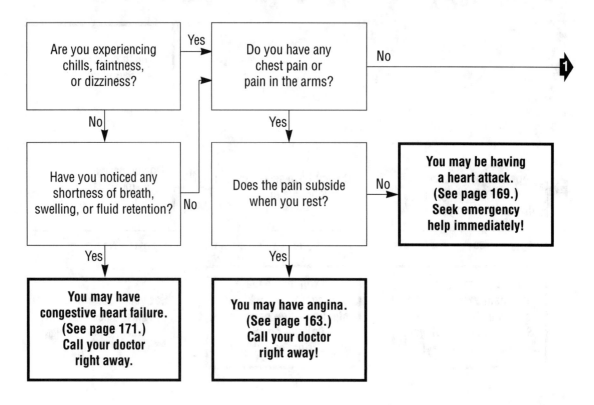

Are you experiencing chills, faintness, or dizziness?

→ Yes → Do you have any chest pain or pain in the arms? → No → **1**

No ↓

Have you noticed any shortness of breath, swelling, or fluid retention? | No

Do you have any chest pain or pain in the arms? → Yes ↓

Does the pain subside when you rest? → No → **You may be having a heart attack. (See page 169.) Seek emergency help immediately!**

Yes ↓

You may have congestive heart failure. (See page 171.) Call your doctor right away.

Yes ↓

You may have angina. (See page 163.) Call your doctor right away!

13. Palpitations

Having a sensation of a more rapid, stronger, or more irregular heartbeat than normal
(Continued)

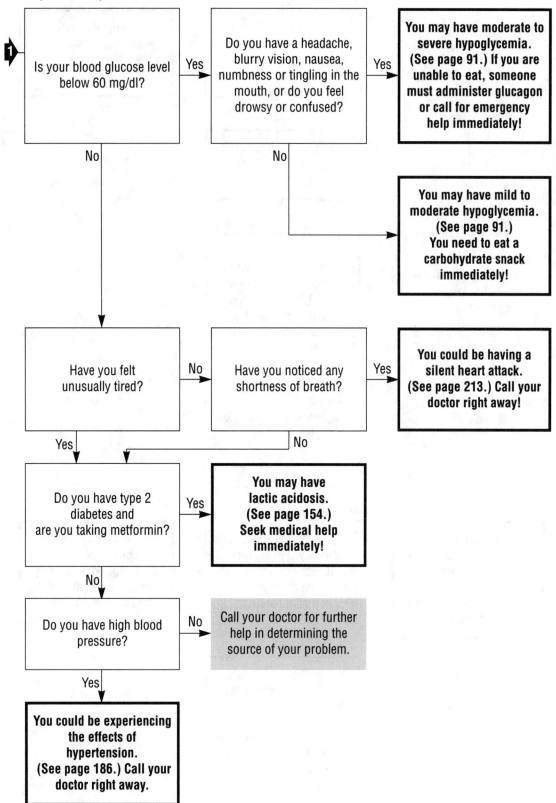

Is your blood glucose level below 60 mg/dl?

Yes → **Do you have a headache, blurry vision, nausea, numbness or tingling in the mouth, or do you feel drowsy or confused?**

Yes → **You may have moderate to severe hypoglycemia. (See page 91.) If you are unable to eat, someone must administer glucagon or call for emergency help immediately!**

No ↓ (from headache question) → **You may have mild to moderate hypoglycemia. (See page 91.) You need to eat a carbohydrate snack immediately!**

No ↓

Have you felt unusually tired?

No → **Have you noticed any shortness of breath?**

Yes → **You could be having a silent heart attack. (See page 213.) Call your doctor right away!**

Yes ↓ / No ↓

Do you have type 2 diabetes and are you taking metformin?

Yes → **You may have lactic acidosis. (See page 154.) Seek medical help immediately!**

No ↓

Do you have high blood pressure?

No → Call your doctor for further help in determining the source of your problem.

Yes ↓

You could be experiencing the effects of hypertension. (See page 186.) Call your doctor right away.

14. Dizziness
The sensation of feeling dizzy, faint, or light-headed

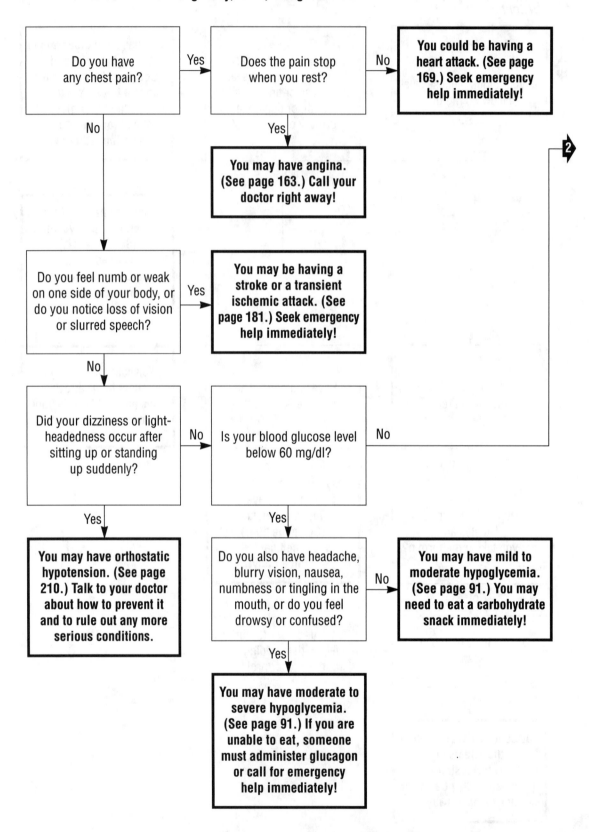

Do you have any chest pain? — Yes → **Does the pain stop when you rest?** — No → **You could be having a heart attack. (See page 169.) Seek emergency help immediately!**

Does the pain stop when you rest? — Yes → **You may have angina. (See page 163.) Call your doctor right away!**

Do you have any chest pain? — No ↓

Do you feel numb or weak on one side of your body, or do you notice loss of vision or slurred speech? — Yes → **You may be having a stroke or a transient ischemic attack. (See page 181.) Seek emergency help immediately!**

Do you feel numb or weak...? — No ↓

Did your dizziness or light-headedness occur after sitting up or standing up suddenly? — No → **Is your blood glucose level below 60 mg/dl?** — No → ▶ 2

Did your dizziness or light-headedness occur...? — Yes → **You may have orthostatic hypotension. (See page 210.) Talk to your doctor about how to prevent it and to rule out any more serious conditions.**

Is your blood glucose level below 60 mg/dl? — Yes → **Do you also have headache, blurry vision, nausea, numbness or tingling in the mouth, or do you feel drowsy or confused?** — No → **You may have mild to moderate hypoglycemia. (See page 91.) You may need to eat a carbohydrate snack immediately!**

Do you also have headache...? — Yes → **You may have moderate to severe hypoglycemia. (See page 91.) If you are unable to eat, someone must administer glucagon or call for emergency help immediately!**

14. Dizziness
The sensation of feeling dizzy, faint, or light-headed *(Continued)*

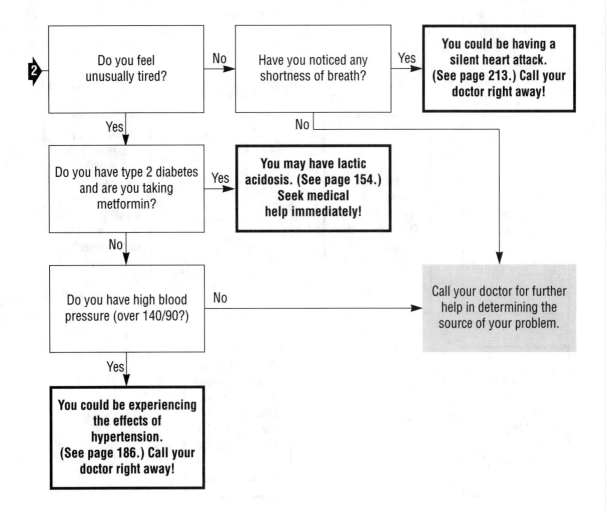

2

Do you feel unusually tired? — **No** → Have you noticed any shortness of breath? — **Yes** → **You could be having a silent heart attack. (See page 213.) Call your doctor right away!**

↓ **Yes**

Do you have type 2 diabetes and are you taking metformin? — **Yes** → **You may have lactic acidosis. (See page 154.) Seek medical help immediately!**

↓ **No**

Do you have high blood pressure (over 140/90?) — **No** →

Shortness of breath → **No** →

Call your doctor for further help in determining the source of your problem.

↓ **Yes**

You could be experiencing the effects of hypertension. (See page 186.) Call your doctor right away!

15. Headache
Feeling pain or pressure in the head

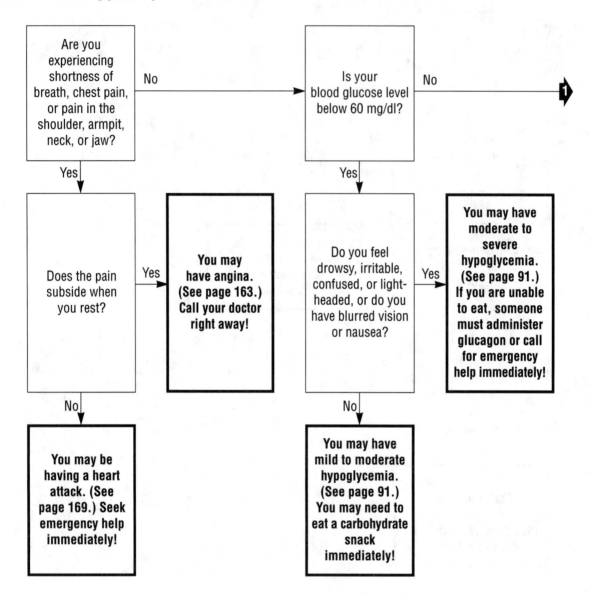

Are you experiencing shortness of breath, chest pain, or pain in the shoulder, armpit, neck, or jaw?

No →

Is your blood glucose level below 60 mg/dl?

No →

Yes ↓

Does the pain subside when you rest?

Yes →

You may have angina. (See page 163.) Call your doctor right away!

No ↓

You may be having a heart attack. (See page 169.) Seek emergency help immediately!

Yes ↓

Do you feel drowsy, irritable, confused, or light-headed, or do you have blurred vision or nausea?

Yes →

You may have moderate to severe hypoglycemia. (See page 91.) If you are unable to eat, someone must administer glucagon or call for emergency help immediately!

No ↓

You may have mild to moderate hypoglycemia. (See page 91.) You may need to eat a carbohydrate snack immediately!

15. Headache

Feeling pain or pressure in the head *(Continued)*

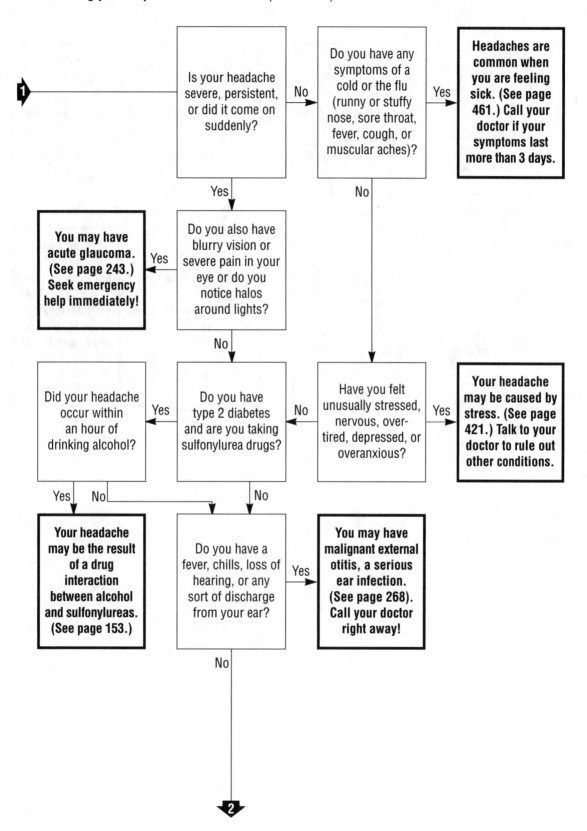

Is your headache severe, persistent, or did it come on suddenly?

No → Do you have any symptoms of a cold or the flu (runny or stuffy nose, sore throat, fever, cough, or muscular aches)?

Yes → **Headaches are common when you are feeling sick. (See page 461.) Call your doctor if your symptoms last more than 3 days.**

Yes (down) → Do you also have blurry vision or severe pain in your eye or do you notice halos around lights?

Yes → **You may have acute glaucoma. (See page 243.) Seek emergency help immediately!**

No (down) →

Did your headache occur within an hour of drinking alcohol?

Yes ← Do you have type 2 diabetes and are you taking sulfonylurea drugs?

No ← Have you felt unusually stressed, nervous, over-tired, depressed, or overanxious?

Yes → **Your headache may be caused by stress. (See page 421.) Talk to your doctor to rule out other conditions.**

Yes / **No** → **Your headache may be the result of a drug interaction between alcohol and sulfonylureas. (See page 153.)**

No → Do you have a fever, chills, loss of hearing, or any sort of discharge from your ear?

Yes → **You may have malignant external otitis, a serious ear infection. (See page 268). Call your doctor right away!**

No (down) → **2**

15. Headache
Feeling pain or pressure in the head *(Continued)*

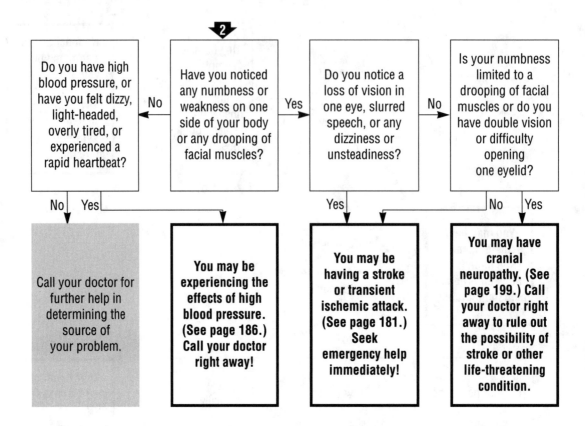

Do you have high blood pressure, or have you felt dizzy, light-headed, overly tired, or experienced a rapid heartbeat?

No ←

Have you noticed any numbness or weakness on one side of your body or any drooping of facial muscles?

Yes →

Do you notice a loss of vision in one eye, slurred speech, or any dizziness or unsteadiness?

No →

Is your numbness limited to a drooping of facial muscles or do you have double vision or difficulty opening one eyelid?

No | Yes

Call your doctor for further help in determining the source of your problem.

Yes

You may be experiencing the effects of high blood pressure. (See page 186.) Call your doctor right away!

Yes

You may be having a stroke or transient ischemic attack. (See page 181.) Seek emergency help immediately!

No | Yes

You may have cranial neuropathy. (See page 199.) Call your doctor right away to rule out the possibility of stroke or other life-threatening condition.

16. Loss of Consciousness
Fainting or losing the ability to respond to stimuli

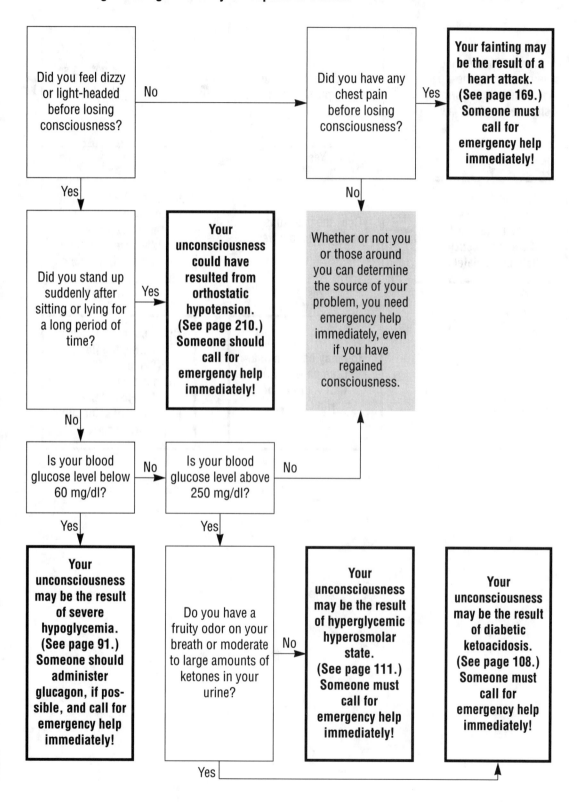

Did you feel dizzy or light-headed before losing consciousness?

No → Did you have any chest pain before losing consciousness?

Yes → **Your fainting may be the result of a heart attack. (See page 169.) Someone must call for emergency help immediately!**

Yes ↓

Did you stand up suddenly after sitting or lying for a long period of time?

Yes → **Your unconsciousness could have resulted from orthostatic hypotension. (See page 210.) Someone should call for emergency help immediately!**

No (from chest pain) → Whether or not you or those around you can determine the source of your problem, you need emergency help immediately, even if you have regained consciousness.

No ↓

Is your blood glucose level below 60 mg/dl?

No → Is your blood glucose level above 250 mg/dl?

No → (to: Whether or not you...)

Yes ↓

Your unconsciousness may be the result of severe hypoglycemia. (See page 91.) Someone should administer glucagon, if possible, and call for emergency help immediately!

Yes ↓

Do you have a fruity odor on your breath or moderate to large amounts of ketones in your urine?

No → **Your unconsciousness may be the result of hyperglycemic hyperosmolar state. (See page 111.) Someone must call for emergency help immediately!**

Your unconsciousness may be the result of diabetic ketoacidosis. (See page 108.) Someone must call for emergency help immediately!

Yes → (to diabetic ketoacidosis box)

17. Chest Pain
Experiencing dull, stabbing, burning, or crushing pain between the neck and abdomen

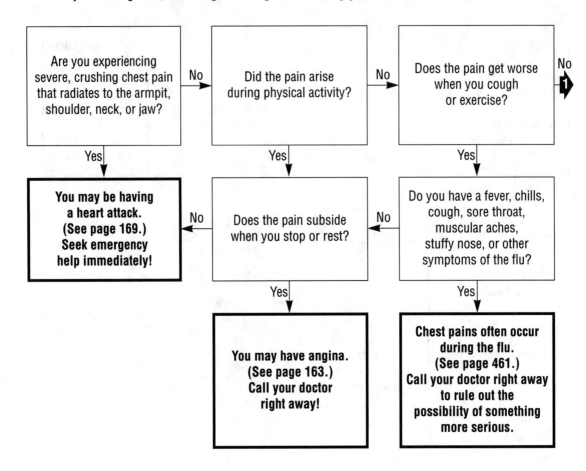

Are you experiencing severe, crushing chest pain that radiates to the armpit, shoulder, neck, or jaw?

No →

Did the pain arise during physical activity?

No →

Does the pain get worse when you cough or exercise?

No → **1**

Yes ↓ (from first box)

You may be having a heart attack. (See page 169.) Seek emergency help immediately!

Yes ↓ (from second box)

Does the pain subside when you stop or rest?

No ← (from angina box pointing left)

Yes ↓

You may have angina. (See page 163.) Call your doctor right away!

Yes ↓ (from third box)

Do you have a fever, chills, cough, sore throat, muscular aches, stuffy nose, or other symptoms of the flu?

No ←

Yes ↓

Chest pains often occur during the flu. (See page 461.) Call your doctor right away to rule out the possibility of something more serious.

17. Chest Pain

Experiencing dull, stabbing, burning, or crushing pain between the neck and abdomen
(Continued)

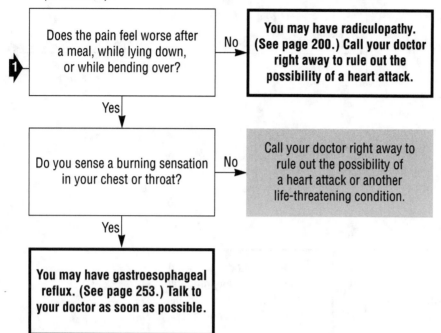

Does the pain feel worse after a meal, while lying down, or while bending over?

No → **You may have radiculopathy. (See page 200.) Call your doctor right away to rule out the possibility of a heart attack.**

Yes ↓

Do you sense a burning sensation in your chest or throat?

No → Call your doctor right away to rule out the possibility of a heart attack or another life-threatening condition.

Yes ↓

You may have gastroesophageal reflux. (See page 253.) Talk to your doctor as soon as possible.

18. Leg and Foot Pain
Feeling any kind of pain in the legs or feet

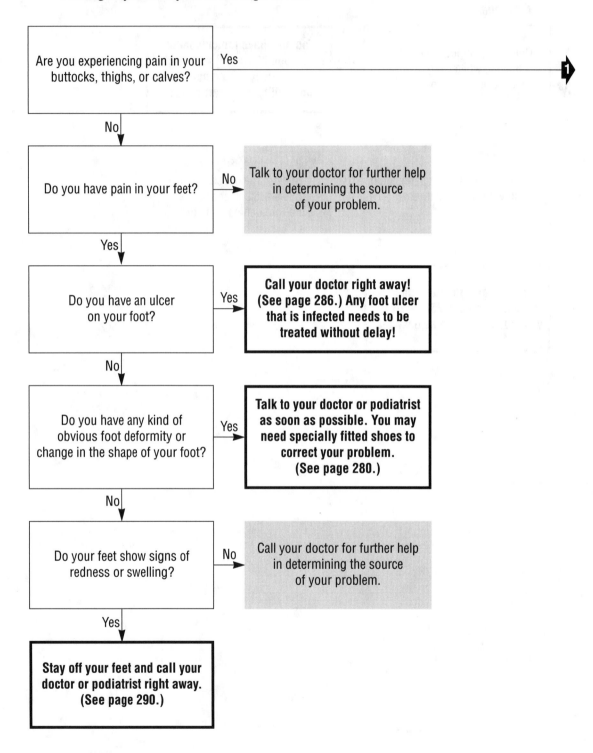

Are you experiencing pain in your buttocks, thighs, or calves? — **Yes** → **1**

No ↓

Do you have pain in your feet? — **No** → Talk to your doctor for further help in determining the source of your problem.

Yes ↓

Do you have an ulcer on your foot? — **Yes** → **Call your doctor right away! (See page 286.) Any foot ulcer that is infected needs to be treated without delay!**

No ↓

Do you have any kind of obvious foot deformity or change in the shape of your foot? — **Yes** → **Talk to your doctor or podiatrist as soon as possible. You may need specially fitted shoes to correct your problem. (See page 280.)**

No ↓

Do your feet show signs of redness or swelling? — **No** → Call your doctor for further help in determining the source of your problem.

Yes ↓

Stay off your feet and call your doctor or podiatrist right away. (See page 290.)

18. Leg and Foot Pain
Feeling any kind of pain in the legs or feet *(Continued)*

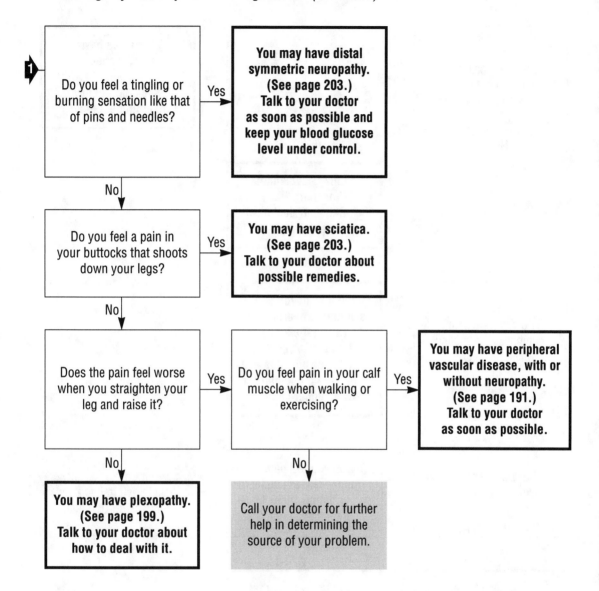

1 Do you feel a tingling or burning sensation like that of pins and needles?

Yes → **You may have distal symmetric neuropathy. (See page 203.) Talk to your doctor as soon as possible and keep your blood glucose level under control.**

No ↓

Do you feel a pain in your buttocks that shoots down your legs?

Yes → **You may have sciatica. (See page 203.) Talk to your doctor about possible remedies.**

No ↓

Does the pain feel worse when you straighten your leg and raise it?

Yes → Do you feel pain in your calf muscle when walking or exercising?

Yes → **You may have peripheral vascular disease, with or without neuropathy. (See page 191.) Talk to your doctor as soon as possible.**

No ↓ (under first question)

You may have plexopathy. (See page 199.) Talk to your doctor about how to deal with it.

No ↓ (under calf muscle question)

Call your doctor for further help in determining the source of your problem.

19. Arm and Hand Pain
Feeling pain in the shoulder, arms, wrist, or hand

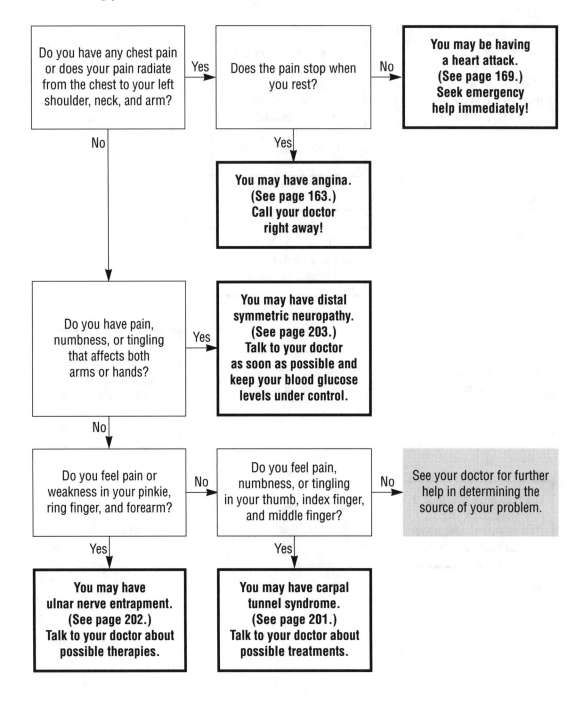

Do you have any chest pain or does your pain radiate from the chest to your left shoulder, neck, and arm?

Yes → Does the pain stop when you rest?

No → **You may be having a heart attack. (See page 169.) Seek emergency help immediately!**

Yes ↓

You may have angina. (See page 163.) Call your doctor right away!

No ↓

Do you have pain, numbness, or tingling that affects both arms or hands?

Yes → **You may have distal symmetric neuropathy. (See page 203.) Talk to your doctor as soon as possible and keep your blood glucose levels under control.**

No ↓

Do you feel pain or weakness in your pinkie, ring finger, and forearm?

No → Do you feel pain, numbness, or tingling in your thumb, index finger, and middle finger?

No → See your doctor for further help in determining the source of your problem.

Yes ↓

You may have ulnar nerve entrapment. (See page 202.) Talk to your doctor about possible therapies.

Yes ↓

You may have carpal tunnel syndrome. (See page 201.) Talk to your doctor about possible treatments.

20. Back Pain
Pain in back or spinal column

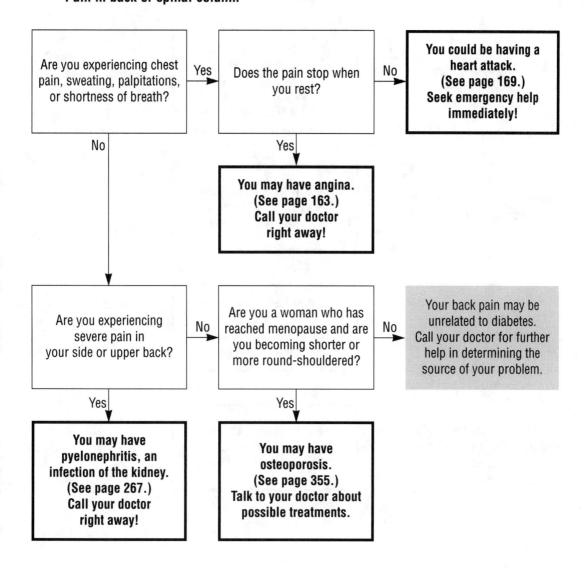

Are you experiencing chest pain, sweating, palpitations, or shortness of breath?

Yes → Does the pain stop when you rest?

No → **You could be having a heart attack. (See page 169.) Seek emergency help immediately!**

Yes → **You may have angina. (See page 163.) Call your doctor right away!**

No ↓

Are you experiencing severe pain in your side or upper back?

No → Are you a woman who has reached menopause and are you becoming shorter or more round-shouldered?

No → Your back pain may be unrelated to diabetes. Call your doctor for further help in determining the source of your problem.

Yes → **You may have pyelonephritis, an infection of the kidney. (See page 267.) Call your doctor right away!**

Yes → **You may have osteoporosis. (See page 355.) Talk to your doctor about possible treatments.**

21. Injection Site Problems
Having skin problems at your injection site

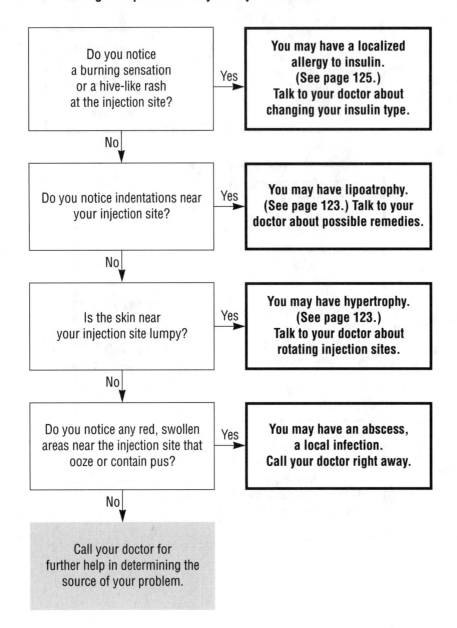

Do you notice
a burning sensation
or a hive-like rash
at the injection site?

Yes → You may have a localized allergy to insulin. (See page 125.) Talk to your doctor about changing your insulin type.

No ↓

Do you notice indentations near your injection site?

Yes → You may have lipoatrophy. (See page 123.) Talk to your doctor about possible remedies.

No ↓

Is the skin near your injection site lumpy?

Yes → You may have hypertrophy. (See page 123.) Talk to your doctor about rotating injection sites.

No ↓

Do you notice any red, swollen areas near the injection site that ooze or contain pus?

Yes → You may have an abscess, a local infection. Call your doctor right away.

No ↓

Call your doctor for further help in determining the source of your problem.

22. Thickening of the Skin
Having areas of skin that have become thicker than normal

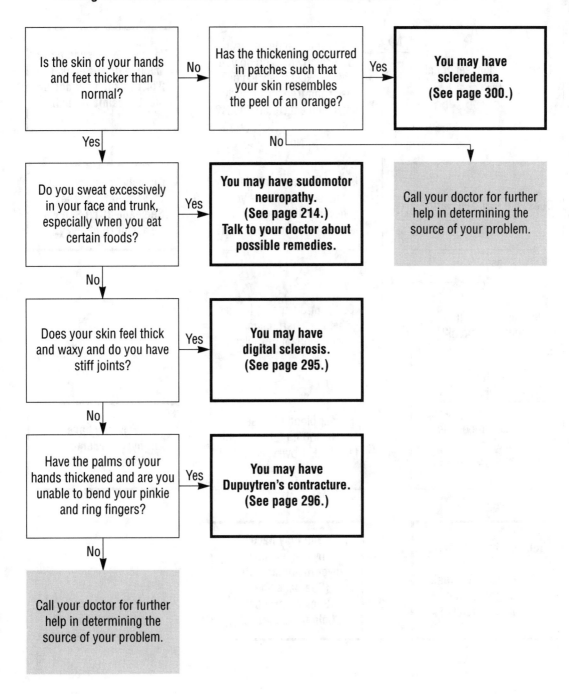

Is the skin of your hands and feet thicker than normal?

No →

Has the thickening occurred in patches such that your skin resembles the peel of an orange?

Yes →

You may have scleredema. (See page 300.)

Yes ↓

No ↓

Do you sweat excessively in your face and trunk, especially when you eat certain foods?

Yes →

You may have sudomotor neuropathy. (See page 214.) Talk to your doctor about possible remedies.

Call your doctor for further help in determining the source of your problem.

No ↓

Does your skin feel thick and waxy and do you have stiff joints?

Yes →

You may have digital sclerosis. (See page 295.)

No ↓

Have the palms of your hands thickened and are you unable to bend your pinkie and ring fingers?

Yes →

You may have Dupuytren's contracture. (See page 296.)

No ↓

Call your doctor for further help in determining the source of your problem.

23. Dry Skin
Having skin that is unusually dry

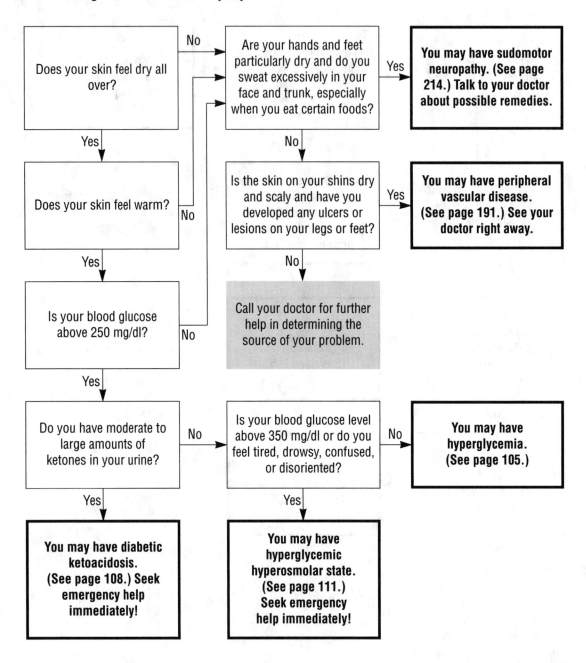

Does your skin feel dry all over?

No → **Are your hands and feet particularly dry and do you sweat excessively in your face and trunk, especially when you eat certain foods?**

Yes → **You may have sudomotor neuropathy. (See page 214.) Talk to your doctor about possible remedies.**

Yes ↓

Does your skin feel warm?

No →

No ↓ **Is the skin on your shins dry and scaly and have you developed any ulcers or lesions on your legs or feet?**

Yes → **You may have peripheral vascular disease. (See page 191.) See your doctor right away.**

Yes ↓

Is your blood glucose above 250 mg/dl?

No →

No ↓ **Call your doctor for further help in determining the source of your problem.**

Yes ↓

Do you have moderate to large amounts of ketones in your urine?

No → **Is your blood glucose level above 350 mg/dl or do you feel tired, drowsy, confused, or disoriented?**

No → **You may have hyperglycemia. (See page 105.)**

Yes ↓

You may have diabetic ketoacidosis. (See page 108.) Seek emergency help immediately!

Yes ↓

You may have hyperglycemic hyperosmolar state. (See page 111.) Seek emergency help immediately!

24. Skin Discoloration
Having any darkening, yellowing, or loss of pigmentation of the skin

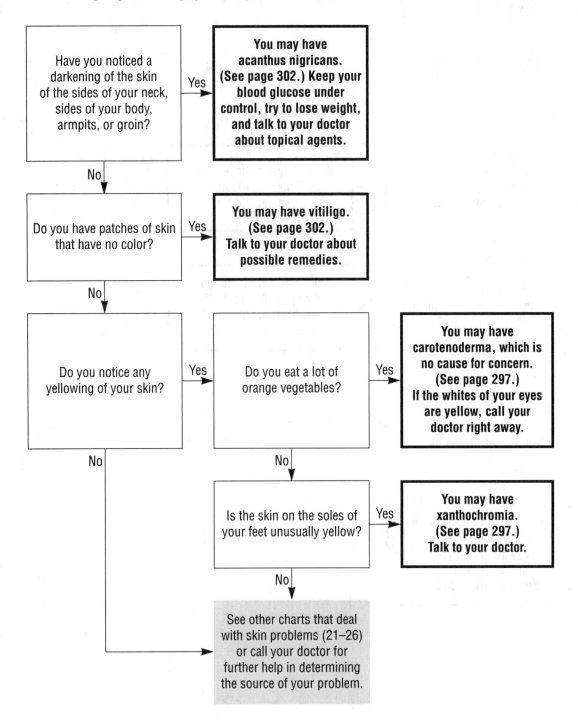

Have you noticed a darkening of the skin of the sides of your neck, sides of your body, armpits, or groin?

Yes → You may have acanthus nigricans. (See page 302.) Keep your blood glucose under control, try to lose weight, and talk to your doctor about topical agents.

No ↓

Do you have patches of skin that have no color?

Yes → You may have vitiligo. (See page 302.) Talk to your doctor about possible remedies.

No ↓

Do you notice any yellowing of your skin?

Yes → Do you eat a lot of orange vegetables?

Yes → You may have carotenoderma, which is no cause for concern. (See page 297.) If the whites of your eyes are yellow, call your doctor right away.

No ↓

Is the skin on the soles of your feet unusually yellow?

Yes → You may have xanthochromia. (See page 297.) Talk to your doctor.

No ↓

See other charts that deal with skin problems (21–26) or call your doctor for further help in determining the source of your problem.

25. Skin Lesions
Having any open sores, ulcers, blisters, boils, swellings, or areas of skin that are red and tender

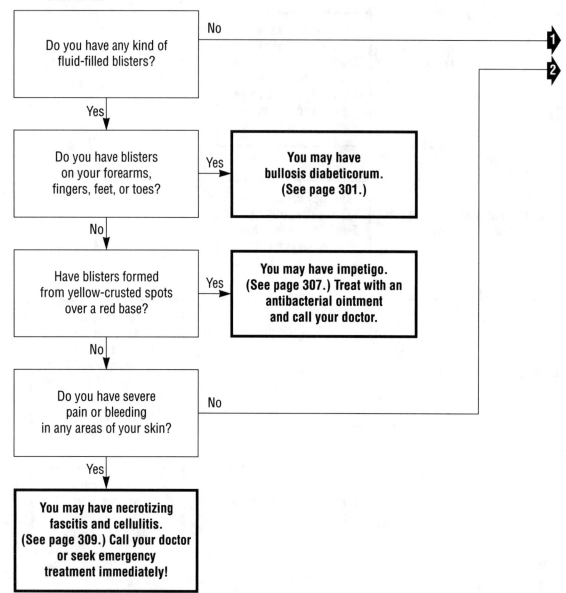

Do you have any kind of fluid-filled blisters?

No → ❶

❷

Yes ↓

Do you have blisters on your forearms, fingers, feet, or toes?

Yes → **You may have bullosis diabeticorum. (See page 301.)**

No ↓

Have blisters formed from yellow-crusted spots over a red base?

Yes → **You may have impetigo. (See page 307.) Treat with an antibacterial ointment and call your doctor.**

No ↓

Do you have severe pain or bleeding in any areas of your skin?

No →

Yes ↓

You may have necrotizing fascitis and cellulitis. (See page 309.) Call your doctor or seek emergency treatment immediately!

25. Skin Lesions

Having any open sores, ulcers, blisters, boils, swellings, or areas of skin that are red and tender *(Continued)*

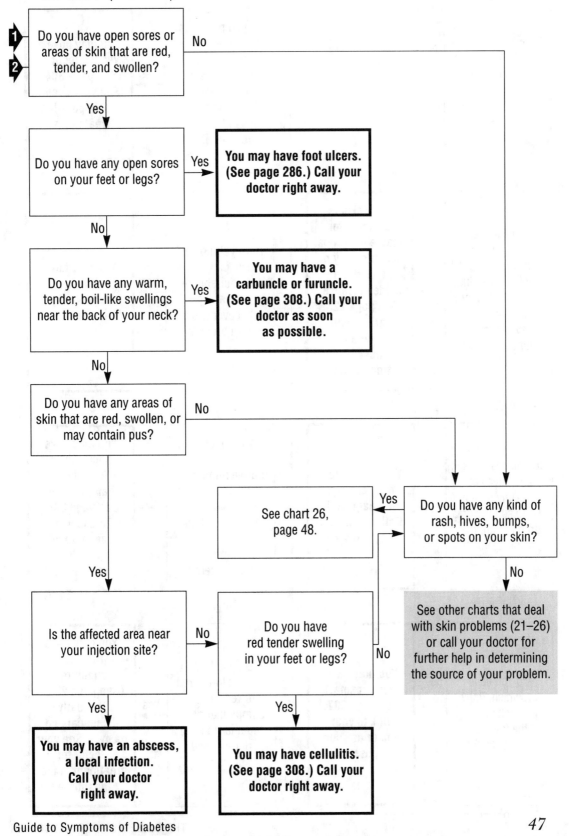

1
2 Do you have open sores or areas of skin that are red, tender, and swollen? — **No** →

↓ **Yes**

Do you have any open sores on your feet or legs? — **Yes** → **You may have foot ulcers. (See page 286.) Call your doctor right away.**

↓ **No**

Do you have any warm, tender, boil-like swellings near the back of your neck? — **Yes** → **You may have a carbuncle or furuncle. (See page 308.) Call your doctor as soon as possible.**

↓ **No**

Do you have any areas of skin that are red, swollen, or may contain pus? — **No** →

↓ **Yes**

Do you have any kind of rash, hives, bumps, or spots on your skin?

Yes → See chart 26, page 48.

No ↓

See other charts that deal with skin problems (21–26) or call your doctor for further help in determining the source of your problem.

Is the affected area near your injection site? — **No** → Do you have red tender swelling in your feet or legs? — **No** →

↓ **Yes** (injection site)

You may have an abscess, a local infection. Call your doctor right away.

↓ **Yes** (red tender swelling)

You may have cellulitis. (See page 308.) Call your doctor right away.

26. Skin Rashes and Itchy Skin
Having any rash, hives, bumps, spots, or itching of the skin

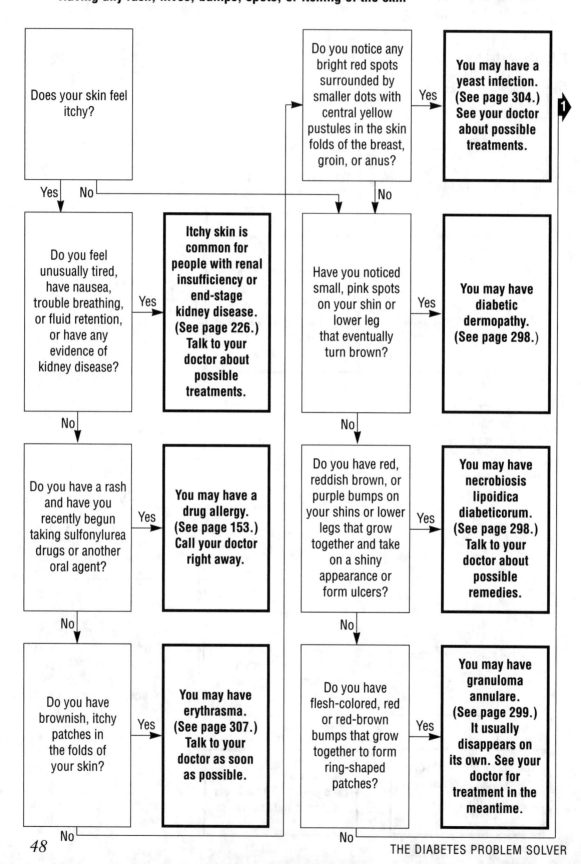

Does your skin feel itchy?

Yes → Do you feel unusually tired, have nausea, trouble breathing, or fluid retention, or have any evidence of kidney disease?

Yes → **Itchy skin is common for people with renal insufficiency or end-stage kidney disease. (See page 226.) Talk to your doctor about possible treatments.**

No → Do you have a rash and have you recently begun taking sulfonylurea drugs or another oral agent?

Yes → **You may have a drug allergy. (See page 153.) Call your doctor right away.**

No → Do you have brownish, itchy patches in the folds of your skin?

Yes → **You may have erythrasma. (See page 307.) Talk to your doctor as soon as possible.**

No →

Do you notice any bright red spots surrounded by smaller dots with central yellow pustules in the skin folds of the breast, groin, or anus?

Yes → **You may have a yeast infection. (See page 304.) See your doctor about possible treatments.** ▷ 1

No → Have you noticed small, pink spots on your shin or lower leg that eventually turn brown?

Yes → **You may have diabetic dermopathy. (See page 298.)**

No → Do you have red, reddish brown, or purple bumps on your shins or lower legs that grow together and take on a shiny appearance or form ulcers?

Yes → **You may have necrobiosis lipoidica diabeticorum. (See page 298.) Talk to your doctor about possible remedies.**

No → Do you have flesh-colored, red or red-brown bumps that grow together to form ring-shaped patches?

Yes → **You may have granuloma annulare. (See page 299.) It usually disappears on its own. See your doctor for treatment in the meantime.**

No →

26. Skin Rashes and Itchy Skin
Having any rash, hives, bumps, spots, or itching of the skin *(Continued)*

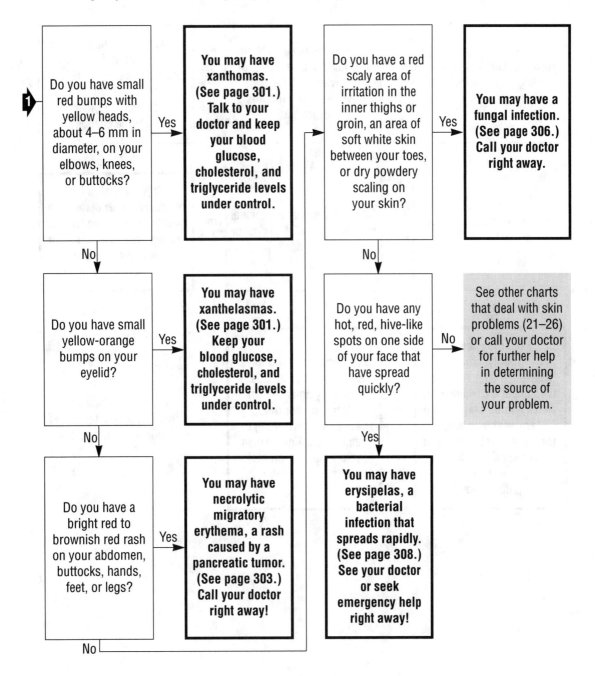

① Do you have small red bumps with yellow heads, about 4–6 mm in diameter, on your elbows, knees, or buttocks?

— Yes → **You may have xanthomas. (See page 301.) Talk to your doctor and keep your blood glucose, cholesterol, and triglyceride levels under control.**

— No ↓

Do you have small yellow-orange bumps on your eyelid?

— Yes → **You may have xanthelasmas. (See page 301.) Keep your blood glucose, cholesterol, and triglyceride levels under control.**

— No ↓

Do you have a bright red to brownish red rash on your abdomen, buttocks, hands, feet, or legs?

— Yes → **You may have necrolytic migratory erythema, a rash caused by a pancreatic tumor. (See page 303.) Call your doctor right away!**

— No

Do you have a red scaly area of irritation in the inner thighs or groin, an area of soft white skin between your toes, or dry powdery scaling on your skin?

— Yes → **You may have a fungal infection. (See page 306.) Call your doctor right away.**

— No ↓

Do you have any hot, red, hive-like spots on one side of your face that have spread quickly?

— No → See other charts that deal with skin problems (21–26) or call your doctor for further help in determining the source of your problem.

— Yes ↓

You may have erysipelas, a bacterial infection that spreads rapidly. (See page 308.) See your doctor or seek emergency help right away!

27. Emotional Problems
Experiencing changes in mood, thoughts, feelings, and behavior

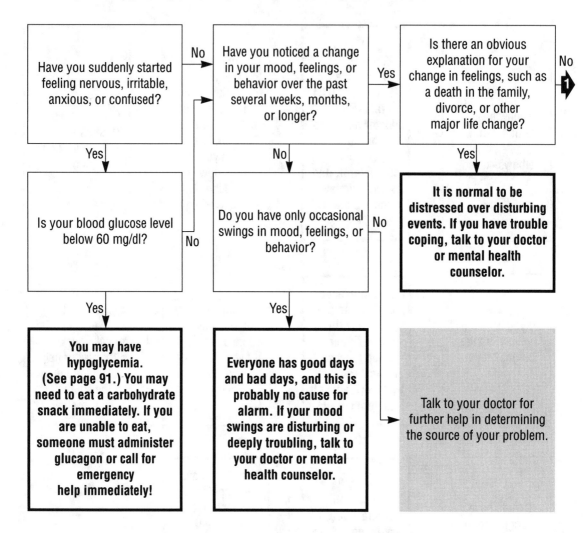

Have you suddenly started feeling nervous, irritable, anxious, or confused?

No → Have you noticed a change in your mood, feelings, or behavior over the past several weeks, months, or longer?

Yes → Is there an obvious explanation for your change in feelings, such as a death in the family, divorce, or other major life change?

No → **1**

Yes ↓ (Have you suddenly started...)

Is your blood glucose level below 60 mg/dl?

No →

No ↓ (Have you noticed a change...)

Do you have only occasional swings in mood, feelings, or behavior?

No →

Yes ↓ (Is there an obvious explanation...)

It is normal to be distressed over disturbing events. If you have trouble coping, talk to your doctor or mental health counselor.

Yes ↓ (Is your blood glucose level...)

You may have hypoglycemia. (See page 91.) You may need to eat a carbohydrate snack immediately. If you are unable to eat, someone must administer glucagon or call for emergency help immediately!

Yes ↓ (Do you have only occasional swings...)

Everyone has good days and bad days, and this is probably no cause for alarm. If your mood swings are disturbing or deeply troubling, talk to your doctor or mental health counselor.

Talk to your doctor for further help in determining the source of your problem.

27. Emotional Problems
Experiencing changes in mood, thoughts, feelings, and behavior *(Continued)*

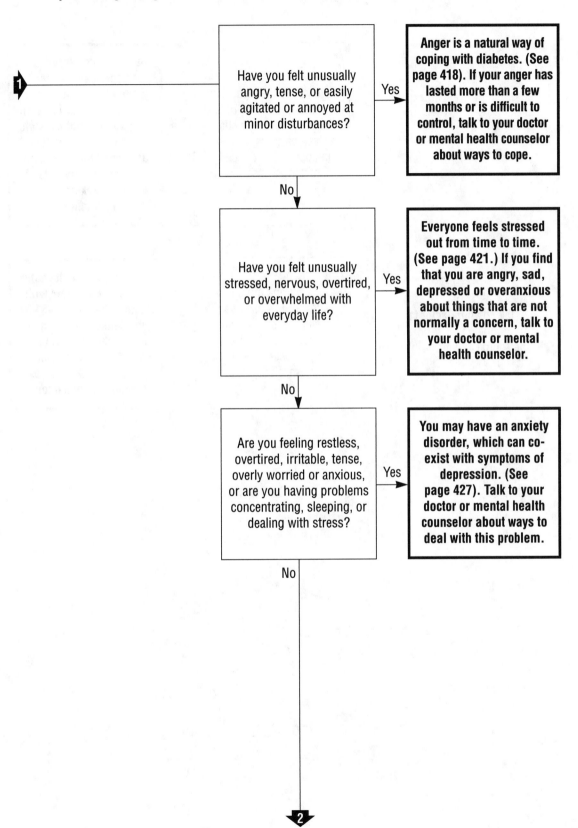

1

Have you felt unusually angry, tense, or easily agitated or annoyed at minor disturbances?

Yes → **Anger is a natural way of coping with diabetes. (See page 418). If your anger has lasted more than a few months or is difficult to control, talk to your doctor or mental health counselor about ways to cope.**

No ↓

Have you felt unusually stressed, nervous, overtired, or overwhelmed with everyday life?

Yes → **Everyone feels stressed out from time to time. (See page 421.) If you find that you are angry, sad, depressed or overanxious about things that are not normally a concern, talk to your doctor or mental health counselor.**

No ↓

Are you feeling restless, overtired, irritable, tense, overly worried or anxious, or are you having problems concentrating, sleeping, or dealing with stress?

Yes → **You may have an anxiety disorder, which can co-exist with symptoms of depression. (See page 427). Talk to your doctor or mental health counselor about ways to deal with this problem.**

No ↓

2

27. Emotional Problems
Experiencing changes in mood, thoughts, feelings, and behavior *(Continued)*

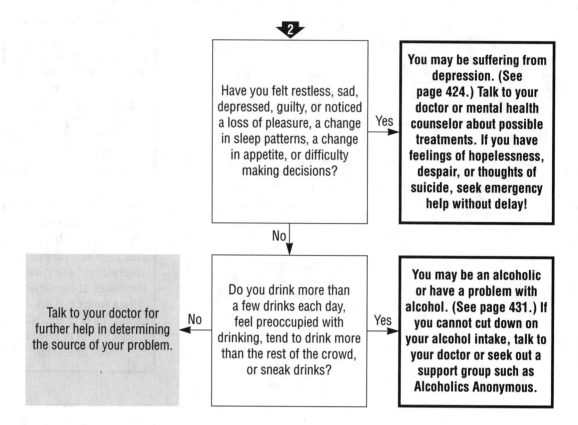

2

Have you felt restless, sad, depressed, guilty, or noticed a loss of pleasure, a change in sleep patterns, a change in appetite, or difficulty making decisions?

Yes → You may be suffering from depression. (See page 424.) Talk to your doctor or mental health counselor about possible treatments. If you have feelings of hopelessness, despair, or thoughts of suicide, seek emergency help without delay!

No ↓

Do you drink more than a few drinks each day, feel preoccupied with drinking, tend to drink more than the rest of the crowd, or sneak drinks?

No → Talk to your doctor for further help in determining the source of your problem.

Yes → You may be an alcoholic or have a problem with alcohol. (See page 431.) If you cannot cut down on your alcohol intake, talk to your doctor or seek out a support group such as Alcoholics Anonymous.

28. Emotional Changes in Women
Having feelings of irritability, unusual sensitivity, or changes in mood

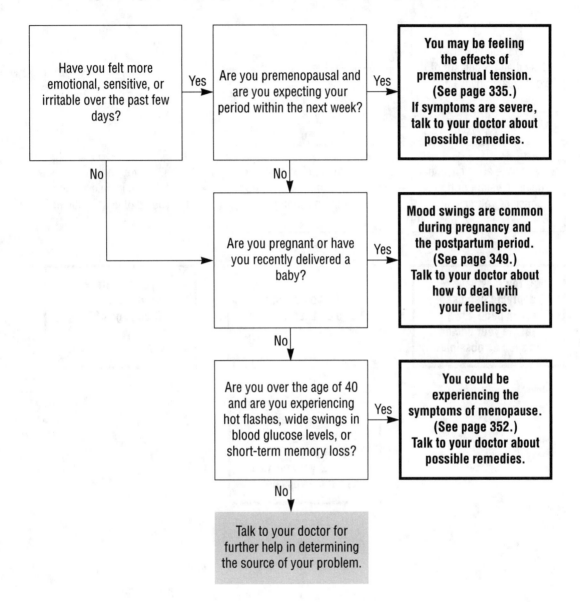

Have you felt more emotional, sensitive, or irritable over the past few days?

Yes → Are you premenopausal and are you expecting your period within the next week?

Yes → **You may be feeling the effects of premenstrual tension. (See page 335.) If symptoms are severe, talk to your doctor about possible remedies.**

No ↓

Are you pregnant or have you recently delivered a baby?

Yes → **Mood swings are common during pregnancy and the postpartum period. (See page 349.) Talk to your doctor about how to deal with your feelings.**

No ↓

Are you over the age of 40 and are you experiencing hot flashes, wide swings in blood glucose levels, or short-term memory loss?

Yes → **You could be experiencing the symptoms of menopause. (See page 352.) Talk to your doctor about possible remedies.**

No ↓

Talk to your doctor for further help in determining the source of your problem.

29. Eating Disorders
Being overly preoccupied with food or losing or gaining weight

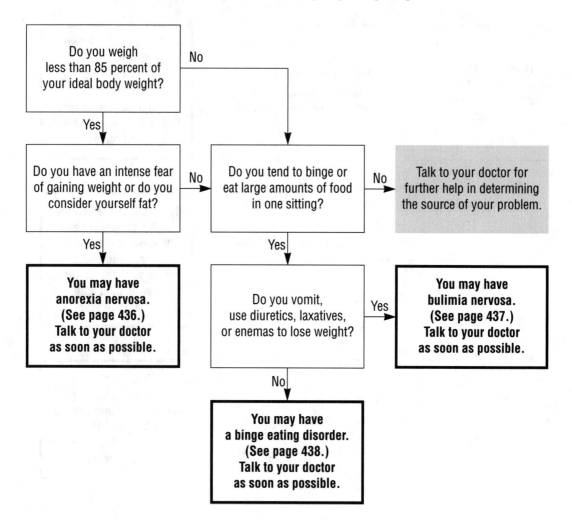

Do you weigh less than 85 percent of your ideal body weight?

No →

Yes ↓

Do you have an intense fear of gaining weight or do you consider yourself fat?

No →

Do you tend to binge or eat large amounts of food in one sitting?

No →

Talk to your doctor for further help in determining the source of your problem.

Yes ↓

You may have anorexia nervosa. (See page 436.) Talk to your doctor as soon as possible.

Yes ↓

Do you vomit, use diuretics, laxatives, or enemas to lose weight?

Yes →

You may have bulimia nervosa. (See page 437.) Talk to your doctor as soon as possible.

No ↓

You may have a binge eating disorder. (See page 438.) Talk to your doctor as soon as possible.

30. Hypoglycemia
Having a blood glucose level below 60 mg/dl or showing symptoms of hypoglycemia

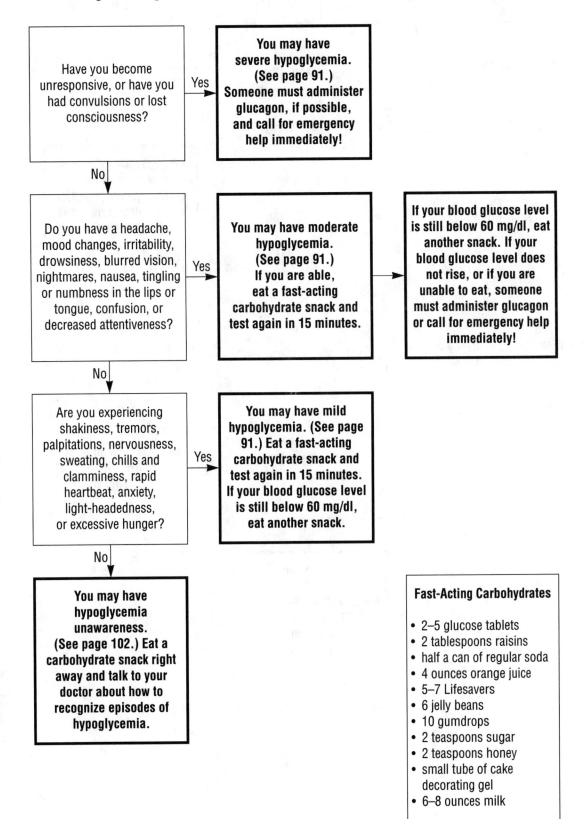

Have you become unresponsive, or have you had convulsions or lost consciousness?

Yes → You may have severe hypoglycemia. (See page 91.) Someone must administer glucagon, if possible, and call for emergency help immediately!

No ↓

Do you have a headache, mood changes, irritability, drowsiness, blurred vision, nightmares, nausea, tingling or numbness in the lips or tongue, confusion, or decreased attentiveness?

Yes → You may have moderate hypoglycemia. (See page 91.) If you are able, eat a fast-acting carbohydrate snack and test again in 15 minutes. → If your blood glucose level is still below 60 mg/dl, eat another snack. If your blood glucose level does not rise, or if you are unable to eat, someone must administer glucagon or call for emergency help immediately!

No ↓

Are you experiencing shakiness, tremors, palpitations, nervousness, sweating, chills and clamminess, rapid heartbeat, anxiety, light-headedness, or excessive hunger?

Yes → You may have mild hypoglycemia. (See page 91.) Eat a fast-acting carbohydrate snack and test again in 15 minutes. If your blood glucose level is still below 60 mg/dl, eat another snack.

No ↓

You may have hypoglycemia unawareness. (See page 102.) Eat a carbohydrate snack right away and talk to your doctor about how to recognize episodes of hypoglycemia.

Fast-Acting Carbohydrates

- 2–5 glucose tablets
- 2 tablespoons raisins
- half a can of regular soda
- 4 ounces orange juice
- 5–7 Lifesavers
- 6 jelly beans
- 10 gumdrops
- 2 teaspoons sugar
- 2 teaspoons honey
- small tube of cake decorating gel
- 6–8 ounces milk

31. Vision Problems
Experiencing any loss, dimness, or distortion of vision, floating spots, or double vision

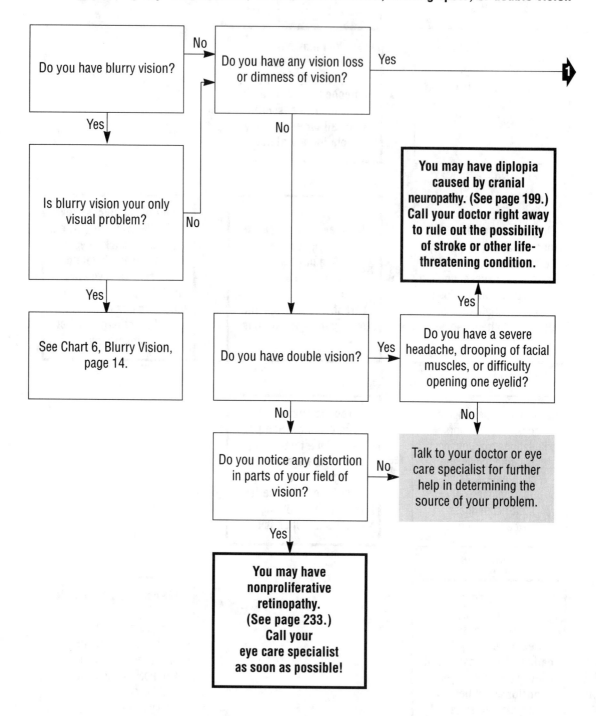

THE DIABETES PROBLEM SOLVER

31. Vision Problems
Experiencing any loss, dimness, or distortion of vision, floating spots, or double vision
(Continued)

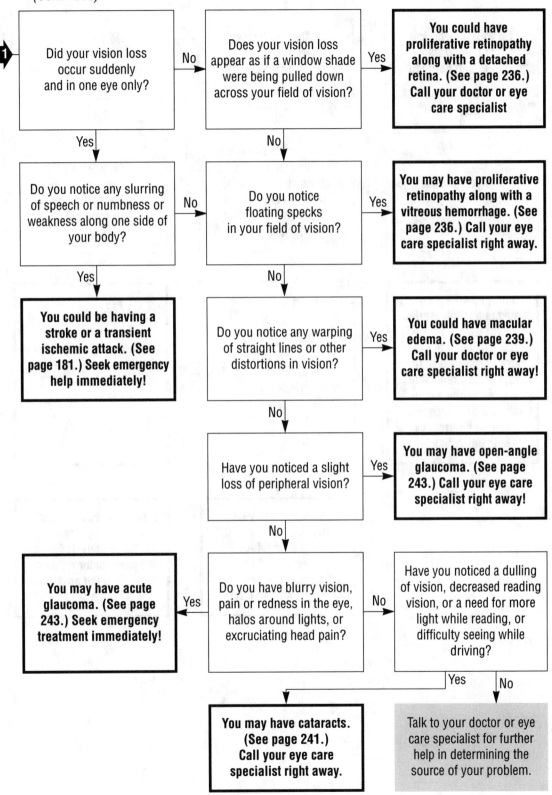

1 Did your vision loss occur suddenly and in one eye only?

→ **No** → Does your vision loss appear as if a window shade were being pulled down across your field of vision? → **Yes** → **You could have proliferative retinopathy along with a detached retina. (See page 236.) Call your doctor or eye care specialist**

↓ **Yes**

Do you notice any slurring of speech or numbness or weakness along one side of your body?

↓ **No** → Does your vision loss appear... **No** ↓

Do you notice floating specks in your field of vision? → **Yes** → **You may have proliferative retinopathy along with a vitreous hemorrhage. (See page 236.) Call your eye care specialist right away.**

↓ **Yes**

You could be having a stroke or a transient ischemic attack. (See page 181.) Seek emergency help immediately!

↓ **No**

Do you notice any warping of straight lines or other distortions in vision? → **Yes** → **You could have macular edema. (See page 239.) Call your doctor or eye care specialist right away!**

↓ **No**

Have you noticed a slight loss of peripheral vision? → **Yes** → **You may have open-angle glaucoma. (See page 243.) Call your eye care specialist right away!**

↓ **No**

You may have acute glaucoma. (See page 243.) Seek emergency treatment immediately! ← **Yes** ← Do you have blurry vision, pain or redness in the eye, halos around lights, or excruciating head pain? → **No** → Have you noticed a dulling of vision, decreased reading vision, or a need for more light while reading, or difficulty seeing while driving?

↓ **Yes**   **Yes** ↓   **No** ↓

You may have cataracts. (See page 241.) Call your eye care specialist right away.

Talk to your doctor or eye care specialist for further help in determining the source of your problem.

32. Numbness and Tingling
Feeling any numbness, tingling, odd sensations, or loss of sensation in any part of the body

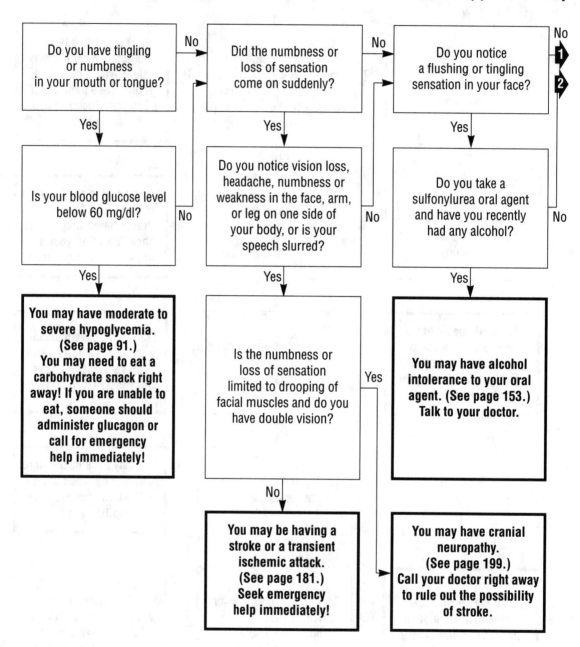

32. Numbness and Tingling
Feeling any numbness, tingling, odd sensations, or loss of sensation in any part of the body *(Continued)*

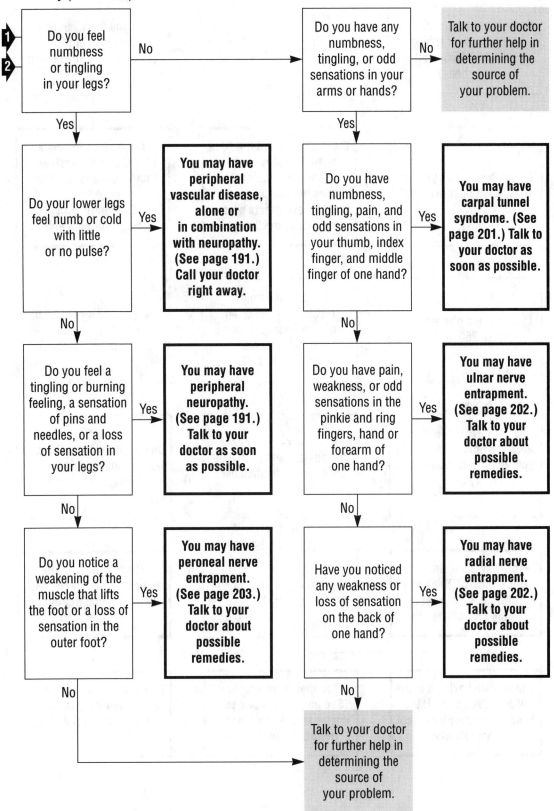

1
2 Do you feel numbness or tingling in your legs? — **No** → Do you have any numbness, tingling, or odd sensations in your arms or hands? — **No** → Talk to your doctor for further help in determining the source of your problem.

Yes ↓

Do your lower legs feel numb or cold with little or no pulse? — **Yes** → **You may have peripheral vascular disease, alone or in combination with neuropathy. (See page 191.) Call your doctor right away.**

Yes ↓

Do you have numbness, tingling, pain, and odd sensations in your thumb, index finger, and middle finger of one hand? — **Yes** → **You may have carpal tunnel syndrome. (See page 201.) Talk to your doctor as soon as possible.**

No ↓

Do you feel a tingling or burning feeling, a sensation of pins and needles, or a loss of sensation in your legs? — **Yes** → **You may have peripheral neuropathy. (See page 191.) Talk to your doctor as soon as possible.**

No ↓

Do you have pain, weakness, or odd sensations in the pinkie and ring fingers, hand or forearm of one hand? — **Yes** → **You may have ulnar nerve entrapment. (See page 202.) Talk to your doctor about possible remedies.**

No ↓

Do you notice a weakening of the muscle that lifts the foot or a loss of sensation in the outer foot? — **Yes** → **You may have peroneal nerve entrapment. (See page 203.) Talk to your doctor about possible remedies.**

No ↓

Have you noticed any weakness or loss of sensation on the back of one hand? — **Yes** → **You may have radial nerve entrapment. (See page 202.) Talk to your doctor about possible remedies.**

No ↓

Talk to your doctor for further help in determining the source of your problem.

33. Muscular Weakness
Feeling tired or weak in muscles anywhere in the body

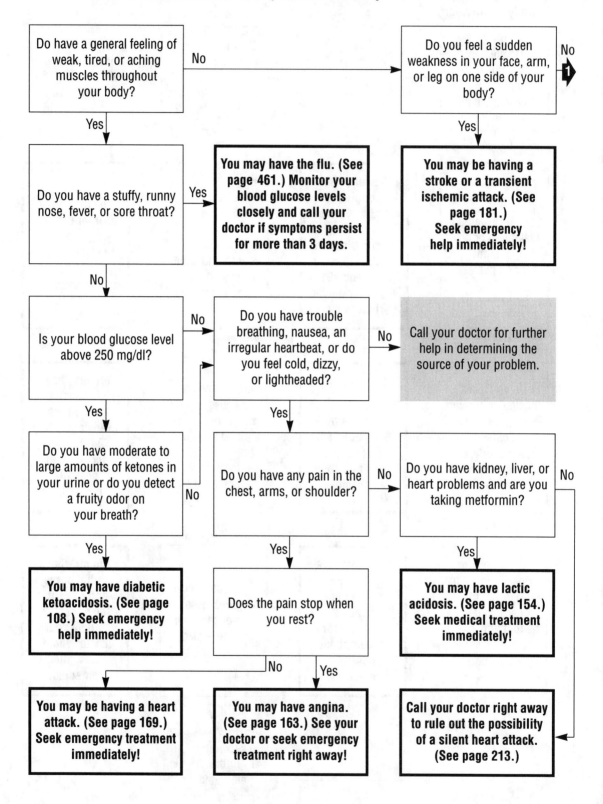

Do have a general feeling of weak, tired, or aching muscles throughout your body?

No →

Do you feel a sudden weakness in your face, arm, or leg on one side of your body?

No → ❶

Yes ↓

Do you have a stuffy, runny nose, fever, or sore throat?

Yes → **You may have the flu. (See page 461.) Monitor your blood glucose levels closely and call your doctor if symptoms persist for more than 3 days.**

Yes ↓ (from sudden weakness) **You may be having a stroke or a transient ischemic attack. (See page 181.) Seek emergency help immediately!**

No ↓

Is your blood glucose level above 250 mg/dl?

No → Do you have trouble breathing, nausea, an irregular heartbeat, or do you feel cold, dizzy, or lightheaded?

No → Call your doctor for further help in determining the source of your problem.

Yes ↓

Do you have moderate to large amounts of ketones in your urine or do you detect a fruity odor on your breath?

Yes ↓ (trouble breathing) Do you have any pain in the chest, arms, or shoulder?

No → Do you have kidney, liver, or heart problems and are you taking metformin?

No →

Yes ↓

You may have diabetic ketoacidosis. (See page 108.) Seek emergency help immediately!

Yes ↓ Does the pain stop when you rest?

Yes ↓ (metformin) **You may have lactic acidosis. (See page 154.) Seek medical treatment immediately!**

No ↓ | **Yes ↓**

You may be having a heart attack. (See page 169.) Seek emergency treatment immediately!

You may have angina. (See page 163.) See your doctor or seek emergency treatment right away!

Call your doctor right away to rule out the possibility of a silent heart attack. (See page 213.)

THE DIABETES PROBLEM SOLVER

33. Muscular Weakness
Feeling tired or weak in muscles anywhere in the body *(Continued)*

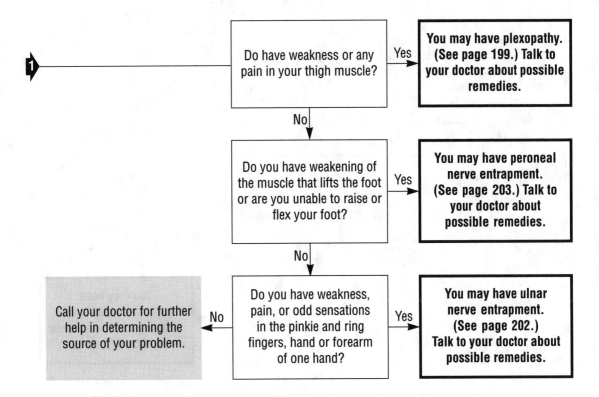

1

Do have weakness or any pain in your thigh muscle? → **Yes** → **You may have plexopathy. (See page 199.) Talk to your doctor about possible remedies.**

No ↓

Do you have weakening of the muscle that lifts the foot or are you unable to raise or flex your foot? → **Yes** → **You may have peroneal nerve entrapment. (See page 203.) Talk to your doctor about possible remedies.**

No ↓

Do you have weakness, pain, or odd sensations in the pinkie and ring fingers, hand or forearm of one hand? → **Yes** → **You may have ulnar nerve entrapment. (See page 202.) Talk to your doctor about possible remedies.**

No → Call your doctor for further help in determining the source of your problem.

34. Foot Problems
Any kind of pain, swelling, or deformity of the foot

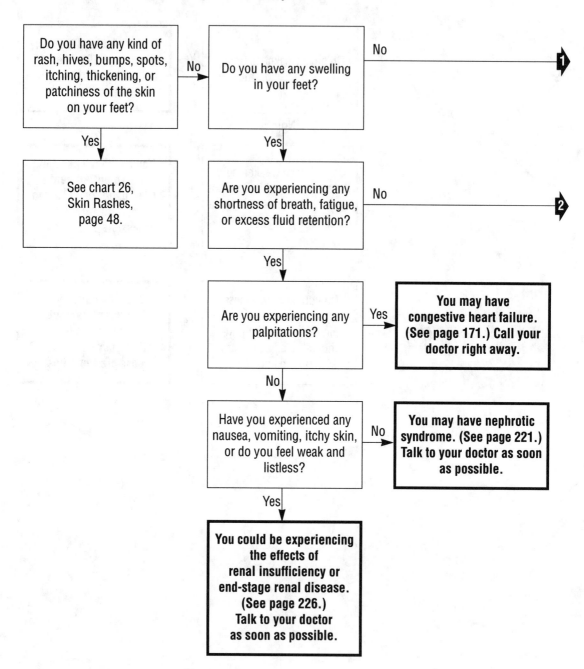

Do you have any kind of rash, hives, bumps, spots, itching, thickening, or patchiness of the skin on your feet?

No →

Do you have any swelling in your feet?

No → 1

Yes ↓

See chart 26, Skin Rashes, page 48.

Yes ↓

Are you experiencing any shortness of breath, fatigue, or excess fluid retention?

No → 2

Yes ↓

Are you experiencing any palpitations?

Yes → You may have congestive heart failure. (See page 171.) Call your doctor right away.

No ↓

Have you experienced any nausea, vomiting, itchy skin, or do you feel weak and listless?

No → You may have nephrotic syndrome. (See page 221.) Talk to your doctor as soon as possible.

Yes ↓

You could be experiencing the effects of renal insufficiency or end-stage renal disease. (See page 226.) Talk to your doctor as soon as possible.

34. Foot Problems
Any kind of pain, swelling, or deformity of the foot *(Continued)*

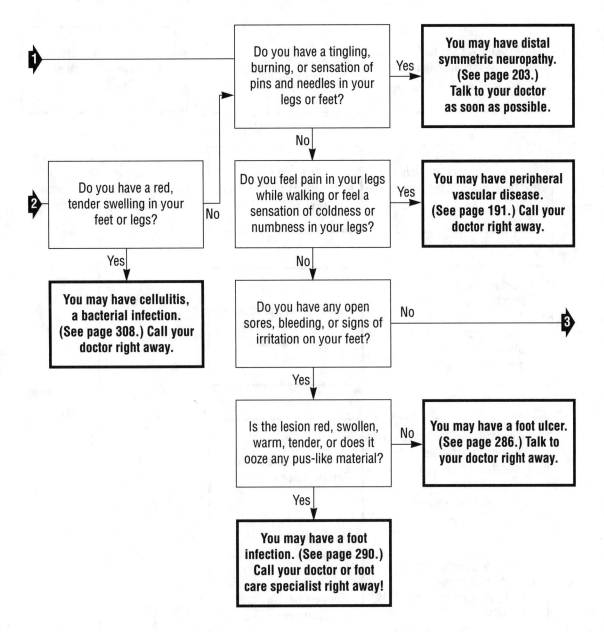

1 → Do you have a tingling, burning, or sensation of pins and needles in your legs or feet? — **Yes** → **You may have distal symmetric neuropathy. (See page 203.) Talk to your doctor as soon as possible.**

No ↓

2 → Do you have a red, tender swelling in your feet or legs? — **No** →

Do you feel pain in your legs while walking or feel a sensation of coldness or numbness in your legs? — **Yes** → **You may have peripheral vascular disease. (See page 191.) Call your doctor right away.**

Yes ↓ (from box 2)

You may have cellulitis, a bacterial infection. (See page 308.) Call your doctor right away.

No ↓ (from leg pain box)

Do you have any open sores, bleeding, or signs of irritation on your feet? — **No** → **3**

Yes ↓

Is the lesion red, swollen, warm, tender, or does it ooze any pus-like material? — **No** → **You may have a foot ulcer. (See page 286.) Talk to your doctor right away.**

Yes ↓

You may have a foot infection. (See page 290.) Call your doctor or foot care specialist right away!

34. Foot Problems
Any kind of pain, swelling, or deformity of the foot *(Continued)*

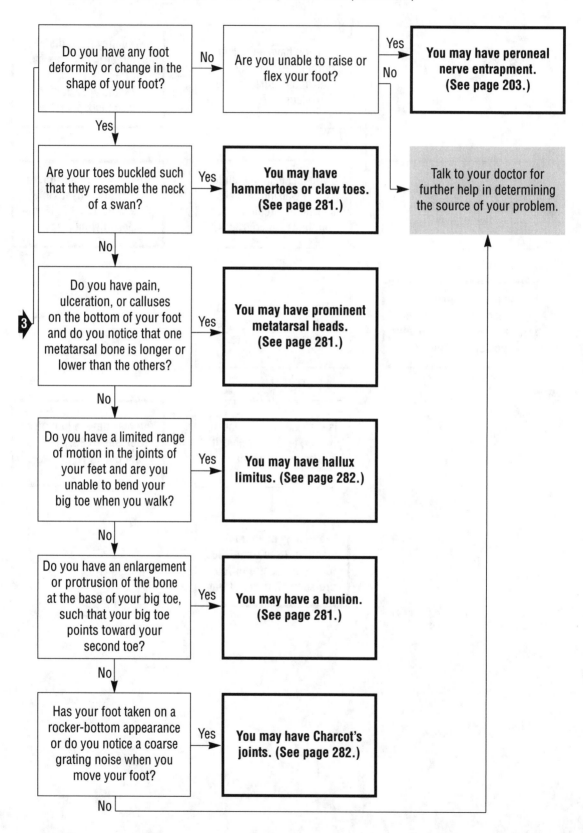

Do you have any foot deformity or change in the shape of your foot?

No → Are you unable to raise or flex your foot?

Yes → **You may have peroneal nerve entrapment. (See page 203.)**

No → Talk to your doctor for further help in determining the source of your problem.

Yes ↓

Are your toes buckled such that they resemble the neck of a swan?

Yes → **You may have hammertoes or claw toes. (See page 281.)**

No ↓

3 Do you have pain, ulceration, or calluses on the bottom of your foot and do you notice that one metatarsal bone is longer or lower than the others?

Yes → **You may have prominent metatarsal heads. (See page 281.)**

No ↓

Do you have a limited range of motion in the joints of your feet and are you unable to bend your big toe when you walk?

Yes → **You may have hallux limitus. (See page 282.)**

No ↓

Do you have an enlargement or protrusion of the bone at the base of your big toe, such that your big toe points toward your second toe?

Yes → **You may have a bunion. (See page 281.)**

No ↓

Has your foot taken on a rocker-bottom appearance or do you notice a coarse grating noise when you move your foot?

Yes → **You may have Charcot's joints. (See page 282.)**

No

35. Hyperglycemia

Having a blood glucose level above 250 mg/dl or showing symptoms of high blood glucose

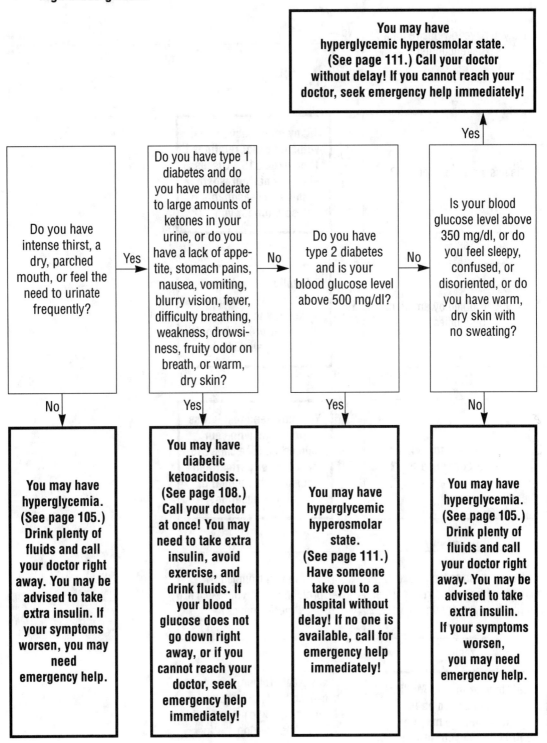

You may have hyperglycemic hyperosmolar state. (See page 111.) Call your doctor without delay! If you cannot reach your doctor, seek emergency help immediately!

Do you have intense thirst, a dry, parched mouth, or feel the need to urinate frequently?

Yes →

Do you have type 1 diabetes and do you have moderate to large amounts of ketones in your urine, or do you have a lack of appetite, stomach pains, nausea, vomiting, blurry vision, fever, difficulty breathing, weakness, drowsiness, fruity odor on breath, or warm, dry skin?

No →

Do you have type 2 diabetes and is your blood glucose level above 500 mg/dl?

No →

Is your blood glucose level above 350 mg/dl, or do you feel sleepy, confused, or disoriented, or do you have warm, dry skin with no sweating?

Yes ↑

No ↓

You may have hyperglycemia. (See page 105.) Drink plenty of fluids and call your doctor right away. You may be advised to take extra insulin. If your symptoms worsen, you may need emergency help.

Yes ↓

You may have diabetic ketoacidosis. (See page 108.) Call your doctor at once! You may need to take extra insulin, avoid exercise, and drink fluids. If your blood glucose does not go down right away, or if you cannot reach your doctor, seek emergency help immediately!

Yes ↓

You may have hyperglycemic hyperosmolar state. (See page 111.) Have someone take you to a hospital without delay! If no one is available, call for emergency help immediately!

No ↓

You may have hyperglycemia. (See page 105.) Drink plenty of fluids and call your doctor right away. You may be advised to take extra insulin. If your symptoms worsen, you may need emergency help.

36. Sexual Problems in Men
Experiencing any difficulties with sexual desire, erections, or orgasm

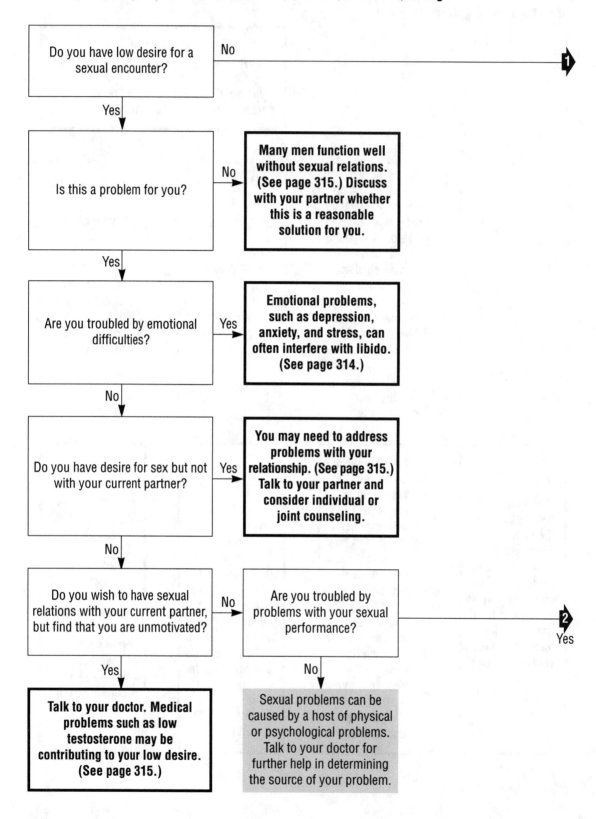

Do you have low desire for a sexual encounter? — No ⟶ **1**

Yes ↓

Is this a problem for you? — No →

Many men function well without sexual relations. (See page 315.) Discuss with your partner whether this is a reasonable solution for you.

Yes ↓

Are you troubled by emotional difficulties? — Yes →

Emotional problems, such as depression, anxiety, and stress, can often interfere with libido. (See page 314.)

No ↓

Do you have desire for sex but not with your current partner? — Yes →

You may need to address problems with your relationship. (See page 315.) Talk to your partner and consider individual or joint counseling.

No ↓

Do you wish to have sexual relations with your current partner, but find that you are unmotivated? — No → Are you troubled by problems with your sexual performance? ⟶ **2** Yes

Yes ↓

Talk to your doctor. Medical problems such as low testosterone may be contributing to your low desire. (See page 315.)

No ↓

Sexual problems can be caused by a host of physical or psychological problems. Talk to your doctor for further help in determining the source of your problem.

36. Sexual Problems in Men
Experiencing any difficulties with sexual desire, erections, or orgasm *(Continued)*

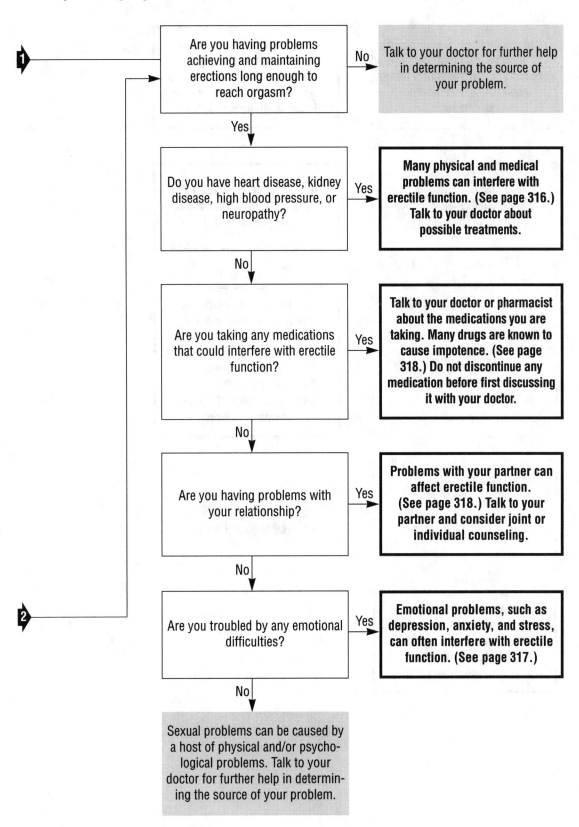

①

Are you having problems achieving and maintaining erections long enough to reach orgasm?

No → Talk to your doctor for further help in determining the source of your problem.

Yes ↓

Do you have heart disease, kidney disease, high blood pressure, or neuropathy?

Yes → **Many physical and medical problems can interfere with erectile function. (See page 316.) Talk to your doctor about possible treatments.**

No ↓

Are you taking any medications that could interfere with erectile function?

Yes → **Talk to your doctor or pharmacist about the medications you are taking. Many drugs are known to cause impotence. (See page 318.) Do not discontinue any medication before first discussing it with your doctor.**

No ↓

Are you having problems with your relationship?

Yes → **Problems with your partner can affect erectile function. (See page 318.) Talk to your partner and consider joint or individual counseling.**

No ↓

②

Are you troubled by any emotional difficulties?

Yes → **Emotional problems, such as depression, anxiety, and stress, can often interfere with erectile function. (See page 317.)**

No ↓

Sexual problems can be caused by a host of physical and/or psychological problems. Talk to your doctor for further help in determining the source of your problem.

37. Problems with Blood Glucose Control in Women

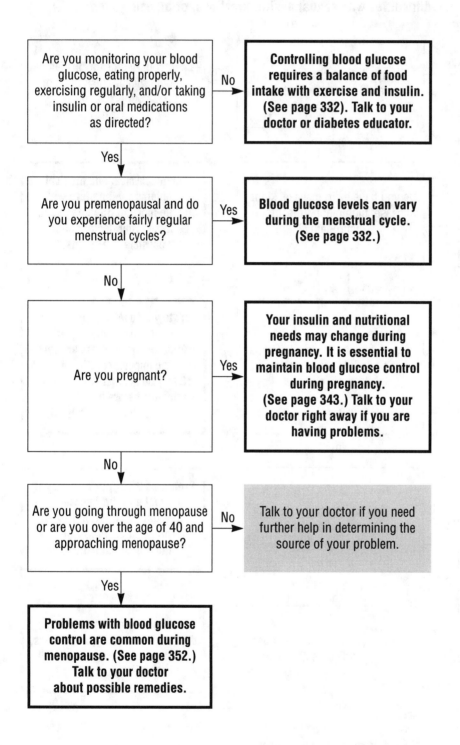

Are you monitoring your blood glucose, eating properly, exercising regularly, and/or taking insulin or oral medications as directed?

No → Controlling blood glucose requires a balance of food intake with exercise and insulin. (See page 332). Talk to your doctor or diabetes educator.

Yes ↓

Are you premenopausal and do you experience fairly regular menstrual cycles?

Yes → Blood glucose levels can vary during the menstrual cycle. (See page 332.)

No ↓

Are you pregnant?

Yes → Your insulin and nutritional needs may change during pregnancy. It is essential to maintain blood glucose control during pregnancy. (See page 343.) Talk to your doctor right away if you are having problems.

No ↓

Are you going through menopause or are you over the age of 40 and approaching menopause?

No → Talk to your doctor if you need further help in determining the source of your problem.

Yes ↓

Problems with blood glucose control are common during menopause. (See page 352.) Talk to your doctor about possible remedies.

38. Pain or Discomfort in Women
Having any symptoms that cause you pain or discomfort

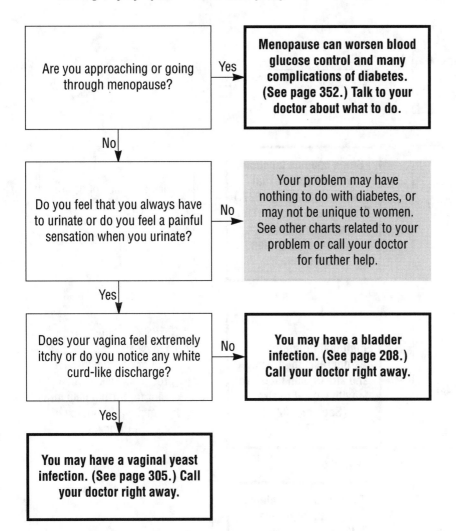

Are you approaching or going through menopause?

Yes → Menopause can worsen blood glucose control and many complications of diabetes. (See page 352.) Talk to your doctor about what to do.

No ↓

Do you feel that you always have to urinate or do you feel a painful sensation when you urinate?

No → Your problem may have nothing to do with diabetes, or may not be unique to women. See other charts related to your problem or call your doctor for further help.

Yes ↓

Does your vagina feel extremely itchy or do you notice any white curd-like discharge?

No → You may have a bladder infection. (See page 208.) Call your doctor right away.

Yes ↓

You may have a vaginal yeast infection. (See page 305.) Call your doctor right away.

39. Sexual Problems in Women
Experiencing any difficulties with sexual desire, arousal, or orgasm

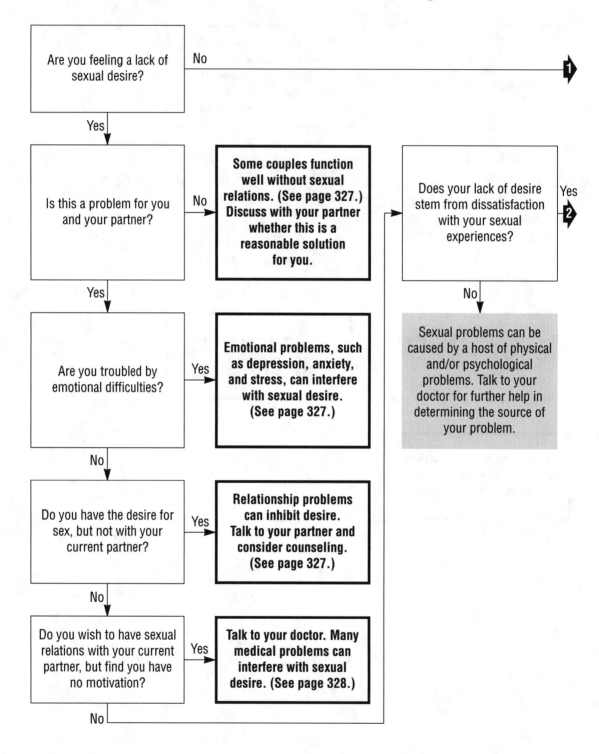

Are you feeling a lack of sexual desire?

No → **1**

Yes ↓

Is this a problem for you and your partner?

No → Some couples function well without sexual relations. (See page 327.) Discuss with your partner whether this is a reasonable solution for you.

→ Does your lack of desire stem from dissatisfaction with your sexual experiences?

Yes → **2**

No ↓

Sexual problems can be caused by a host of physical and/or psychological problems. Talk to your doctor for further help in determining the source of your problem.

Yes ↓

Are you troubled by emotional difficulties?

Yes → Emotional problems, such as depression, anxiety, and stress, can interfere with sexual desire. (See page 327.)

No ↓

Do you have the desire for sex, but not with your current partner?

Yes → Relationship problems can inhibit desire. Talk to your partner and consider counseling. (See page 327.)

No ↓

Do you wish to have sexual relations with your current partner, but find you have no motivation?

Yes → Talk to your doctor. Many medical problems can interfere with sexual desire. (See page 328.)

No

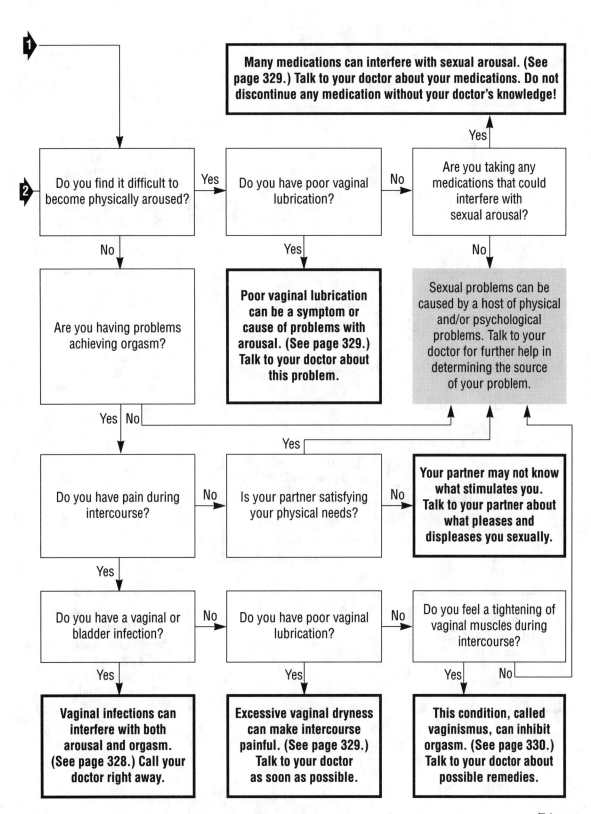

Many medications can interfere with sexual arousal. (See page 329.) Talk to your doctor about your medications. Do not discontinue any medication without your doctor's knowledge!

Do you find it difficult to become physically aroused?

Do you have poor vaginal lubrication?

Are you taking any medications that could interfere with sexual arousal?

Are you having problems achieving orgasm?

Poor vaginal lubrication can be a symptom or cause of problems with arousal. (See page 329.) Talk to your doctor about this problem.

Sexual problems can be caused by a host of physical and/or psychological problems. Talk to your doctor for further help in determining the source of your problem.

Do you have pain during intercourse?

Is your partner satisfying your physical needs?

Your partner may not know what stimulates you. Talk to your partner about what pleases and displeases you sexually.

Do you have a vaginal or bladder infection?

Do you have poor vaginal lubrication?

Do you feel a tightening of vaginal muscles during intercourse?

Vaginal infections can interfere with both arousal and orgasm. (See page 328.) Call your doctor right away.

Excessive vaginal dryness can make intercourse painful. (See page 329.) Talk to your doctor as soon as possible.

This condition, called vaginismus, can inhibit orgasm. (See page 330.) Talk to your doctor about possible remedies.

40. Urinary Problems

Frequent urination, painful urination, abnormal looking urine, incomplete voiding, or problems with bladder control

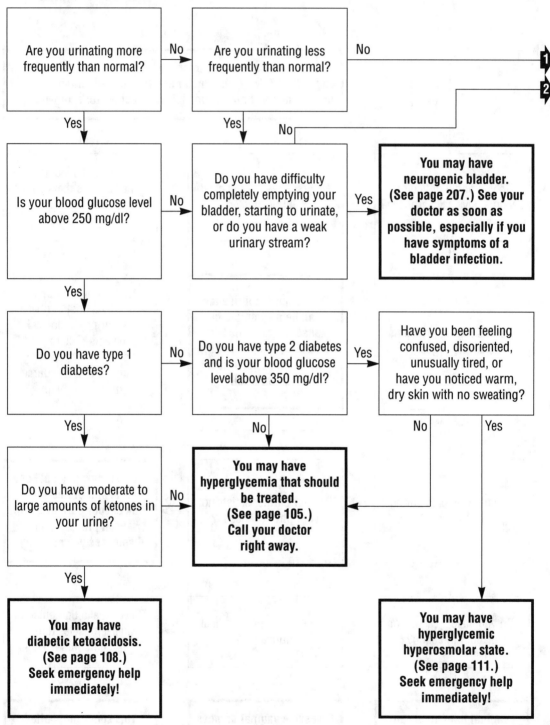

40. Urinary Problems

Frequent urination, painful urination, abnormal looking urine, incomplete voiding, or problems with bladder control *(Continued)*

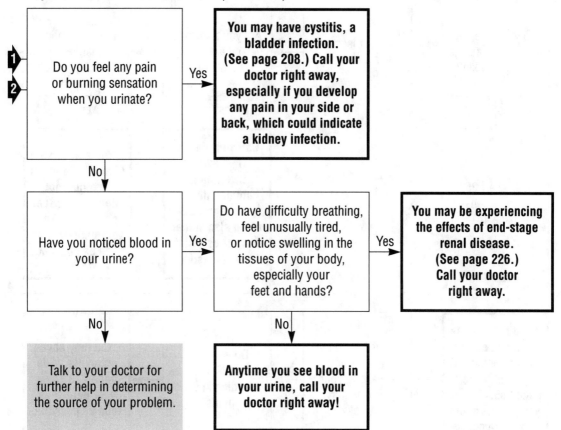

1
2
Do you feel any pain or burning sensation when you urinate?

Yes → **You may have cystitis, a bladder infection. (See page 208.) Call your doctor right away, especially if you develop any pain in your side or back, which could indicate a kidney infection.**

No ↓

Have you noticed blood in your urine?

Yes → Do have difficulty breathing, feel unusually tired, or notice swelling in the tissues of your body, especially your feet and hands?

Yes → **You may be experiencing the effects of end-stage renal disease. (See page 226.) Call your doctor right away.**

No ↓

Talk to your doctor for further help in determining the source of your problem.

No ↓

Anytime you see blood in your urine, call your doctor right away!

41. Swelling
Having any kind of swelling, swollen joints, fluid retention, or fluid accumulation

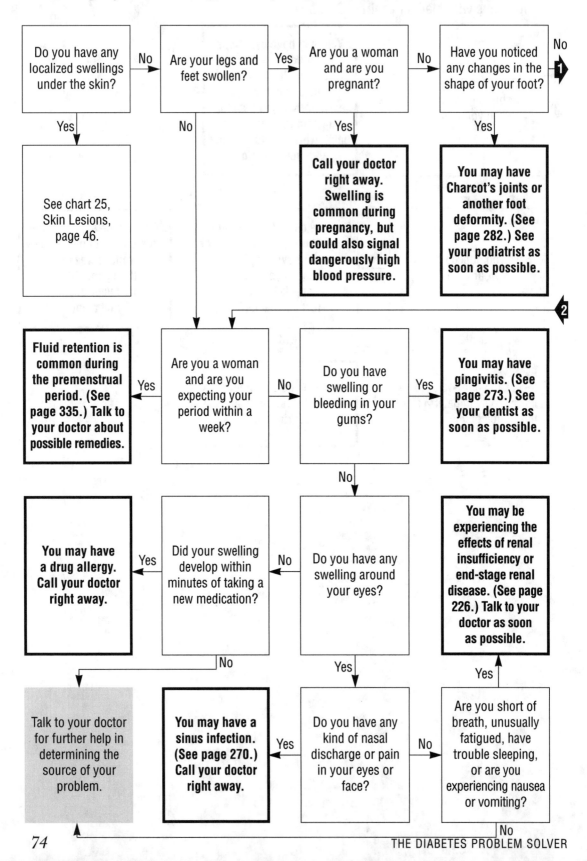

Do you have any localized swellings under the skin? — No → Are your legs and feet swollen? — Yes → Are you a woman and are you pregnant? — No → Have you noticed any changes in the shape of your foot? — No → ❶

Do you have any localized swellings under the skin? — Yes → See chart 25, Skin Lesions, page 46.

Are your legs and feet swollen? — No →

Are you a woman and are you pregnant? — Yes → **Call your doctor right away. Swelling is common during pregnancy, but could also signal dangerously high blood pressure.**

Have you noticed any changes in the shape of your foot? — Yes → **You may have Charcot's joints or another foot deformity. (See page 282.) See your podiatrist as soon as possible.**

❷

Fluid retention is common during the premenstrual period. (See page 335.) Talk to your doctor about possible remedies. ← Yes — Are you a woman and are you expecting your period within a week? — No → Do you have swelling or bleeding in your gums? — Yes → **You may have gingivitis. (See page 273.) See your dentist as soon as possible.**

Do you have swelling or bleeding in your gums? — No ↓

You may have a drug allergy. Call your doctor right away. ← Yes — Did your swelling develop within minutes of taking a new medication? — No → Do you have any swelling around your eyes? — No →

You may be experiencing the effects of renal insufficiency or end-stage renal disease. (See page 226.) Talk to your doctor as soon as possible.

Did your swelling develop within minutes of taking a new medication? — No ↓

Talk to your doctor for further help in determining the source of your problem.

You may have a sinus infection. (See page 270.) Call your doctor right away. ← Yes — Do you have any kind of nasal discharge or pain in your eyes or face? — No → Are you short of breath, unusually fatigued, have trouble sleeping, or are you experiencing nausea or vomiting? — Yes ↑

Do you have any swelling around your eyes? — Yes ↓

Do you have any kind of nasal discharge or pain in your eyes or face? (from "Do you have any swelling around your eyes?" Yes)

Are you short of breath, unusually fatigued, have trouble sleeping, or are you experiencing nausea or vomiting? — No →

THE DIABETES PROBLEM SOLVER

41. Swelling
Having any kind of swelling, swollen joints, fluid retention, or fluid accumulation
(Continued)

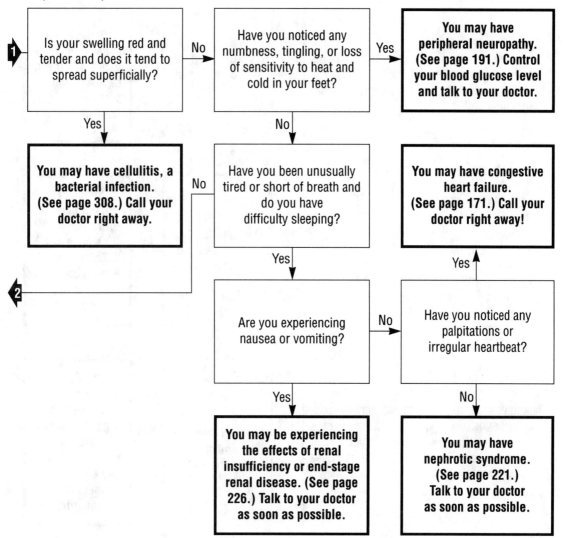

1 Is your swelling red and tender and does it tend to spread superficially?

No → Have you noticed any numbness, tingling, or loss of sensitivity to heat and cold in your feet?

Yes → You may have peripheral neuropathy. (See page 191.) Control your blood glucose level and talk to your doctor.

Yes ↓ You may have cellulitis, a bacterial infection. (See page 308.) Call your doctor right away.

No → Have you been unusually tired or short of breath and do you have difficulty sleeping?

2

Yes ↓ Are you experiencing nausea or vomiting?

No → Have you noticed any palpitations or irregular heartbeat?

Yes ↑ You may have congestive heart failure. (See page 171.) Call your doctor right away!

Yes ↓ You may be experiencing the effects of renal insufficiency or end-stage renal disease. (See page 226.) Talk to your doctor as soon as possible.

No ↓ You may have nephrotic syndrome. (See page 221.) Talk to your doctor as soon as possible.

42. Intestinal Problems
Having diarrhea, loose bowels, constipation, or other signs of abdominal distress

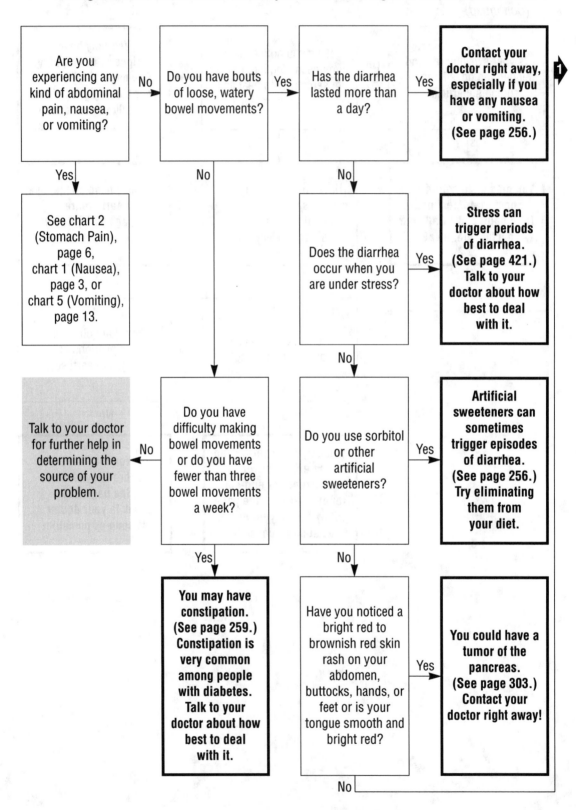

Are you experiencing any kind of abdominal pain, nausea, or vomiting?

— No → Do you have bouts of loose, watery bowel movements?

— Yes → Has the diarrhea lasted more than a day?

— Yes → **Contact your doctor right away, especially if you have any nausea or vomiting. (See page 256.)** ➊

Are you experiencing any kind of abdominal pain, nausea, or vomiting? — Yes ↓

See chart 2 (Stomach Pain), page 6, chart 1 (Nausea), page 3, or chart 5 (Vomiting), page 13.

Has the diarrhea lasted more than a day? — No ↓

Does the diarrhea occur when you are under stress?

— Yes → **Stress can trigger periods of diarrhea. (See page 421.) Talk to your doctor about how best to deal with it.**

— No ↓

Talk to your doctor for further help in determining the source of your problem.

← No — Do you have difficulty making bowel movements or do you have fewer than three bowel movements a week?

Do you use sorbitol or other artificial sweeteners?

— Yes → **Artificial sweeteners can sometimes trigger episodes of diarrhea. (See page 256.) Try eliminating them from your diet.**

Do you have difficulty making bowel movements...? — Yes ↓

You may have constipation. (See page 259.) Constipation is very common among people with diabetes. Talk to your doctor about how best to deal with it.

Do you use sorbitol or other artificial sweeteners? — No ↓

Have you noticed a bright red to brownish red skin rash on your abdomen, buttocks, hands, or feet or is your tongue smooth and bright red?

— Yes → **You could have a tumor of the pancreas. (See page 303.) Contact your doctor right away!**

— No

42. Intestinal Problems
Having diarrhea, loose bowels, constipation, or other signs of abdominal distress
(Continued)

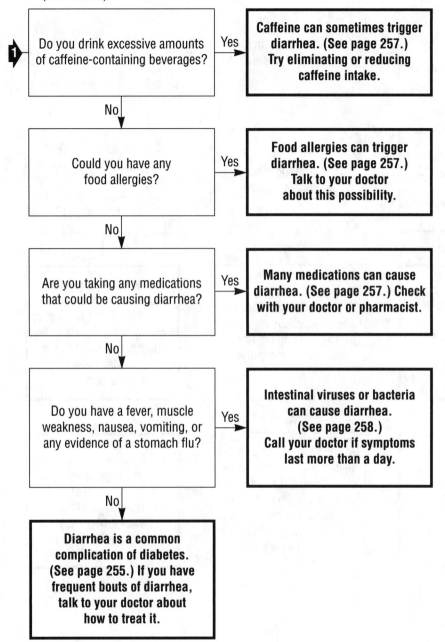

Do you drink excessive amounts of caffeine-containing beverages?

Yes → Caffeine can sometimes trigger diarrhea. (See page 257.) Try eliminating or reducing caffeine intake.

No ↓

Could you have any food allergies?

Yes → Food allergies can trigger diarrhea. (See page 257.) Talk to your doctor about this possibility.

No ↓

Are you taking any medications that could be causing diarrhea?

Yes → Many medications can cause diarrhea. (See page 257.) Check with your doctor or pharmacist.

No ↓

Do you have a fever, muscle weakness, nausea, vomiting, or any evidence of a stomach flu?

Yes → Intestinal viruses or bacteria can cause diarrhea. (See page 258.) Call your doctor if symptoms last more than a day.

No ↓

Diarrhea is a common complication of diabetes. (See page 255.) If you have frequent bouts of diarrhea, talk to your doctor about how to treat it.

43. Problems with the Mouth

Having any kind of soreness, discomfort, sour taste, or odd sensations that affect the mouth, teeth, gums, or tongue

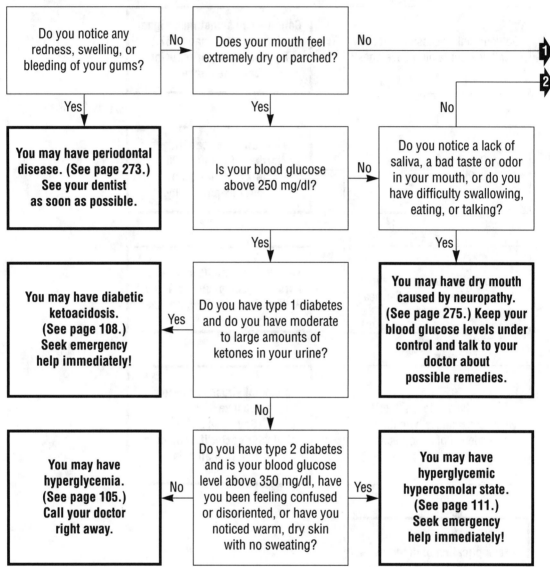

Do you notice any redness, swelling, or bleeding of your gums? —No→ Does your mouth feel extremely dry or parched? —No→ **1**

2

Yes↓ (from first box)

You may have periodontal disease. (See page 273.) See your dentist as soon as possible.

Yes↓ (from dry mouth box)

Is your blood glucose above 250 mg/dl? —No→ Do you notice a lack of saliva, a bad taste or odor in your mouth, or do you have difficulty swallowing, eating, or talking?

You may have diabetic ketoacidosis. (See page 108.) Seek emergency help immediately! ←Yes— Do you have type 1 diabetes and do you have moderate to large amounts of ketones in your urine?

Yes↓ (from blood glucose box)

Yes↓ (from saliva box)

You may have dry mouth caused by neuropathy. (See page 275.) Keep your blood glucose levels under control and talk to your doctor about possible remedies.

No↓ (from ketones box)

You may have hyperglycemia. (See page 105.) Call your doctor right away. ←No— Do you have type 2 diabetes and is your blood glucose level above 350 mg/dl, have you been feeling confused or disoriented, or have you noticed warm, dry skin with no sweating? —Yes→ **You may have hyperglycemic hyperosmolar state. (See page 111.) Seek emergency help immediately!**

43. Problems with the Mouth

Having any kind of soreness, discomfort, sour taste, or odd sensations that affect the mouth, teeth, gums, or tongue *(Continued)*

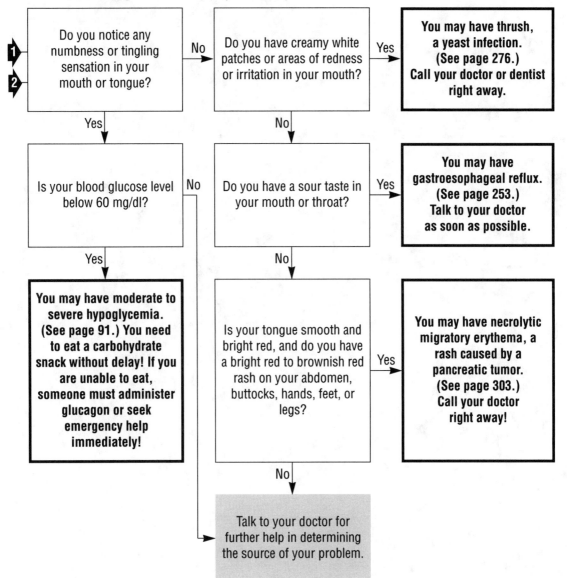

1
2

Do you notice any numbness or tingling sensation in your mouth or tongue?

No →

Do you have creamy white patches or areas of redness or irritation in your mouth?

Yes →

You may have thrush, a yeast infection. (See page 276.) Call your doctor or dentist right away.

Yes ↓

No ↓

Is your blood glucose level below 60 mg/dl?

No →

Do you have a sour taste in your mouth or throat?

Yes →

You may have gastroesophageal reflux. (See page 253.) Talk to your doctor as soon as possible.

Yes ↓

No ↓

You may have moderate to severe hypoglycemia. (See page 91.) You need to eat a carbohydrate snack without delay! If you are unable to eat, someone must administer glucagon or seek emergency help immediately!

Is your tongue smooth and bright red, and do you have a bright red to brownish red rash on your abdomen, buttocks, hands, feet, or legs?

Yes →

You may have necrolytic migratory erythema, a rash caused by a pancreatic tumor. (See page 303.) Call your doctor right away!

No ↓

Talk to your doctor for further help in determining the source of your problem.

Chapter 1
Solving Monitoring and Testing Problems

The key to managing your diabetes and living a normal life is to keep your blood glucose levels as close to normal as possible. By controlling blood glucose levels, you can prevent many of the complications of diabetes, and you can also prevent emergency situations from arising. In the past, it was difficult to gauge how well you were doing and difficult to predict when an emergency would arise until you were right in the middle of it. Today, you can keep close tabs on your blood glucose control by testing.

Two types of tests are especially important to you. With a blood glucose meter, you can monitor your blood glucose levels several times a day. This will tell you whether you are meeting your blood glucose target goals on a daily basis. With test strips, you can test your urine for ketones, chemicals that can appear in your blood when your blood glucose level is too high. By testing your blood regularly and your urine when you have to, you'll be able to better manage your diabetes.

Blood Glucose Monitoring

Whether you have type 1, type 2, or gestational diabetes, your goal is to keep your blood glucose levels as close to normal as possible, with a plan that works for you. The only way to know for sure whether you are meeting your goal is to test your blood glucose levels. Testing also helps tell you when problems arise—when you are having a low blood glucose reaction or when you are at risk for ketoacidosis or hyperglycemic hyperosmolar state, for example. And monitoring can tell you whether you need to make any adjustments in your eating, exercise, or insulin schedule.

When to Test

When you test and how often you test depends on your reasons for testing. If you use insulin and are testing so that you can adjust your next insulin injection or want to know what you should eat at your next meal, then you need to check your blood glucose every time you plan an injection or a meal. This would mean you would need to test three to four times a day. If you exercise regularly, you may also want to add another test to see whether you need to eat anything before you begin.

If you are aiming for tight control, you need to monitor at least four and perhaps five times a day. You should test before each meal and before bedtime every day, and in the middle of the night (around 3 a.m.) at least once a week. When you monitor less than four times a day, glucose control worsens.

On the other hand, maybe you are just trying to prevent hyperglycemia and diabetic ketoacidosis and aren't so concerned about keeping your blood glucose levels close to normal all the time. If you have adopted a more relaxed schedule and are taking insulin once or twice a day, then you may opt to monitor twice a day.

If you have type 2 diabetes, then your blood glucose level is probably somewhat stable over the course of the day and you don't have to monitor quite as often. If you are taking oral medications to control your blood glucose, you don't have to monitor as often as someone who is taking insulin. When you first begin taking an oral agent, you may need to monitor more frequently as you and your health care team try to figure out the right dose. You may also need to monitor frequently whenever you need to change your dose or when there is a change in your care plan (such as a new exercise routine). In addition to testing before breakfast and dinner, you may also want to test 2 hours after breakfast and dinner to see how well your plan is working and whether any changes are needed. Once your blood glucose levels are under control, testing only once or twice a day may be all you need.

If you have type 2 or gestational diabetes and you manage without any insulin or medications, then you may opt to test less often once your blood glucose levels are under control. This could be as often as once or twice a day or as little as three or four times a week. On certain occasions, you might want to test more often, such as after a special dinner or an extra-strenuous workout.

You should also consider testing whenever you are not feeling quite right and you don't know why. If you are not feeling well, you need to test more often. If you are feeling a little shaky after your normal 2-mile run, you need to know why. Maybe you suspect hypoglycemia and take an extra dose of carbohydrate. But your glucose levels may actually be high and something else might be going on. The only way to tell for sure is to monitor your blood glucose.

You should discuss when and how often to test with your diabetes health care team. Suggested times to test include:

- before breakfast, lunch, dinner, or an especially big snack
- before you go to bed
- 1 to 2 hours after breakfast, lunch, dinner, or an especially big snack
- at 2 or 3 a.m.

You should do extra tests:

- when you're ill
- if you suspect hypoglycemia
- before you drive (if you take insulin or sulfonylureas)
- when you are physically active
- if you start taking a non-diabetes or an over-the-counter medication that could affect your blood glucose level or your ability to recognize hypoglycemia (talk to your doctor or pharmacist about these possibilities)
- if you have frequent insulin reactions overnight or wake up with high blood glucose levels (over 180 mg/dl)
- whenever you change your insulin injection plan, your oral medication dose, your eating plan, or your exercise plan
- when you have lost or gained weight
- when you are pregnant, thinking about becoming pregnant, or think you may be pregnant

- when you have trouble recognizing the warning signs of hypoglycemia

- when your blood glucose levels have been dangerously high or low (outside your acceptable range)

- when you are on intensive insulin therapy

How to Test

First, make sure you have the following supplies at hand. (For more information on particular supplies and brand names, see the American Diabetes Association Buyer's Guide to Diabetes Supplies published every October in *Diabetes Forecast* magazine.)

- lancet (blood-letting device)

- clean test strip

- cotton ball or tissue

- a watch or other timer

- a blood glucose meter or color chart for determining blood glucose level

To test your blood glucose level, follow these steps. (Check the manufacturer's directions for your particular blood glucose meter.)

- Make sure your hands are clean and dry. Any soap or lotion on your hands can cause inaccurate test results.

- Using the lancet, puncture the skin of a finger, toe, or earlobe. Most people use the side of a finger.

- Squeeze out a large drop of blood.

- Let the drop fall onto the pad of a test strip (or onto the sensor if your meter already has the test strip inside it). Wait the instructed amount of time for the test strip to develop.

- Wipe excess blood from the test strip, if the manufacturer's instructions say to do so. Then insert the test strip into the meter, or compare the test strip to the color chart on the vial. With some meters, it is not necessary to wipe off the blood and a smaller drop of blood will do.

- Dispose of the lancet safely.

- Record your numbers.

Problems with Testing

Expense

Blood glucose testing can be expensive. Before buying any meter, check with your diabetes center, insurance plan, HMO, or company health program. They may pay for only specific meters or have a limited cost allowance. Also find out if you are covered for test strips and the quantity allowed. When you purchase a meter, bear in mind the cost of the test strips. The meter that seemed like a great bargain may be a major burden if the test strips are too expensive. If you want to use generic strips, which are cheaper, make sure that you buy a meter that can use them.

Lancing

The trick is getting a drop of blood that is big enough for your meter without causing you too much pain. Automatic lancets are the quickest and easiest to use. With an automatic lancet you can better produce a uniform size drop of blood from either hand. Automatic lancets also allow you to adjust how deeply you poke your finger. The shallowest poke hurts less and causes less scarring of your fingers.

When you purchase an automatic lancing device, you will need to purchase the lancets separately. Make sure that you can get replacement lancets to fit your device. Consider the cost of the replacement lancets when buying your lancing device. Also make sure that the lancet you use produces a drop of blood big enough to get an accurate reading on your blood glucose meter.

Dexterity

If you have trouble with small hand and finger movements you may want to consider using a larger meter. Some glucose meters are about the size of a credit card and some are even as small as a pen, but these can be difficult to use if you have dexterity problems. If you choose a larger meter, make sure it will not be too cumbersome to carry around. Some strips come individually wrapped in foil. If you find this type of wrapping difficult to remove, avoid brands that use this type of strip. Also, lancets can pose dexterity problems. You will probably want to use an automatic lancing device that resets easily with a simple push-pull movement.

Vision

Consider how well you can see the readings before you buy any meter. Two companies sell meters that store 20 readings, feature displays and literature in large print, and offer audiocassette training materials. Touch-n-Talk II, a voice synthesizer, works with LifeScan's One Touch II meter. The talking device reads your results aloud to you and stores data. Accu-Check II Freedom system guides you with verbal cues and audible beeps. You can also look for a meter with a large digital display if you have any problems seeing.

If you have any vision loss, try to enlist the help of a family member to help you read and record your results. Make sure they know how to use all your diabetes supplies and equipment.

If you have any degree of color blindness, try out different models to make sure you can read the digital display. Some meters have black and gray displays while others feature red or green numbers that may be difficult to read.

Accuracy

What happens if you open a new batch of test strips and suddenly all your readings are much higher or lower than they used to be? The problem may be due to miscalibration. Whenever you open a new batch of strips, you need to standardize or calibrate your meter to make up for variations from batch to batch. Some machines calibrate all by themselves. Make sure you know how your machine works and recalibrate according to manufacturer's instructions if necessary.

Another thing you can do to ensure meter accuracy is check your meter each month to see that it is measuring glucose levels accurately. Meters themselves can sometimes drift. To do this, place a drop of a standard "control" solution of glucose (this should come with your meter or can be purchased at your pharmacy). The reading on the meter should match the concentration of glucose in the control solution. If not, call the manufacturer of your meter. Make sure that the problem is not caused by old or damaged test strips. Check with the manufacturer to see if your strips have expired, and check them for damage before you use them.

To further ensure accurate readings, bring your glucose test system with you to your doctor's appointment or meeting with your diabetes educator. Perform the test in front of her and have her verify that you are doing it right. You may also want to have your doctor test your glucose using her equipment and compare results. Also, when your blood glucose levels are measured in the laboratory, compare your results to the lab test results. For some meters, your results should be within 15 percent of the lab results. For example, if the lab measures your blood glucose level as 150 mg/dl, your own measurement should be within 127 to 173 mg/dl. If your result is out of this range, then you may want to go over your techniques with your diabetes educator or doctor.

Record Keeping

All the finger-poking in the world won't do you any good unless you keep a good record of your test results. Record all your test results in the logbook that came with your glucose meter, or ask your diabetes educator for a new logbook if you don't have one. Or consider creating your own customized logbook. You will want to make sure you have room to record the date, time, actual meter reading, and any unusual circumstances or notes about your general well-being. Bring your logbook to your regular medical appointments. You and your health care team will find the logbook helpful when reviewing your progress, especially if you have been experiencing any problems.

You can also go high-tech to log your blood glucose readings. Instead of buying a standard meter, you may want to consider a data management system, which not only measures your blood glucose, but also stores test results and information on the time, date, insulin doses, exercise, and food intake. Some systems will even allow you to download the information into your computer or your doctor's computer. Before you buy a system, see if your health care team recommends one and make sure your system is compatible with theirs. You can also buy computer programs that take data management a step further. Such programs allow you to download your data and then will give you a detailed analysis of your diabetes management plan, complete with averages, printouts, graphs, and more. However, don't forget the value of a good logbook and piece of graph paper, which some people find more helpful to get a measurable handle on their overall blood glucose control.

Ketone Testing

When you don't have enough insulin available to use the glucose in your blood, your body burns fat instead of glucose. When your body burns fat, it produces toxic substances known as ketones. It is important to keep ketones from building to high levels. This can lead to a life-threatening situation known as diabetic ketoacidosis (see Chapter 3). By testing for ketones, you can prevent diabetic ketoacidosis from becoming a threat to you.

■ SYMPTOMS

The first warning that your body may be producing ketones is a consistently high blood glucose level—250 mg/dl or above. You may also experience a lack of appetite, stomach pains, nausea, vomiting, blurry vision, fever, a sensation of feeling flushed, difficulty breathing, feelings of weakness, drowsiness, a fruity odor on your breath, intense thirst, dry mouth, or the need to urinate frequently.

■ RISKS

High levels of ketones in the urine can be a sign that you are developing diabetic ketoacidosis. This is an extremely serious situation that can lead to seizures, coma, and even death. People with type 1 diabetes are more likely than people with type 2 diabetes to develop diabetic ketoacidosis.

■ WHAT TO DO

You should always test for ketones:

- when your blood glucose readings are over 240 mg/dl on more than one occasion
- when you are ill, especially when you have a high fever, bouts of vomiting, or diarrhea
- during any kind of acute stress, whether it is physical (such as surgery or trauma) or psychological (such as work or family problems)
- when you are chronically tired
- when you have fruity breath, vomiting, breathing difficulties, or are having a hard time concentrating

To test for ketones, you will need a sample of urine. Blood samples are not used to test ketones at home. You will need to buy special ketone test strips, available at most pharmacies. Dip a ketone test strip in a urine sample or pass it directly in a stream of urine. Time the test according to the directions on the package. If ketones are present, the strip will change colors. Compare the test strip to the color chart on the package, and record the results in your daily log. Ketone levels are not reported in units such as milligrams or deciliters. Instead, the chart will tell you whether you have trace to small, moderate, or large amounts of ketones in your urine. Ask your health care team in advance what to do if you have ketones in your urine.

■ TREATMENT

If you have high urine ketones, along with high blood glucose levels, you need to take action to lower them immediately. Talk to your health care team about what specific action you should take. They may suggest that you:

- Take extra insulin. Consult with your health care team about how much insulin you should take.

- Drink plenty of water to prevent dehydration.

- Avoid exercise. Exercise will make your body burn more fat and produce more ketones, because there isn't any insulin to let glucose into your cells. If you continue to exercise, you could counteract the effect of taking extra insulin.

■ PREVENTION

To prevent ketones in your urine, make sure to monitor your blood glucose levels and know what to do if your blood glucose climbs too high. Never skip an insulin dose, and always test for ketones and blood glucose whenever you are ill or under stress.

Chapter 2
Solving Hypoglycemia Problems

Hypoglycemia occurs when there is too little glucose in the blood. This is more likely to happen when something happens to make insulin act more rapidly, when you don't eat enough food or don't eat at the right time, if your exercise or activity burns up too much glucose, or if you use alcohol or other drugs. In people without diabetes, the body stops releasing insulin before glucose levels fall too low. In addition, other hormones kick in that counteract insulin and cause glucose to be released into the bloodstream to prevent low blood glucose. But if you have diabetes, especially if you use insulin or oral medications that lower blood glucose, such as sulfonylureas, you can't put a stop to the insulin that has already been injected or released. And because the counterregulatory hormones may not be acting as they should, your body can't get blood glucose levels up to normal.

Hypoglycemia (Low Blood Glucose)

The level of glucose that produces symptoms of hypoglycemia varies from person to person and for the same person under different circumstances. Ask your doctor about your safe range of blood glucose values. Mild and moderate reactions to hypoglycemia can be easily treated by eating extra carbohydrate, if recognized in time. But if left untreated, severe hypoglycemia can cause unconsciousness and send you to the emergency room. The best way to prevent a hypoglycemic reaction is to know what causes it, recognize when it is occurring, and treat it promptly.

If you experience only mild episodes of hypoglycemia and treat them promptly, you may notice only a minimal disruption to your daily life. However, frequent moderate or severe attacks can have more threatening consequences. Because moderate and severe hypoglycemia affects your brain's ability to function, anything that requires you to think and concentrate can be affected. For example, hypoglycemia could make it difficult to concentrate while taking an exam in school or making a presentation to a new client. If you drive a car, ride a bike, or operate any kind of heavy machinery, hypoglycemia could be extremely dangerous. If you have frequent moderate or severe episodes, your central nervous system could become damaged. This is especially true in young children.

Some patients develop a fear of hypoglycemia that could lead to chronic overeating, undertreatment with insulin or other medications, or both. This is risky because it will increase the chance of hyperglycemia, which can also be life-threatening. It can also increase the risk of developing diabetes complications over time (see Chapter 3). Other patients develop a lack of concern over hypoglycemia and maintain blood glucose levels that put them at risk for recurrent bouts of hypoglycemia.

If you have heart disease, hypoglycemia poses an additional risk. When your blood glucose level gets too low, your heart beats faster than normal. Talk to your doctor about this and discuss whether you need to modify your blood glucose goals to reduce the risk of hypoglycemia and the effect it may have on your heart condition.

Anyone with diabetes can develop hypoglycemia. People with type 1 diabetes are especially prone to this condition. On average, people with type 1 have one or two episodes of hypoglycemia each week. People with type 2 diabetes experience hypoglycemia less frequently. It is also common in the elderly, among people who drink alcohol, and among those who are managing their diabetes with intensive therapy. Any situation that causes your body to use up glucose faster than you can release it into the bloodstream can make hypoglycemia more likely. That is why you have to be especially careful about timing your diet, exercise, and insulin injections to avoid hypoglycemia.

When you don't have enough glucose in your blood, you may experience the symptoms (what you feel) and signs (what others notice) of hypoglycemia. There are two kinds of signals that tell you a hypoglycemic reaction is occurring: those that are caused by the effect of low blood glucose on the autonomic nervous system (the nerves that work without you even realizing it) and those that are caused by the effect of low blood glucose on the brain. Symptoms of hypoglycemia usually appear when blood glucose levels fall below 50–60 mg/dl. However, some people may not feel any symptoms at this level, and others may feel symptoms at even higher glucose levels.

You may not feel all the symptoms of hypoglycemia, but it is important that you learn to recognize the signs and symptoms *you* experience during hypoglycemia. The only sure way to know whether you have hypoglycemia is to test your blood glucose level. However, you may not always have the time or the opportunity to test your blood glucose during a bout of hypoglycemia. If you already know you are prone to hypoglycemia, you may want to measure your blood glucose level when you suspect an episode, so you know how you feel when your blood glucose begins to drop. Once you know how your own body reacts to low blood glucose, you can learn to identify the symptoms and treat early to prevent a mild episode from becoming a severe one.

Mild Hypoglycemia

During an episode of mild hypoglycemia, you may experience any of the following symptoms: shakiness, tremors, palpitations, nervousness, sweating, chills and clamminess, rapid heartbeat, anxiety, light-headedness, and excessive hunger. These are all due to effects on the autonomic nervous system. Mild hypoglycemia will probably not affect your brain, and you should be able to recognize the symptoms and treat yourself.

Moderate Hypoglycemia

If you have a moderate hypoglycemic reaction, you will experience both autonomic and cognitive symptoms caused by effects on the brain. In addition to the symptoms listed above, you may also experience headache, mood changes, irritability, drowsiness, blurred vision, nightmares, nausea, tingling or numbness in the lips or tongue, confusion, and decreased attentiveness.

Severe Hypoglycemia

If the early warning signs of hypoglycemia go unnoticed or ignored, then severe hypoglycemia can occur. If your brain has too little glucose for too long, you may become unresponsive, have convulsions, or lose consciousness. This is an emergency situation that requires *immediate* attention.

■ WHAT TO DO

If you suspect an episode of hypoglycemia, test your blood glucose level right away. Talk to your health care team about the level at which you should begin treatment. If you are unable to test, but recognize the symptoms, do not wait until you are able to test your blood. Instead, treat right away. Never wait until you get home, especially if you have to drive.

■ TREATMENT

Mild Hypoglycemia

In general, if your blood glucose level is less than 70 mg/dl, or if you are experiencing symptoms of hypoglycemia, you should eat 10–15 grams of a fast-acting carbohydrate. Each of the suggested snacks below has 10–15 grams of carbohydrate.

- 2–5 glucose tablets
- 2 tablespoons raisins
- 4 ounces regular soda
- 4 ounces fruit juice
- 5–7 Lifesavers
- 6 jelly beans
- 10 gumdrops
- 2 teaspoons sugar
- 2 teaspoons honey
- 1 tube (0.68 ounces) Cake Mate decorator gel
- 6–8 ounces fat-free or 1% milk

The easiest carbohydrate to keep on hand is probably glucose, sold in tablet or gel form at most pharmacies. Two to five glucose tablets or one package of glucose gel will most likely relieve your symptoms if you are having a mild reaction of hypoglycemia. After taking your pocket carbohydrate, wait 10 to 15 minutes and test again. If your blood glucose levels are still under 70 mg/dl, you may need an additional dose of carbohydrate. Talk to your health care team about what blood glucose levels you should aim for after treatment.

Moderate Hypoglycemia

If your symptoms are more severe and longer lasting, you may be having a moderate episode of hypoglycemia. Because you may also experience some confusion or impaired judgment, you may require assistance in treating yourself. You may even become belligerent and refuse treatment. Make sure those close to you know what to do if you have hypoglycemia. If you have taken one dose of carbohydrate (10–15 grams), test your blood glucose level again in 15 minutes. If after 15 minutes your blood glucose is still too low for you, or if you are still experiencing hypoglycemic symptoms, then take another 10–15 grams of carbohydrate and retest your blood glucose 15 minutes later. If you are being uncooperative and refuse to eat any carbohydrate snacks, you may need to be injected with glucagon, a hormone that causes the liver to release glucose and shuts down insulin release.

Severe Hypoglycemia

If you do not respond to the above treatment or you have waited too long to treat low blood glucose, you will probably require assistance. Make sure those people who spend a lot of time with you know what to do during a severe hypoglycemic episode. If you have severe hypoglycemia, you may refuse help, be unable to swallow, or be unconscious. In this case you may require intravenous glucose or a shot of glucagon. If these are not available, your helper may be advised to apply a glucose gel between your cheek and gum.

If you are having a severe episode of hypoglycemia and medical personnel are available, intravenous glucose will be given to you. Most likely, you will be given 10–25 grams of glucose in the form of a 50% dextrose solution (dextrose is the optically pure chemical form of glucose used by the body). This will be given over a 1- to 3-minute period. After that, intravenous glucose will be given at a rate of 5–10 grams per hour until you have fully recovered and are ready to eat.

If you are unable to get emergency help right away, which is often the case, glucagon should be injected. If you are prone to hypoglycemia, always keeps a supply of glucagon nearby. Make sure anyone you spend time with—your parents, spouse, older children, siblings, roommates, friends, coach, teammates, or teachers—knows how to mix, draw up, and administer glucagon and how to recognize when glucagon treatment is necessary. Talk to your doctor or diabetes educator about whether to buy a glucagon kit, which is available by prescription. Have your diabetes educator teach you and your helpers how to use it.

A glucagon kit contains a syringe filled with a diluting solution and a bottle of powdered glucagon. Before injecting, the powder must be mixed with the diluting fluid. Instructions for mixing and injecting glucagon are included in the kit. Make sure you go over the directions ahead of time with someone who can inject glucagon if you need it. The directions are not difficult, but at the moment you need help, it might be hard for your loved one to concentrate on learning how to do it. So practice beforehand!

Glucagon should be injected the same way as insulin. Choose a site with fatty tissue, such as the upper thigh, back of the arm, abdomen, or buttocks. Make sure your hands and the injection site are clean and dry. Gently pinch a fold of skin between thumb and forefinger and inject straight in. Push the needle through the skin quickly. Push the plunger in to inject glucagon and pull the needle straight out. You may need to apply pressure with a piece of gauze or cotton ball to prevent bleeding.

The usual dose of glucagon to treat a child less than 5 years old is 0.25–0.5 mg. For children 5 to 10 years old, 0.5–1.0 mg is recommended, and for those over the age of 10, 1.0 mg is recommended. Glucagon should be injected intramuscularly (into the muscle) or subcutaneously (under the skin) into the shoulder or thigh. Make sure you or your child's helper has been shown how and where to inject glucagon.

After you have been given glucagon you are likely to vomit, so your helper should keep your head elevated above your stomach. You should respond to glucagon within 5 to 20 minutes. Once you are awake enough to chew and swallow, drink a clear fluid, such as ginger ale or 7-Up. This should help settle your stomach. Then try to eat a substantial snack such as bread and peanut butter or a half of a cheese sandwich. If you do not respond to the glucagon within 20 minutes, your helper should give you another dose and call for emergency help right away.

■ PREVENTION

If you have frequent episodes of hypoglycemia, it is important to figure out what causes them and take steps to prevent them from happening in the first place. Even if you experience hypoglycemia only occasionally, make sure you know what to do to keep a mild episode from becoming life-threatening.

Insulin Irregularities

Sometimes, errors in insulin use can lead to hypoglycemia. Check that you have not reversed your morning and evening doses. Make sure you have not mixed up your short- and intermediate-acting insulins. Also, make sure that you time your insulin injections with your meals. Don't wait too long to eat after injecting insulin if you are prone to hypoglycemia. In addition, don't give yourself extra insulin without talking to your doctor first about the circumstances for which this would be necessary. Check your injection site. If you have a hypertrophied injection site (a lumpy area caused by an overgrowth of fat cells), your insulin absorption could be unpredictable (see pages 123–124). Also, if you inject into an exercising muscle, insulin will be absorbed more rapidly than you might expect and could be contributing to low blood glucose. If you are following an intensive insulin therapy program you are more prone to hypoglycemia and may need to monitor your blood glucose more frequently.

Nutrition

If you skip meals or eat less food than you normally do after an insulin injection, hypoglycemia is more likely to occur. Also, if you delay your meals and snacks for too long after an insulin injection, hypoglycemia is more likely. Even if you don't take insulin, you may invite an occasional episode of hypoglycemia if you don't eat regularly. Talk to your dietitian about how to better coordinate your meals with your medication, insulin, and daily activities.

Exercise

Any time you exercise when you did not intend to, or exercise longer or more strenuously than you usually do, you may develop hypoglycemia.

Always have a pocket carbohydrate available when exercising. If you experience any early warning signs during exercise, don't continue. Stop and test your blood glucose if you are able to. If you can't test or if your blood glucose level is low, eat a 15-gram portion of a fast-acting carbohydrate. If you have become hypoglycemic during a similar exercise or activity in the past, plan ahead and eat an extra snack either before, during, or after the activity, depending on when the episode occurred. Or, you could make adjustments in your insulin schedule to accommodate your exercise. Talk to your doctor first.

Sexual Activity

If you tend to develop hypoglycemia when you sleep or when you exercise, then you may also have a low blood glucose reaction following sexual activity, especially if you are intimate at night. Talk to your doctor about how to adjust for this. Because some of the symptoms of hypoglycemia—sweating, rapid heartbeat, chills and clamminess, and shakiness—occur naturally during orgasm, it may be difficult in the middle of sexual ecstasy to tell whether you are having a low blood glucose reaction. And it may be less than desirable to stop in the middle of a sexual encounter and test your blood glucose. Therefore, it is especially important to take preventive steps in advance. You may want to change the timing of your insulin or you may need a snack before or after any sexual activity. If you try testing yourself after an act of intimacy to see whether hypoglycemia is a problem for you, then you can develop a plan for preventing it in the future. Be especially careful if you are combining sexual activity with alcohol.

Nighttime Hypoglycemia

You can become hypoglycemic during the night without even knowing it. This is especially true if you have been adjusting your insulin and meals to avoid morning hypoglycemia. The problem is that sometimes you end up with low blood glucose in the middle of the night. Sometimes when this happens, the body compensates by releasing more glucose and you become hyperglycemic (see the Somogyi Effect, page 115).

To prevent nighttime hypoglycemia, try monitoring your blood glucose at bedtime and again at 2 or 3 a.m. If you are indeed having hypoglycemic episodes during the night, talk to your doctor about what to do. You may want to add extra food at bedtime. Consider a snack that contains protein, which stimulates glucagon production, which in turn releases glucose from the liver. A snack is especially important when you think you might develop hypoglycemia, such as when you have exercised intensely during the day or when your bedtime glucose is less than 100 mg/dl.

Also, consider using an insulin that does not peak between 1 and 3 a.m. If you are taking insulin twice a day, taking your intermediate-acting insulin at bedtime or substituting a long-acting insulin for it may do the trick. If you are using an insulin pump, you may consider programming it to give less insulin during the predawn hours. Talk to your doctor about the strategy that works best for you.

Sleeping Late

You can probably sleep an extra 30 to 45 minutes without having to change your eating or insulin schedule. If you sleep more than 45 minutes past when you normally get up, then you may need to make some adjustments. Talk to your health care team about what to do if you oversleep. If you oversleep accidentally, test your blood glucose immediately when you wake up and take a dose of fast-acting carbohydrate if you are hypoglycemic. If you know you are going to sleep in the next morning, you may need to make some changes in your nighttime schedule. For example, you may try reducing your nighttime dose of intermediate- or long-acting insulin by 10 to 15 percent. This increases the risk of high blood glucose in the morning, however. Or you could eat a little more before you go to bed at night. But again, you have to be careful you don't end up hyperglycemic. It is probably safest to wake up at your normal time, test your blood glucose level, take insulin or oral medication, eat breakfast, and then go back to sleep. Don't wake up and take insulin without eating under any circumstances. Talk to your health care team about how to best plan for those days when you need to sleep in.

Alcohol

Alcohol indirectly lowers blood glucose levels, so it is especially important to prevent hypoglycemia if you are drinking alcohol. Normally, when blood glucose levels start to drop, your body signals the liver to release more glucose. This gives you some time to recognize and treat hypoglycemia before it becomes severe. But alcohol interferes with that process and you can have a severe episode of hypoglycemia with little warning. Alcohol also affects your judgment, and so it might become even more difficult to recognize the warning signs and to act appropriately.

But that doesn't mean that you can never have an alcoholic drink. If you do drink, do so in moderation. For women, this means no more than one drink a day, and for men, two drinks a day. One drink is defined as 12 ounces of beer, 5 ounces of wine, or 1 1/2 ounces of 80 proof distilled spirits. Make sure you never drink alcohol on an empty stomach, especially if you take insulin or sulfonylurea drugs. Make sure those around you know how to recognize a hypoglycemic episode, since the signs of hypoglycemia are similar to those of intoxication. Also keep in mind that you need to be able to think clearly enough to recognize the signs of low blood glucose and to know how to treat it.

Talk to your doctor or dietitian about the best way to incorporate alcohol into your meal plan and how best to accommodate an alcoholic beverage you may want to have even if you haven't planned ahead. You may want to test your blood glucose before you have a drink to make sure it isn't on the low side. If your blood glucose is below 100 mg/dl, make sure to have a snack. You may want to have a small snack anytime you drink alcohol to counteract any glucose-lowering effect.

Check with your doctor about the advisability of drinking alcohol. Some medications limit alcohol use. You may also be advised not to drink alcohol if you have pancreatitis, high triglyceride levels, stomach problems, neuropathy, kidney disease, certain kinds of heart disease, or other medical conditions.

Hypoglycemia in the Elderly

If you are elderly, you are at high risk for developing hypoglycemia, especially if you have any complicating conditions, take insulin or oral agents, or receive any other medications. If you have physical limitations that interfere with your ability to monitor blood glucose, give yourself insulin, or even manage day-to-day living, then keeping your blood glucose within the optimal range may be even more challenging. It is important that you and those around you be aware of the signs of hypoglycemia and know what to do should it occur.

If you are older, but in good general health, you and you health care team may want to aim for a plan that gives you good blood glucose control but does not put you at risk for hypoglycemia. For example, you may want to keep your fasting glucose level at 115 mg/dl and your after-meal glucose level at around 180 mg/dl. However, if you have any complicating factors or medical conditions or are prone to hypoglycemia, you may want to take a more conservative approach. Some older patients find it more appropriate to aim for fasting glucose levels of less than 140 mg/dl and after-meal glucose levels under 200–220 mg/dl. Talk to the members of your health care team about what works for you.

If you have mobility problems, make sure to keep a source of fast-acting glucose near you at all times—in your pocket or on a bedside table, for example. If you have problems testing your blood glucose or administering insulin, try to get someone to help you carry out these tasks at specific times. Also, make sure you don't skip meals, medications, or insulin injections. If you tend to forget, set an alarm to go off at designated times to remind you to eat or take insulin. Try to enlist the help of your health care team and those around you to help you control your blood glucose so that hypoglycemia does not occur. Also make sure your friends, family, or caregivers know what to do during a hypoglycemic episode.

Hypoglycemia and Intensive Therapy

If you are managing your diabetes with intensive therapy, then you are at high risk for hypoglycemia. This is especially true if you are male, an adolescent, have had diabetes for a long time, had a high glycated hemoglobin level before beginning intensive therapy and have a low glycated hemoglobin reading during therapy, or if you have a history of hypoglycemia.

■ WHAT TO DO

Make sure you know the warning signs and symptoms of a hypoglycemic episode and know what blood glucose level triggers these symptoms for you. Be especially careful during exercise and physical activity. Even a routine activity such as household chores or climbing stairs may cause blood glucose levels to drop. Any vigorous exercise could provoke hypoglycemia for as long as 12–24 hours after exercising. Talk to your doctor about how you might modify your current program to incorporate both routine and vigorous activities.

If you are under intensive therapy, make sure you test your blood glucose more frequently. In addition to testing four times a day, as recommended, also test 2 hours after eating. If your blood glucose level is under 100 mg/dl, you have a higher than usual chance of developing hypoglycemia before your next meal and may need an additional snack. If you are under intensive therapy and have experienced repeated episodes of hypoglycemia, test your blood glucose before driving an automobile.

■ PREVENTION

Whenever you develop hypoglycemia, try to figure out what happened. Did you just engage in sexual activity? Did you skip part of your meal because it was too salty? Did you swim a few extra laps in the pool or end up vacuuming the whole house because your teenager neglected his chores? Think about what events could have precipitated the attack and make a note of it. If you exercised a little more, you may need to eat a little more or alter the timing of your insulin. If your schedule changes, you may need to test more often and make adjustments in insulin doses or timing or in what you eat. By becoming aware of what activities and actions trigger hypoglycemia, you can prevent it from happening in the future. Make sure to go over your plan with your health care team.

Hypoglycemia Unawareness

An important aspect of dealing with hypoglycemia is to recognize an episode and take immediate steps to prevent it from becoming severe. But for many people, hypoglycemia occurs without apparent symptoms. This phenomenon, called hypoglycemia unawareness, seems to be much more common than previously realized. In the Diabetes Control and Complications Trial, a 10-year study of the effects of intensive therapy, one-third of all episodes of severe hypoglycemia occurred in patients who had no evident symptoms.

■ SYMPTOMS

If you have hypoglycemia unawareness, you are experiencing hypo-glycemia without any symptoms. The first sign may in fact be impaired thinking, which makes it even more difficult to know when you are having a low blood glucose reaction. You may find yourself in the middle of a severe episode without any warning at all.

■ RISKS

Hypoglycemia is fairly common in people who tightly control their blood glucose levels. It is also common in pregnant women and in people who have been recently diagnosed with diabetes. People who have repeated episodes of hypoglycemia are also at risk for hypo-glycemia unawareness.

■ WHAT TO DO

If you have blood glucose readings below 55 mg/dl without any symptoms, either on occasion or frequently, talk to your doctor or health care team right away. You and your doctor should devise a plan for changing your blood glucose goals to prevent hypoglycemia.

If you are in the middle of an episode without warning, make sure those around you know what to do. If you are able, test your blood glucose level. If it is below 50–60 mg/dl, take 10–15 grams of a fast-acting carbohydrate. If you are unable to test, eat a fast-acting carbohydrate snack anyhow. Wait 15 minutes, then test again. You will probably need a second dose of carbohydrate. If you are having a severe hypoglycemic reaction, which is often the case with hypoglycemic unawareness, you will require assistance or emergency treatment.

If you have hypoglycemia unawareness, make sure those around you know the signs. Carry a supply of pocket carbohydrate and a glucagon kit with you at all times and make sure your helpers know how to use it.

■ TREATMENT

If you fail to respond to eating fast-acting carbohydrates or if you have become unresponsive, are having convulsions, or have lost consciousness, then you will need emergency assistance. Those around you should call for help immediately. If possible, you should be given an injection of glucagon. If medical help arrives and glucagon has not been administered, you will be given intravenous glucose.

■ PREVENTION

If you have hypoglycemia unawareness, talk to your health care team about what you can do to prevent it. By preventing even mild hypoglycemia, you may be able to restore at least some of your ability to detect the symptoms of hypoglycemia. You may want to change your blood glucose goals. For example, if you had been aiming for a between-meal blood glucose level of 120 mg/dl, then 140 mg/dl may be a more appropriate target. You may also be advised to monitor your blood glucose levels more frequently. This is especially important before you drive and after strenuous exercise. Also monitor any time that you do something that in the past has triggered hypoglycemia. If you seem to develop hypoglycemia every time you clean the house or argue with your boss before lunch, then test your blood glucose level whenever this occurs. Also, make sure those around you know how to detect hypoglycemia and know what to do if you are having an episode.

Chapter 3
Solving Hyperglycemia Problems

If you have diabetes, your body either doesn't produce enough insulin or doesn't respond to insulin as it should. Insulin helps glucose get into the cells that need it. Without it, glucose remains in your blood and your blood glucose levels climb too high. This can result in a host of problems. High blood glucose levels over time can affect the way the blood does its job. As a result, you can develop many of the complications of diabetes, such as heart disease, eye disease, and kidney disease. In the short term, having high blood glucose levels can make you feel bad. If your glucose levels remain too high for too long and you fail to recognize what is happening, life-threatening situations can develop. It is important to recognize the warning signs of hyperglycemia so you can take action to get your blood glucose levels down to normal.

Hyperglycemia (High Blood Glucose)

No matter how hard you try, it is unlikely you can maintain perfect blood glucose control. There will be times when your blood glucose level may rise a little above normal or fall too low. But if your blood glucose level is always or often higher than it should be or if you frequently have abnormally high blood glucose levels, you will be more likely to develop diabetes complications and you could put yourself at risk for life-threatening situations, including seizures, coma, or even death.

■ SYMPTOMS

The symptoms of high blood glucose may be subtle. You may feel unusually thirsty or feel the need to urinate more frequently. You may even experience blurry vision. Sometimes if your blood glucose levels are too high, you just don't feel quite right. You may feel tired and have no energy. The only way to know for sure is to test your blood glucose level. If it is higher than 250 mg/dl, you have hyperglycemia. (Some people will experience symptoms at lower blood glucose levels.)

■ RISKS

Chronically high blood glucose levels over time can trigger and worsen many of the complications of diabetes. These include retinopathy (eye disease), heart disease, nephropathy (kidney disease), neuropathy (nerve disease), and infection. In the short term, extremely high levels of blood glucose could lead to two especially dangerous conditions, diabetic ketoacidosis or hyperglycemic hyperosmolar state. Both of these conditions, if left untreated, can cause coma and even death.

■ WHAT TO DO

If you feel any of the symptoms listed above, test your blood glucose level. If it is above 350 mg/dl, call a member of your health care team right away. If your blood glucose levels are lower (250–350 mg/dl), and you have any symptoms of diabetic ketoacidosis or hyperglycemic hyperosmolar state (see below), call your health care team immediately. If your blood glucose level is over 500 mg/dl, call for emergency help or have someone drive you to an emergency room at once.

■ TREATMENT

What to do about your hyperglycemia depends on the severity of the situation and whether you have ketones in your urine. If your blood glucose is borderline high and you have no other symptoms, you may be advised to exercise a little or just wait out the situation and focus on preventing it from happening in the future. If your blood glucose levels are above 250 mg/dl, your health care team member may advise taking extra insulin and drinking plenty of fluids. You should discuss with your health care team in advance what steps to take should your blood glucose levels fall within this range. If your blood glucose levels are dangerously high (over 500 mg/dl), you will require emergency treatment.

■ PREVENTION

To prevent hyperglycemia, you need to identify the events that caused it and take steps to ensure that it doesn't happen again. Eating too much food, taking too little insulin, skipping insulin doses or oral agents, or delaying insulin injections are likely culprits.

Unexplained Hyperglycemia

If you don't know what caused your hyperglycemia, you may have unexplained hyperglycemia. Sometimes you know why your blood glucose levels are high (over 250 mg/dl). Maybe you ate too much of a high-carbohydrate meal. Or maybe you skipped a dose of insulin because you weren't feeling well. It is important to figure out why your blood glucose levels may rise unexpectedly, especially if this happens often.

Preventing unexplained hyperglycemia requires a little detective work. After all, if you knew the cause, it wouldn't be happening in the first place. If your bouts of hyperglycemia occur frequently, you may first want to track your patterns of eating, activity, and insulin or medication use to see how they affect your blood glucose levels. If your hyperglycemia occurs an hour after your meal, then you may want to allow more time between your insulin injection and eating. If your blood glucose levels are high before mealtime, you may want to exercise before you eat. If your blood glucose levels are high when you wake up, you may be experiencing the dawn phenomenon or the Somogyi effect (see below). To prevent this, your health care team may suggest eating less at breakfast or the night before, or adjusting your insulin dose.

Unexplained hyperglycemia can also be due to problems with insulin and insulin delivery, especially if you are using an insulin pump. First, check your insulin. If it has expired or has been subjected to extremes in temperature, it may be inactive and unable to do its job. Check the bottle to see if it looks clumped or filled with little particles. If the vial is nearly empty or you have used it for more than 1 month, it may be time to open a fresh bottle.

Problems with the insertion site or injection site can also affect insulin action. If you placed the needle near a scar or mole, or into an area that is red and swollen, insulin absorption could be delayed. This can result in high blood glucose levels. If you are using an insulin pump, check to make sure that the needle has not come out of the infusion site and that the infusion line has not come loose from the pump. If insulin is leaking, it cannot get to where it needs to go. Also check for blood, air, or kinks in the infusion line. If you have noticed any of these things or if the infusion set has been in place for more than 2 days, think about changing the infusion line.

Also, check to see that the basal rate is set correctly on your insulin pump. Check the battery. If it has run down, insulin cannot be pumped efficiently. Make sure the insulin cartridge is not empty and has been placed correctly. Always make sure to prime the pump with insulin when inserting a fresh cartridge. If the pump is not working correctly, insulin will not be delivered at the correct dose and blood glucose levels will rise.

Other factors can also affect blood glucose levels. Illness, stress, medications, level of physical activity, or any change in your normal routine can also lead to changes in hormonal action and blood glucose levels. If you are female, your blood glucose may be more difficult to control at certain phases of your menstrual cycle. If you are going through menopause, this could also affect your blood glucose levels. If you still can't figure out what is causing your hyperglycemia, check with a member of your health care team.

Diabetic Ketoacidosis

Diabetic ketoacidosis (also known as DKA) is a life-threatening condition that usually occurs in people with type 1 diabetes. However, people with type 2 diabetes can also develop diabetic ketoacidosis. Diabetic ketoacidosis begins when there is too little insulin in the blood and too much of the hormones that increase glucose levels in the blood. When this happens, the body can't use the glucose in the blood for energy and instead starts to break down fat and protein. When fat breaks down, ketones are produced that can accumulate and lead to difficulty in breathing, shock, pneumonia, seizures, coma, and even death.

■ SYMPTOMS

If you regularly monitor your blood glucose levels, the most important warning signs of diabetic ketoacidosis are consistently high blood glucose levels—250 mg/dl or above. You may also experience a lack of appetite, stomach pains, nausea, vomiting, blurry vision, fever, a sensation of feeling flushed, difficulty breathing, feelings of weakness, drowsiness, a fruity odor on your breath, intense thirst, dry mouth, or the need to urinate frequently.

▓ RISKS

Twenty percent of all people hospitalized for diabetes have diabetic ketoacidosis. The actual incidence of diabetic ketoacidosis among people with diabetes is even higher, because milder cases can be treated outside the hospital. Diabetic ketoacidosis is more likely to develop in females and in those under the age of 15. However, because there are more older people with diabetes, doctors are seeing more episodes of diabetic ketoacidosis in people over the age of 45.

Diabetic ketoacidosis is more likely to occur in people with diabetes who have not yet been diagnosed than in people who are aware they have diabetes and are taking insulin and keeping their blood glucose levels under control. If you already know you have diabetes, diabetic ketoacidosis can be triggered if you stop taking your insulin for one reason or another. Teenagers who may be embarrassed about having diabetes may not adhere to diet and insulin schedules. Young women with eating disorders who may skip meals and insulin injections are especially prone to diabetic ketoacidosis.

Diabetic ketoacidosis is also more likely to occur during periods of emotional or physical stress or illness. You may not feel like eating and think it's okay to skip your insulin injection. But this is the worst thing you could do. When you have an infection, for example, or find yourself in a stressful situation, your body releases hormones that cause the liver to release stored glucose. This increases the glucose levels in your blood. Even if your insulin levels are normal, if your blood glucose shoots up, you may not have enough insulin to handle the available glucose. People with diabetes who abuse alcohol are also at high risk for developing diabetic ketoacidosis.

Diabetic ketoacidosis is a life-threatening condition that should be taken seriously. If untreated, it could result in coma and even death. Cerebral edema, a rare complication of diabetic ketoacidosis in young children, can also occur. Warning signs include headache, drowsiness, and lethargy, which can lead to seizures and sometimes even death. Adults may develop hypoxemia, a condition marked by low oxygen levels in the blood. This is thought to occur as a result of water accumulation in the lungs and decreased lung function, which can lead to respiratory distress. This is more likely to occur in people with other complicating conditions, such as infection.

■ WHAT TO DO

If you have any of the signs of diabetic ketoacidosis listed above, check your blood glucose level *immediately*. If your blood glucose level is over 250 mg/dl, call a member of your health care team *at once*. You should also test your urine for the presence of ketones. Trace amounts of ketones are probably no cause for alarm, but if your urine has moderate or large amounts of ketones, call your health care team immediately. You will first want to take action to lower your blood glucose and ketone levels. You will probably need to take fast-acting insulin, but check with your health care team to figure out how much and what kind of insulin to take. You should also drink plenty of water to prevent dehydration. Also, avoid exercise. Exercise counters the effects of taking extra insulin and just causes the body to burn more fat. Keep checking your blood glucose and ketone levels. If the levels of ketones in your urine do not decrease right away or if you are vomiting, *get emergency help at once*.

■ TREATMENT

If you require emergency care, you will be given insulin to bring blood glucose levels and urine ketone levels within normal range. How a patient responds to insulin can vary widely, but blood glucose levels should decrease from 600 mg/dl to 250–300 mg/dl in 4 to 6 hours. Once glucose levels are in this range, insulin administration should continue. Even with continued insulin administration, it can take as much as 12 hours to treat diabetic ketoacidosis.

In addition to insulin therapy, you will also be given fluids to treat dehydration and replace all the water you have lost. How much fluid you are given will depend on how much you have lost. Your health care team will carefully monitor fluid intake and urine output. In addition to fluids, you will also need to get your electrolytes back in balance and will most likely be given potassium. Usually potassium therapy is not begun until you are producing a normal amount of urine. You may also be given other salts and electrolytes to bring everything back into balance.

Most patients hospitalized for diabetic ketoacidosis will recover in 24 hours. However, depending on the severity of the episode, the underlying causes, and any other complicating factors, you may need hospitalization for several days or weeks. Once you leave the hospital, your doctor will most likely want to follow up your progress at frequent intervals.

■ PREVENTION

Given the severity of diabetic ketoacidosis, it is critical to prevent it from happening in the first place. The most important tool for preventing diabetes is to monitor blood glucose levels regularly and maintain good blood glucose control. Ask your health care team members how to make adjustments in your meal plan and insulin should your blood glucose levels rise unexpectedly. If you are taking insulin, *never* skip an insulin dose. Make sure your insulin has not expired and that it is properly stored. If you are using a pump, check that your pump is working properly and is free of clogs.

If you are sick or under stress, monitor your blood glucose frequently and test your urine for ketones. Do both tests every 4 hours, at least, until you are feeling better. Any time you are feeling queasy or are vomiting, check your urine for ketones. Make sure to do this even if your blood glucose levels are normal. Also, be prepared: discuss in advance with your health care team what you should look for as early warning signs of diabetic ketoacidosis and what you should do if an episode occurs. Make sure that those close to you also know how to recognize the warning signs of diabetic ketoacidosis and know what they can do to help.

Hyperglycemic Hyperosmolar State

Hyperglycemic hyperosmolar state (also known as Hyperglycemic Hyperosmolar Nonketotic Syndrome, HHNS) is similar in some ways to diabetic ketoacidosis, but is much more likely to affect people with type 2 diabetes. Both conditions occur when blood glucose levels climb too high. If you have type 2 diabetes, you can be at risk for hyperglycemic hyperosmolar state whether you manage your diabetes through diet and exercise alone, take oral agents, or use insulin. However, most cases of hyperglycemic hyperosmolar state occur in people who don't use insulin. In many instances, hyperglycemic hyperosmolar state develops in people who don't even realize they have diabetes.

Hyperglycemic hyperosmolar state begins when your blood glucose levels rise too high. Your body produces more urine to get rid of excess glucose and dehydration sets in. This process can go on for days and even weeks. As dehydration continues, you can become confused and disoriented. This makes it even more difficult for you to get a needed drink of water, make it to a toilet, or even recognize that hyperglycemic hyperosmolar state is occurring. If unchecked, the severe dehydration in hyperglycemic hyperosmolar state can lead to seizures, coma, and death.

■ SYMPTOMS

Unlike diabetic ketoacidosis, the body does not produce ketones during hyperglycemic hyperosmolar state and so the symptoms are not as recognizable. If you have hyperglycemic hyperosmolar state, you might not even realize what is happening until it is too late. The symptoms of hyperglycemic hyperosmolar state include dry parched mouth, extreme thirst (although this can disappear during the course of hyperglycemic hyperosmolar state), sleepiness, feeling confused or disoriented, warm dry skin with no sweating, and high blood glucose levels (over 350 mg/dl). If you experience any of these symptoms, check your blood glucose level at once and call your doctor.

■ RISKS

Hyperglycemic hyperosmolar state occurs almost exclusively in people with type 2 diabetes. Elderly people with type 2 diabetes, especially those in nursing homes, are at an especially high risk for developing hyperglycemic hyperosmolar state. One-third of all cases of hyperglycemic hyperosmolar state happen to people in nursing homes. People who have diabetes but have not yet been diagnosed are also prime targets for hyperglycemic hyperosmolar state, because their blood glucose can rise to high levels without them even knowing it.

Hyperglycemic hyperosmolar state is most likely to occur during times of illness or infection. Any kind of physical or psychological trauma or stress can increase your risk for hyperglycemic hyperosmolar state. Certain medications can also make an episode of hyperglycemic hyperosmolar state more likely. If you are undergoing peritoneal dialysis or intravenous feedings, you will be given large amounts of glucose, and this increases your chances for developing hyperglycemic hyperosmolar state. Any circumstances that make you stop taking insulin or skip an insulin dose can also put you at high risk for hyperglycemic hyperosmolar state. Alcohol abuse also makes hyperglycemic hyperosmolar state more likely.

■ WHAT TO DO

If your blood glucose level is over 350 mg/dl, call your doctor or a member of your health care team *right away*. If your blood glucose is over 500 mg/dl, have someone take you to a hospital immediately. If no one is available, call for emergency help *at once*.

■ TREATMENT

The treatment for hyperglycemic hyperosmolar state is similar to that for diabetic ketoacidosis. If you have severe hyperglycemic hyperosmolar state and require emergency treatment, you will be given insulin, fluids, and electrolytes. You may be given an initial dose of insulin that depends on your weight and then a smaller continuous dose of insulin, depending on how fast your glucose levels fall. Once your blood glucose levels fall below 200 mg/dl, you will be given an infusion of glucose solution and your insulin dose will be lowered further. It may take as long as 4 to 6 hours for glucose levels to fall to safe levels.

Dehydration is a big problem if you have hyperglycemic hyperosmolar state. It is not uncommon to lose fluids in an amount equal to 15 percent of your body weight. If you have hyperglycemic hyperosmolar state, you will be given normal saline solution for several hours until your fluid volume approaches normal. Once this is achieved, saline will continue to be given at a reduced level and perhaps a lower concentration. Fluid input and urine output will be carefully monitored. In addition to fluid, several electrolytes will need replenishing. It is most important to replace lost potassium, and this will be given to you throughout the first 24 hours, as long as urine output is sufficient.

■ PREVENTION

The best way to prevent hyperglycemic hyperosmolar state or any form of hyperglycemia from occurring is to monitor blood glucose levels regularly. If you test your blood glucose once or twice a day, you will be alerted to the problem before it gets out of control. If you notice a high reading, don't ignore it. Talk to the members of your health care team in advance about what action to take if your blood glucose reaches a high level (greater than 250 mg/dl). Even if you don't take insulin on a regular basis, you may need to take it if your blood glucose levels rise too high. If you are ill or have an infection, monitor your blood glucose 3 to 4 times a day. You may also want to monitor more frequently if you are feeling stressed out, either physically or emotionally. If you do take insulin regularly, don't skip any doses, even if you are feeling sick and have to force yourself to eat. Also, make sure to drink plenty of fluids and avoid the use of caffeine or alcohol, especially when you are not feeling well. Most importantly, develop a plan of action with the members of your health care team to handle any swings in your blood glucose level.

Dawn Phenomenon

What's going on here? You go to bed at night and wake up the next morning hungry and with an empty stomach. You would expect your blood glucose levels to be low. But instead, you find them to be quite high. This seeming paradox is a result of the dawn phenomenon. It is the body's way of giving you a boost of energy to start the day by building up glucose while you sleep.

In the early hours of the morning, your body produces certain growth hormones. These hormones repress the action of insulin and allow blood glucose levels to rise between 4 and 8 a.m. The dawn phenomenon is a natural process and in itself is not a problem. But if your blood glucose levels climb too high during these hours, you may want to make adjustments to keep your blood glucose levels on an even keel.

■ SYMPTOMS

If your blood glucose levels rise too high because of the dawn phenomenon, you may wake up feeling some of the symptoms of hyperglycemia: excessive thirst, frequent urination, or blurry vision. Or you may feel no symptoms at all. The surest way to find out if the dawn phenomenon is creating problems for you is to test your blood glucose level at 2 a.m. and again when you wake up. If it is higher than 200 mg/dl, talk to the members of your health care team about how to make adjustments in your nighttime routine to prevent this from occurring.

■ RISKS

Any time your blood glucose levels rise too high, you are at risk for all the problems associated with hyperglycemia. Just how great the risk is depends on how high your blood glucose levels rise and how often this happens. High blood glucose levels over time can increase the risk of all the complications of diabetes: eye disease, kidney disease, nerve disease, heart disease, and infections. Extremely high blood glucose levels (over 500 mg/dl) can trigger emergency situations such as diabetic ketoacidosis and hyperglycemic hyperosmolar state. The dawn phenomenon on its own is unlikely to cause blood glucose levels to rise high enough to trigger such episodes. However, any time your blood glucose goes too high and you don't make the necessary adjustments to bring it back down, other actions such as eating too much or forgetting to take your insulin or oral medication can greatly increase the risk of severe hyperglycemia.

■ WHAT TO DO

If your blood glucose levels are too high when you wake up, you may need to take a higher dose of insulin than you normally take. Talk to your health care team in advance about the best way to deal with morning episodes of hyperglycemia.

■ PREVENTION

The best way to deal with hyperglycemia due to the dawn phenomenon is to prevent it from happening in the first place. You might consider decreasing your food intake at night or increasing your physical activity. Adjusting the timing or dose of your insulin may also do the trick. For example, some people find that moving the evening insulin dose from 8 p.m. to 11 p.m. prevents the dawn phenomenon.

However, it is important to distinguish the dawn phenomenon from the Somogyi effect (see below). This condition, which results in high blood glucose, is triggered by low blood glucose levels. Thus, if you think you are affected by the dawn phenomenon, but really have the Somogyi effect, anything that results in lower blood glucose (such as taking more insulin the evening before) could actually worsen your situation. If your 2 a.m. blood glucose level is less than 60 mg/dl and then rises above 180 mg/dl at 7 a.m., you may have the Somogyi effect. Talk to the members of your health care team about the best way to diagnose and prevent your early morning hyperglycemia.

Somogyi Effect

The Somogyi effect, or rebound hyperglycemia, is another one of your body's reactions to hypoglycemia. In most people, whenever blood glucose gets too low, certain hormones called counterregulatory hormones kick in and cause blood glucose levels to rise. In individuals without diabetes, this effect is quickly counteracted by an increase in insulin, which lowers blood glucose. If you have diabetes, your body may not make enough insulin or may not respond to insulin and you may become hyperglycemic due to these hormones.

■ SYMPTOMS

If you are experiencing the Somogyi effect, you may not even notice the episode of hypoglycemia that triggers the hyperglycemia. Or, you may first notice the symptoms of hypoglycemia (shakiness, nervousness, moodiness, sweating, irritability, chills, clamminess, rapid heartbeat, anxiety, light-headedness, dizziness, hunger, blurred vision, nausea, or tingling or numbness in your lips or tongue) followed by symptoms of hyperglycemia (dry parched mouth, extreme thirst, and the need to urinate frequently). Eating too much food to treat the hypoglycemia can cause an even greater rise in blood glucose levels, which can increase the symptoms of hyperglycemia. Only careful blood glucose monitoring will tell you and your doctor if you are experiencing rebound hyperglycemia. If your blood glucose levels fall below 65 mg/dl and then rise above 200 mg/dl within a few hours, you may be experiencing the Somogyi effect (the exact blood glucose values may vary). This can occur during waking hours or while you sleep at night.

■ RISKS

Swings in blood glucose levels can increase the likelihood and severity of the complications of diabetes over time. The Somogyi effect is a natural mechanism to counteract severe episodes of hypoglycemia. The greatest risk is that blood glucose levels may rise too high, especially if the initial hypoglycemia is treated too aggressively. The trick is to eat just enough carbohydrate to treat the hypoglycemia (probably 15 grams), but not enough to trigger hyperglycemia.

■ WHAT TO DO

The problem in treating rebound hyperglycemia is that you might not know that it was triggered by an episode of hypoglycemia. Aggressive attempts to lower blood glucose could end up causing another episode of hypoglycemia, which in turn causes another bout of hyperglycemia. If you have attempted to treat hyperglycemia with increased doses of insulin and you end up with recurring episodes of hyperglycemia, the Somogyi effect may be responsible.

The only sure way to know is to carefully monitor your blood glucose. If you notice that your blood glucose level falls below 65 mg/dl and then rises to over 200 mg/dl a few hours later, then this may be occurring. Talk to your health care team about the best approach to take in the middle of an episode and what your individual blood glucose values indicating an episode may be. If your hypoglycemia is mild, you may be advised to take a small amount of carbohydrate (about 15 grams) to bring your glucose levels to within normal range. If your blood glucose levels rise above 200 mg/dl, you may be advised to reduce your food intake or increase your physical activity. However, increasing your dose of insulin is not advised if you indeed have rebound hyperglycemia, because it may trigger another round of hypoglycemia and hyperglycemia. If your blood glucose level rises above 250 mg/dl, check for ketones and call a member of your health care team. If it rises above 500 mg/dl, seek emergency treatment immediately.

■ PREVENTION

The best way to treat rebound hyperglycemia is to determine what is causing the initial episode of hypoglycemia and prevent this from occurring in the future. If your episodes are occurring during the day, measure your blood glucose levels several times throughout the day and make note of your exact mealtimes and physical activity. You and your health care team should develop a plan based on your pattern of activity. If you are exercising on an empty stomach, for example, you may need to have a snack before you work out, but check your blood glucose to be sure. If you are taking insulin, you may need to make adjustments in the timing of injections and your meals. If you are experiencing rebound hyperglycemia in the early morning, then try measuring your blood glucose levels between 2 and 4 a.m. and then again at 7 a.m. If blood glucose levels fall below 60 mg/dl between 2 and 4 a.m. but then rise above 180 mg/dl at 7 a.m., you may want to consider a change in your bedtime snack or postponing your evening dose of insulin. Talk to your health care team about the approach that will work best for you.

Brittle Diabetes

Brittle diabetes refers to wide, unpredictable swings in blood glucose levels. In the past, many patients felt frustrated because they didn't always know what was causing these drastic changes in blood glucose levels. The term is used less commonly now, because widespread use of self-monitoring of blood glucose has given people a better handle on controlling their blood glucose levels. By frequently testing your blood glucose, you have a clue to what causes your blood glucose to go up and down and you are better able to keep it under control. However, some people still have a hard time controlling blood glucose levels because their bodies have exaggerated responses to food, medication, physical activity, and stress. If you are one of these people, especially if you take insulin, you may eat about the same amount of food every day at the same time, inject the same amount of insulin at the designated times each day, and even exercise regularly. But you may find that one day your blood glucose levels are high and the next day they are low for no apparent reason. If this is the case, it may take some detective work to figure out what is causing these wide swings in blood glucose.

■ SYMPTOMS

If you have brittle diabetes, you may frequently experience symptoms of both hypoglycemia (low blood glucose) and hyperglycemia (high blood glucose). Symptoms of hypoglycemia include shakiness, nervousness, sweating, irritability, impatience, chills and clamminess, rapid heartbeat, anxiety, light-headedness, hunger, sleepiness, anger, stubbornness, sadness, lack of coordination, blurred vision, nausea, tingling or numbness in the lips or tongue, nightmares, crying out during sleep, headaches, any change in behavior or personality, delirium, confusion, and, in severe cases, unconsciousness. Symptoms of hyperglycemia include a dry, parched mouth, excessive thirst, and frequent urination. Untreated hyperglycemia could lead to diabetic ketoacidosis or hyperglycemic hyperosmolar state. Your body may not show all of the symptoms of hypoglycemia or hyperglycemia. The only way to know for sure whether your blood glucose levels are swinging one way or another is to measure them.

RISKS

In the short term, both extreme high or low blood sugar levels that go untreated could lead to unconsciousness, seizures, coma, and even death. It is important to be aware of the symptoms of both high and low blood glucose levels and know what to do if yours swing too widely. Over time, the Diabetes Control and Complications Trial showed that wide swings in blood glucose can greatly increase the likelihood and severity of the complications of diabetes, including eye disease, kidney disease, nerve disease, heart disease, and infections.

WHAT TO DO

If you are prone to wide swings in blood glucose levels, talk to members of your health care team in advance about what to do if your levels fall too low or rise too high. The first thing you should do is test your blood glucose. If your blood glucose levels are below 60–70 mg/dl or are near 60–70 mg/dl and you are experiencing any of the symptoms of hypoglycemia, you probably need to take a quick fix of carbohydrate. If you are unable to test your blood glucose, but feel any of the symptoms, don't wait to test. Take 10–15 grams of a fast-acting carbohydrate, then retest in 15 minutes. If your glucose level is still low, eat another 10–15 grams of carbohydrate.

If your blood glucose levels are above 250 mg/dl and/or if you are feeling any of the symptoms of diabetic ketoacidosis or hyperglycemic hyperosmolar state, call your health care team immediately. Talk to your health care team in advance about what to do if your blood glucose goes too high. You may need to take an extra dose of insulin, for example. If your blood glucose level is above 500 mg/dl, get emergency treatment immediately.

TREATMENT

You may be able to adjust your blood glucose levels on your own. Talk to your health care team about specific actions you can take. If your blood glucose levels are too high or too low, you may require emergency treatment.

To prevent brittle diabetes from causing further problems, you need to figure out what is causing the wide swings in blood glucose levels. Carefully monitor your blood glucose and keep a log of your daily activities, food intake, medications, insulin, and make a note of your general feelings of physical and emotional health. In tracking down the possible culprit, consider the following possibilities.

Timing of Insulin Injections

Are you allowing a full 30 to 45 minutes to give your regular insulin time to kick in before eating meals? You may need to alter the timing of insulin injections and mealtimes.

Insulin Dose

Check that you are measuring your insulin dose accurately. If you are taking too much insulin at one time, it may take varying amounts of time to work. Consider using an insulin pump to spread out an insulin dose over time.

Injection Sites

Make sure you are rotating your injection sites regularly. Insulin is absorbed at the most consistent rate from the abdomen. (See Chapter 4 for more information on insulin absorption.)

Injection Depth

Make sure that you inject your insulin at the same depth each time.

Blood Flow

Working muscles and warm temperatures speed up insulin absorption. Cool temperatures and tobacco slow it down. Think about whether you are injecting insulin near working muscles or whether your home and office are different temperatures.

Neuropathy

Damage to nerves can affect the absorption of food. (See Chapter 10 for more information on neuropathy.)

Dehydration

If you are dehydrated from high blood glucose levels, it may be harder for insulin to flow into your tissues.

Talk to your doctor or diabetes educator about other things you can do to better control your blood glucose levels.

Impaired Glucose Tolerance

If you take a test for diabetes called a glucose tolerance test and your test results do not indicate diabetes, but are not normal either, you have impaired glucose tolerance. Most of the time, your blood glucose levels are probably normal. But the test shows that your blood glucose levels remained higher than someone without diabetes. What this diagnosis really means is that you may be at risk for developing type 2 diabetes. People with impaired glucose tolerance are also at greater risk for heart attacks.

■ SYMPTOMS

If you have impaired glucose tolerance, you may show few of the symptoms of diabetes under normal living conditions, and you are probably unaware that you even have it. However, it is possible that some symptoms may appear in certain situations, such as when you are under stress, feel ill, or consume large amounts of carbohydrate. Even if you don't have any of the classic symptoms of diabetes on a daily basis (excessive thirst, frequent urination, and blurry vision), if you find that you "feel funny" when you eat a lot of candy or drink a lot of sugar-laden soft drinks, you may want to ask your doctor for a glucose tolerance test. This will tell you whether you have impaired glucose tolerance and whether you may be at risk for developing diabetes in the future.

During an oral glucose tolerance test, you will be asked to drink a high-glucose solution. Two hours after the glucose drink, people without diabetes will have a blood glucose level of less than 140 mg/dl. People with diabetes will have a blood glucose level above 200 mg/dl. If you have a blood glucose level between 140 and 200 mg/dl, you may have impaired glucose tolerance.

■ RISKS

If you are diagnosed with impaired glucose tolerance, you are up to seven times more likely to develop diabetes within 7 to 8 years than someone with normal glucose tolerance. You are also at a greater risk of developing cardiovascular disease. If you are female, you are more likely to develop gestational diabetes during pregnancy.

■ PREVENTION

If you have been diagnosed with impaired glucose tolerance, don't panic. You don't have diabetes, but you are at risk. Despite this increased risk, many people with impaired glucose tolerance never develop diabetes. Talk to your doctor or a diabetes educator about the best ways to prevent diabetes from occurring. Since type 2 diabetes occurs most frequently in individuals who are overweight and inactive, the best approach is to adopt a healthy lifestyle. Keep your weight down, exercise regularly, and avoid eating too much fat in your diet. You may want to talk to a nutritional counselor about ways to modify your diet to prevent diabetes and eat more healthy foods, without entirely giving up all the foods you love. Or talk to an exercise physiologist or personal trainer to find ways to incorporate physical activities that you enjoy into your lifestyle. The trick is to make lifestyle choices that you can live with.

Chapter 4
Solving Insulin
Delivery Problems

Insulin is a hormone that the body produces to do many jobs. One of its most important jobs is to act as a key to let glucose into cells, where it is used for energy. Without glucose, cells die and the body cannot survive. If you have diabetes, insulin somehow can't do its job. If you have type 1 diabetes, your body doesn't make the insulin it needs and you will have to give yourself insulin. If you have type 2 diabetes, your body probably makes insulin, but it may not make enough or it may not respond to insulin the way it should. Even though your body makes insulin, you may find that you have to take extra insulin to keep your diabetes under control. Most of the problems with insulin involve delivery. Getting it to the right place at the right time in the amount needed is not always an easy task.

Injection Site Problems

Several types of problems can occur at injection sites. *Lipoatrophy* results from a loss of fat at the injection site and appears as dents in the skin. *Hypertrophy* is caused by an overgrowth of fat cells and gives the skin a lumpy appearance. The key to overcoming these types of problems is to rotate the injection site. In addition to these two common skin problems, some people experience burning, itching, or a rash at the injection site. This may be due to a local insulin allergy (see below) that is not helped by rotating the injection site.

■ SYMPTOMS

If you notice indentations, or dents, in the skin near your injection site, then you may have lipoatrophy. This condition is thought to be caused by an immune reaction to insulin that results in a loss of fat under the skin where you inject insulin.

If you notice lumps in the skin around your injection site, then you may have hypertrophy, also know as lipohypertrophy. Your skin may resemble scar tissue. This is thought to occur when fat cells grow inappropriately and make the skin look lumpy.

■ RISKS

Injection site problems can occur in anyone who injects insulin. Lipoatrophy is more common in young women and is more likely to occur in people who use less purified forms of insulin, especially beef insulin. Hypertrophy is not an immune or allergic reaction and is not affected by the type of insulin used. However, it is more common in people who do not regularly rotate injection sites. Lipoatrophy and hypertrophy pose no health risks in and of themselves. Irregularities in insulin absorption can occur when insulin is injected into lumpy skin, though, so it is best to try to prevent them from occurring in the first place.

■ WHAT TO DO

If you already have lipoatrophy, you may want to switch to a more highly purified and less immunogenic form of insulin, such as pork or, preferably, human insulin. To get rid of the dents that are already there, you can try injecting human insulin into the margins of the dented area. This can build up fat deposits in the area and fill in the dents. However, this procedure is not a cure-all and it could be several months before you see any noticeable improvement. Talk to your doctor or diabetes educator about the best way to go about this.

If you have hypertrophy, switching to human insulin will not help. Your best bet is to avoid injecting into existing lumps and to rotate injection sites to prevent the further formation of skin lumps.

■ PREVENTION

To prevent lipoatrophy, try switching to human insulin if you haven't already done so. Both lipoatrophy and hypertrophy can be prevented by rotating the injection site. Where you decide to inject insulin is up to you. Whatever you decide, the important thing is to inject at different sites within the body to prevent skin problems. Some people find that rotating all injections within one general area such as the abdomen works well. Other people get better results by doing all morning injections in one general area such at the buttocks and all evening injections in another area such as the abdomen.

Within these general areas, it is best to change the exact site of injection from day to day. Divide the body area into sites about the size of a quarter. Try to make each new injection at least a finger-width away from the last shot. You may want to figure out a way to remember where you injected your last shot. Once you have used all the available injection sites, you can then start over in the same body area.

In rotating sites, keep in mind that insulin is absorbed differently from different parts of the body. The abdomen is frequently used because insulin is absorbed most quickly and consistently from this site. It is absorbed more slowly from the arms and slower still in the legs and buttocks. However, if you are actively working your muscles in these areas, insulin may be absorbed more quickly. Every person is different, with different amounts of muscle and fat in the various areas of the body. Try to develop an awareness of how your own body absorbs insulin.

Insulin Allergy

With so many people turning to human insulin, insulin allergy is becoming less and less common. However, some people may still experience an allergic response to an insulin preparation. Insulin allergies can be local (confined to the area around the injection site) or systemic (affecting the whole body). If you do have an allergic reaction, you may be allergic to the insulin itself or to ingredients used in the insulin preparation, such as the protamine in NPH or the zinc used in lente insulins. And what may appear to be a local allergic reaction may really be due to an improper injection technique. It is important to consult with your health care team to figure out the source of your allergy.

■ SYMPTOMS

Burning, itching, redness, swelling, hives, or rash at the insulin injection site could indicate a local allergic reaction. Depending on the cause of the allergic reaction, symptoms can occur within 30 minutes after injection or over the course of several hours. Delayed allergic reactions may appear over the course of 24 hours. In rare cases, insulin can trigger a severe asthmatic or anaphylactic response, due to a systemic allergy. These symptoms, which occur within minutes, include difficulty in breathing, respiratory distress, vomiting, abdominal distress, and even shock. However, this response is extremely rare, especially with the wide use of human insulin.

■ RISKS

Insulin allergies are usually local and systemic responses are very rare. You are more likely to have an insulin allergy if you are allergic to penicillin or have a history of other allergies, have been on insulin intermittently, or are overweight.

Local insulin allergies are not life-threatening and usually clear up on their own after a few months. However, in rare cases, a life-threatening systemic allergic reaction can occur.

■ WHAT TO DO

Local allergic responses usually appear during the first 2 weeks of therapy and clear up on their own within a month or two. Make sure you are injecting insulin properly and that your cleansing alcohol contains no contaminants. Also make sure that there are no signs of infection (extreme tenderness and redness, pus formation or anything that oozes) at the injection site. If there is an infection you may need to be treated with an antibacterial agent.

If your symptoms are mild and produce only minor discomfort, you may want to just wait it out and see if the allergy clears up on its own. However, if the allergic reaction persists for more than a month and is making you uncomfortable, talk to your doctor about what steps to take. You may want to switch to human insulin if you have not already done so. If you see no improvement in 2 to 14 doses, your doctor may conduct a skin test to see which insulin preparations are least reactive. You may be advised to switch to the least reactive form of insulin. If you continue to have a persistent, severe allergy to the least reactive insulin, your doctor may recommend treatment by insulin desensitization. You may also want to be tested for an allergy to zinc, protamine, preservatives, or the rubber stopper used to cap the insulin vial.

If you have a general, or systemic, reaction to insulin, call your doctor right away or seek emergency medical treatment if your symptoms are severe. These symptoms include loss of color, clamminess of the skin, a drop in blood pressure, rapid but weak pulse, restlessness, difficulty breathing, anxiety, and sometimes unconsciousness. If you have type 2 diabetes, your doctor may want you to discontinue insulin and treat you with an aggressive low-calorie diet, exercise, and oral agents. If you have type 1 diabetes and require insulin, you will need to be desensitized in a hospital setting.

■ TREATMENT

If you require insulin and are having a general, or systemic, insulin reaction, you will need to be treated in an intensive care unit that is prepared to deal with anaphylactic shock. After skin testing for the least reactive insulin, you will need to undergo insulin desensitization. If you are having a local insulin allergic reaction, you may still need to undergo desensitization, but will probably not require hospitalization.

To do this, you will be given low doses of the least reactive insulin at periodic intervals. The dose of insulin will be increased until you receive 1 unit of insulin or until a skin reaction occurs. If a skin reaction occurs, the dose will be dropped and again increased at periodic intervals until plasma glucose is under satisfactory control. You may be given a dose of steroid or antihistamine if desensitization is not occurring. The amount of insulin will then be increased until you can tolerate a therapeutic level of insulin without an allergic reaction.

Inactive Insulin

The insulin you buy is a protein that comes as a solution in buffered water. Under normal conditions it can last a month stored at room temperature, and even longer in the refrigerator. Insulin is fairly stable stored this way, but extremes of temperature or excessive agitation can cause the protein to denature, or unfold, and become inactivated. Often, protein denaturation causes a change in the visible appearance of a protein solution or suspension. However, different preparations of insulin look a little different to begin with. Some are clear, some are a little cloudy. It is important to know what your particular insulin should look like. If there is a change in the appearance of your insulin preparation, it could mean the insulin is no longer active. Using inactive insulin could cause you to lose control of your blood glucose level and even lead to emergency situations. Any time your blood glucose level rises unexpectedly and you have not forgotten an insulin injection, or altered your diet or exercise pattern, check for changes in your insulin.

■ SYMPTOMS

If you are controlling your blood glucose level with insulin, any unexplained episode of hyperglycemia could mean that your insulin has gone bad. A sure sign of hyperglycemia is a high blood glucose reading (anything above 250 mg/dl). Other signs of hyperglycemia include intense thirst, a dry mouth, and the need to urinate frequently. If your blood glucose rises too high for too long, life-threatening situations such as diabetic ketoacidosis or hyperglycemic hyperosmolar state can occur (see Chapter 3). Symptoms of diabetic ketoacidosis include nausea and vomiting, weakness, abdominal pain, warm dry skin, loss of consciousness, or a fruity odor on the breath.

■ RISKS

Using any insulin that has changed in appearance or has expired could lead to hyperglycemia, diabetic ketoacidosis, or hyperglycemic hyperosmolar state. Repeated episodes of hyperglycemia over time can increase your risk of many of the complications of diabetes.

■ WHAT TO DO

If you are experiencing any of the symptoms of hyperglycemia, you need to treat this right away. First, measure your blood glucose level. If it is higher than 250 mg/dl, also check for ketones. If you have ketones in your urine and show any of the signs of diabetic ketoacidosis, call your doctor right away. If your blood glucose level is higher than 300 mg/dl, seek emergency treatment at once.

If your doctor tells you to take an additional dose of insulin, do not use insulin from the same container if there is a visible change in the insulin. Open a fresh bottle that has not expired.

■ PREVENTION

To prevent using a spoiled container of insulin, it is important to store it properly and check its visual appearance before each use. Also check the expiration date. Do not use any vial of insulin that has expired. Unopened and unused bottles of insulin can be stored in the refrigerator until needed, as long as they have not expired. When you open a bottle of insulin, write the date that you opened it clearly on the label. Opened bottles of insulin that are stored in the refrigerator should be discarded after 3 months. Opened bottles of insulin are best kept at room temperature, but should be discarded after 1 month.

Also check for changes in the appearance of your bottle of insulin. Never use insulin if it looks abnormal. Regular and lispro insulins are clear. Always check for any floating or settled particles, cloudiness, or change in color. Other types of insulin, such as NPH or lente, come as suspensions. With suspensions, the insulin is never completely dissolved, even when new, and may have a cloudy appearance due to tiny particles floating in the liquid. However, in these preparations, the cloudiness should be uniform. You should not see any large clumps of material. If you see any sort of clumpiness, discard the bottle and open a new one. If you dilute your insulin, use only the diluent recommended by the manufacturer. Diluted insulin can be safely stored for 4 to 6 weeks in the refrigerator.

If you find something wrong with newly purchased insulin, return it to where you bought it right away. If anything develops later on, try to figure out what might have caused it. Did you shake it too much or store it in a hot glove compartment? Did you leave it out in the cold, causing it to freeze or thaw? Any excessive agitation or extremes of temperature can cause insulin to denature and lose its strength.

Adjusting to Human Insulin

If you have insulin allergies or problems with animal insulins, you'll probably appreciate the widespread availability of human insulins. In addition, synthetic modified insulins can provide you with even greater flexibility in developing a treatment plan that works for you. Maybe you need the fast action of lispro to accommodate changes in food intake or exercise, for example. Human insulins, in general, tend to peak faster than their animal counterparts, so you may need to adjust your insulin dose and schedule when you switch to human insulin.

■ SYMPTOMS

Some people experience more bouts with hypoglycemia when switching to human insulin from animal insulin. Any of the symptoms of hypoglycemia or hyperglycemia could mean that you are having a problem adjusting to human insulin. Symptoms of hypoglycemia include hunger, shakiness, nervousness, sweating, irritability, impatience, chills and clamminess, rapid heartbeat, anxiety, light-headedness or dizziness, blurred vision, nausea, sleepiness, tingling or numbness in the lips or tongue, and confusion. Symptoms of hyperglycemia include dry parched mouth, extreme thirst, sleepiness, confusion, and warm dry skin with no sweating.

■ WHAT TO DO

If you have recently switched to human insulin from an animal insulin and are experiencing any of the symptoms of hypoglycemia or hyperglycemia, test your blood glucose level right away. If your blood glucose level is low, your insulin may have kicked in too early, according to how you have timed your meal and your injection. If this is the case, you may need to eat something right away. If your meal is not ready, eat a fast-acting carbohydrate. It is less likely that you will experience hyperglycemia when adjusting to human insulin. Should this occur, it will probably be mild (a blood glucose level between 200 and 300 mg/dl). If this is the case, consider going for a brisk walk or other moderate activity. If your blood glucose level climbs over 300 mg/dl, something else may be contributing and you may need to treat it more aggressively (see Chapter 3).

■ PREVENTION

When switching to human insulin or any other kind of insulin, it is best to plan ahead to prevent swings in blood glucose from occurring in the first place. Talk to your doctor or diabetes educator about how to best make adjustments in your schedule. Bear in mind that all human insulins enter the bloodstream more quickly, start acting earlier, peak earlier, and last for a shorter period of time than their animal counterparts. The synthetic human insulin lispro, for example, is active within 15 minutes of injection and peaks in about an hour. This form may be handy if you don't know exactly how much you will eat at a meal, because you can inject it when you eat or even after you have eaten.

In general, you will inject human insulin closer to the start of your meal. You may need to experiment to figure out which timing works best for you and the insulin you are taking. If your insulin is kicking in too soon and triggering hypoglycemia, eat your meal closer to the time of injection or consider lowering your insulin dose. If you are finding that your long-acting insulin is not lasting through the night, you may want to take your insulin a little later. Also take into account where in your body you are injecting the insulin and how this affects the absorption time. If you need your insulin to last longer, consider injecting into your arms, or better yet, your thighs or buttocks, where it will be absorbed more slowly.

While you are adjusting to human insulin, monitor your blood glucose level frequently. This will tell you whether your insulin is kicking in too soon and whether you need to change the timing, dose, or site of injection. Your health care team can help you interpret your blood glucose readings and figure out how to change your insulin injection schedule, if necessary.

Timing of Insulin Injections

In people who don't have diabetes, the pancreas puts out a steady amount of insulin throughout the day and night. This basal level of insulin helps to keep the cells of the body supplied with the glucose the body needs for energy to carry on daily living. Your body needs more glucose during the day when you are active. The meals you eat supply the needed glucose. After you eat a meal, your glucose level is high and your body makes more insulin, which helps glucose enter the cells that need it. At night when you are inactive, you need less glucose and your insulin levels are low. If you don't have diabetes, your body responds to the amount of glucose in your blood automatically. But if you have diabetes, you face a great challenge: trying to match the insulin in your blood with the amount of glucose in your blood. Most insulin plans are designed to mimic what the body does naturally.

■ SYMPTOMS

If you are on insulin and experiencing swings in blood glucose, you may be having problems with the timing of your injections. An occasional high or low blood glucose reading is probably no cause for concern. But if you find that your blood glucose readings are often too high (above 250 mg/dl) or too low (below 60 mg/dl) throughout the day, or if you frequently experience any of the symptoms of hypoglycemia or hyperglycemia, talk to your doctor or diabetes educator. You may want to change your insulin injection plan altogether, or you may need to work out ways to make occasional changes in your injection schedule to accommodate changes in your meal or exercise schedule as they arise.

■ WHAT TO DO

Any episode of hypoglycemia or hyperglycemia should be treated right away. If your blood glucose levels fall too low, you could develop hypoglycemia, which, if left untreated, can lead to unconsciousness. If your glucose level climbs too high, you will develop hyperglycemia, which can progress to diabetic ketoacidosis, a life-threatening condition that can cause seizures, unconsciousness, coma, and even death.

If you have hypoglycemia, you need to increase the amount of glucose in your blood as soon as possible. This is best done by eating a fast-acting carbohydrate snack. If your hypoglycemia is more severe and you become confused, you may need to have someone give you a glucagon injection. (For more on what to do if you are hypoglycemic, see Chapter 2.)

If your blood glucose is over 250 mg/dl, you may need to treat your hyperglycemia. This can be accomplished with an extra dose of insulin. (For more on what to do if you are hyperglycemic, see Chapter 3.) Talk to your doctor or a member of your health care team about what to do in an emergency situation should your blood glucose levels swing too high or too low. If your levels are chronically high or low, talk to your doctor about how you might change your insulin injection schedule to help you better control your blood glucose levels.

■ PREVENTION

To prevent swings in blood glucose, you may need to make changes in your insulin injection schedule. Most insulin plans will try mimic the function of a normal pancreas. The pancreas puts out a steady stream of insulin throughout the day and night. This is known as the basal or baseline level of insulin. When you eat a meal, your blood glucose level rises. A normally functioning pancreas will put out more insulin in response to the increase in blood glucose. When blood glucose levels fall, the pancreas puts out less insulin. If you use an insulin pump, your pump puts out a steady stream of insulin throughout the day and night.

You can program it to pump extra insulin before meals or you can manually control it to put out extra insulin.

If you are injecting insulin, then you most likely will want a plan that will accomplish the same thing. Most people use combination insulin plans. By using a combination of long-acting insulin to provide basal levels of insulin and shorter-acting insulin to act as a bolus, or booster, dose to cover the rise in glucose with your meals, you can mimic the action of a normal pancreas. The trick is finding the schedule that works for you.

When you develop an insulin schedule or when you make changes in your existing schedule, it helps to know when different types of insulin will take effect. This information is summarized in the chart below.

Sample Insulin Plans

Some sample plans are summarized in the graphs below. It is best to talk to your doctor about the plan that will work best for you.

Graph 1 shows a single shot of intermediate-acting insulin injected in the morning. This plan provides adequate coverage over much of the day, but it will leave you uncovered for breakfast and for most of the

WHEN WILL INSULIN TAKE EFFECT?

Type of Insulin	When Taken	When It's Active	Blood Test That Shows Its Effect
Short acting	Before a meal	Between that meal and the next meal	After that meal and before next meal
Intermediate acting	Before breakfast	Between lunch and dinner	Before dinner
Intermediate acting	Before dinner or bedtime	Overnight	Before breakfast
Long acting	Before breakfast or before dinner or half dose at each time	Overnight, because short-acting insulin hides its effect during the day	Before breakfast

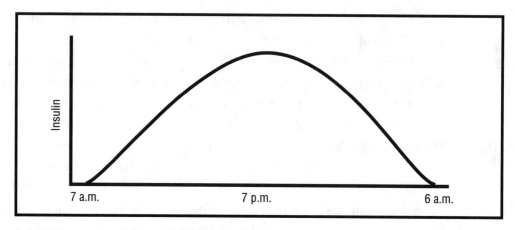

GRAPH 1: One shot of intermediate-acting insulin.

night. Also, high insulin levels when the insulin peaks may leave you susceptible to hypoglycemia.

Graph 2 splits intermediate-acting insulin into two shots taken at breakfast and dinnertime. This is better than a single shot, but may leave you uncovered from 3 to 10 a.m. In Graph 3, long-acting insulin is split into two shots, which provides basal level coverage around the clock. However, this plan does not provide the bolus dose of insulin to cover your meals.

Most people who need to take insulin will benefit the most by mixing different types of insulin in multiple shots. In Graph 4, regular and intermediate-acting NPH insulins are split and mixed in two shots given

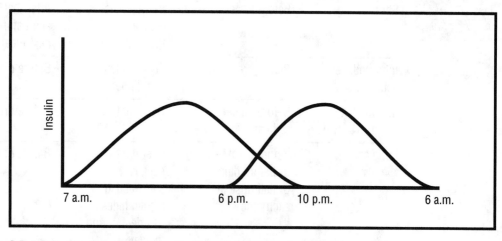

GRAPH 2: Intermediate-acting insulin split into two shots.

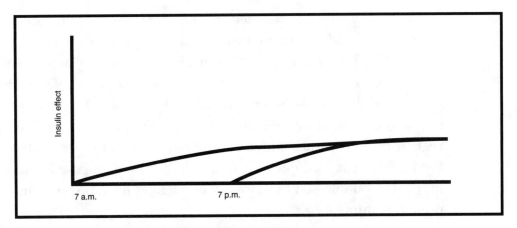

GRAPH 3: Long-acting insulin split into two shots.

30 minutes before breakfast and dinner. Regular insulin goes to work 30 minutes after injection, in time to cover breakfast. As regular insulin decreases, NPH insulin starts to work. Just before dinnertime, when the intermediate insulin starts to wear off, another mixed dose is given. Regular insulin will kick in to cover your dinner meal, while NPH will carry you through the night.

This type of plan can be modified by using a faster-acting insulin, such as lispro instead of regular insulin. The advantage of lispro is that it can be given at breakfast, or even just after breakfast, and the dose can be tailored to accommodate the amount of food you eat.

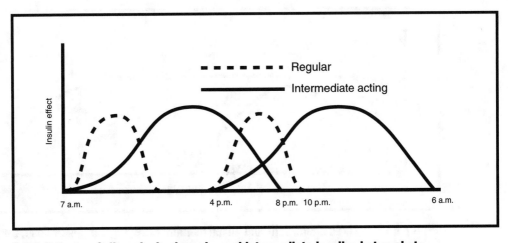

GRAPH 4: Split and mixed regular and intermediate insulins in two shots.

You may need to experiment to find the right combinations of intermediate and fast-acting insulins. You may want to start out with a 2-to-1 ratio of intermediate-acting insulin to regular or lispro insulin (two parts NPH, one part regular or lispro). You may prefer a premixed formula, such as a 70/30 mixture of NPH/regular. Or you may want to split and mix the dose yourself. This way you can change the amount of regular or NPH insulin independently to account for activity level and food intake. For example, if you have high blood glucose levels in the morning, you may want to move your evening insulin shot from dinner-time to bedtime.

If you find that the two-shot plan is too rigid, you may prefer a three-shot plan. This will allow you more opportunities to make changes to accommodate your activity and food schedule. For example, if you find that your blood glucose level dips too low in the early morning hours, you may want to take a shot of regular insulin at dinnertime and delay the intermediate shot until bedtime. This is shown in Graph 5. The more often you inject insulin, the more chances you have to make changes in your dose to fine-tune your control.

Other three-shot plans can also work for you. Graph 6 shows a split and mixed morning dose, a regular dose, and a split and mixed evening dose. This plan incorporates long-acting and regular insulins given at breakfast, regular insulin at lunch, and long-acting and regular insulins given at dinnertime. The long-acting doses provide coverage through the day and evening, and the regular doses provide meal

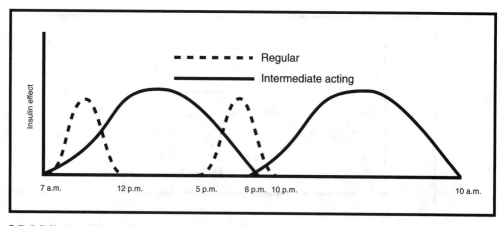

GRAPH 5: Three shots: split and mixed morning dose, regular dinner dose, and intermediate evening dose.

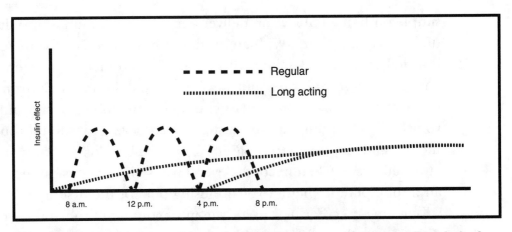

G R A P H   6 :   Three shots: split and mixed morning dose, regular dose, split and mixed evening dose.

coverage. This plan can also take advantage of the faster-acting lispro, and it allows you to make changes in doses as your activity and food schedule demand. For example, if you exercise in the afternoon, you may want to decrease your evening or noontime dose of regular insulin. If you plan to eat a bigger dinner, you can increase your evening dose of regular insulin.

With any insulin plan, especially one that incorporates multiple shots, it is important to monitor your blood glucose levels frequently. That will provide you and your doctor with important information. If your blood glucose level rises too high or goes too low between injections, you may need to change your insulin dose, the timing of your injections, your activity level, or your food intake. Your blood glucose level is especially important in figuring out how to coordinate the timing of your injection and your next meal. For example, if your blood glucose level is low, you may want to wait until after you eat to inject insulin. If your level is high, take your insulin before you eat. Frequent monitoring can also give you and your doctor a good idea about how your overall plan is working and how to fine-tune your injection schedule, if necessary. Talk to your doctor about whether any changes are needed.

Insulin Pumps

An insulin pump is a convenient technological device that can help you take the insulin you need when you need it with minimum intrusion. A simple push of a button can deliver a measured amount of insulin any time of day, anywhere. With an insulin pump, a needle or catheter is inserted under the skin and left in place for several days before you change the insertion site. Your insulin pump delivers insulin from a pre-filled syringe, through thin plastic tubing to the insertion site and into your body. The pump delivers a steady basal level of insulin throughout the day and allows you to program or manually deliver a bolus of insulin at mealtimes or when needed. Several types of problems can occur with an insulin pump, whether you are using one for the first time or you are a long-time user. For new users, the most common problems have to do with finding the right dose of basal insulin and mealtime bolus dose. Others may find that problems can develop at the injection site. Probably the most common problem with using an insulin pump occurs when clogs and kinks in the line end up stopping or slowing down the flow of insulin into your body. Fortunately, most of these problems are easily fixed.

Adjusting to the Pump

■ SYMPTOMS

When you first start using an insulin pump or if you are making changes in your meal plan, exercise level, or insulin doses, you may experience swings in blood glucose levels. You might observe this directly by measuring your blood glucose level and finding that some-times it is too high (over 250 mg/dl) and sometimes it is too low (under 60 mg/dl). Or you may experience some of the symptoms of hypo-glycemia or hyperglycemia. If this is the case, then you will need to make adjustments in your insulin delivery rates.

■ WHAT TO DO

Talk to your doctor or diabetes educator about the best way to figure out what your basal and bolus insulin doses should be. If you have been injecting insulin, you know what your total insulin dose over the course of the day has been. Add up the total number of units of insulin you have been taking in a day. (In general, if you are within 20 percent of your ideal body weight, your total daily insulin dose will be 0.5 to 1.0 unit per kilogram of body weight.) Your total basal dose of insulin using an insulin pump should be some percentage of that total dose, usually about 40 to 50 percent. The other 50 to 60 percent of your daily insulin dose can be divided into before-meal bolus doses. The biggest doses will be given at breakfast and dinner, with smaller doses at lunch and bedtime. For example, you might take 15 to 25 percent of your insulin before breakfast, 15 percent before lunch, 15 to 20 percent before dinner, and up to 10 percent to cover your bedtime snack. Exactly how big the insulin bolus is will depend on your eating and activity pattern.

As you get used to your pump, you will most likely have to take the time to figure out the best basal rates and bolus doses that work for you. During this period especially, frequent blood glucose monitoring is essential. If your blood glucose levels are consistently high throughout the day, you may need to increase your basal rate. If they are too low, you may need to lower your basal rate. You may even want to change the basal rate at night, to keep your blood glucose levels in check. For example, if you experience low blood glucose at night, you might want to lower your basal rate during the nighttime hours. If you have hyperglycemia in the morning due to the dawn phenomenon (see page 114), think about increasing your basal rate in the early morning hours.

If you are using regular insulin in your pump, you should activate the bolus dose 30 minutes before your meal. If you are using lispro insulin in your pump, the bolus should be given immediately before eating a meal. If you are finding that your level climbs too high after a meal, you may need to eat less carbohydrates during the next meal or take more insulin. You may also find it helpful to count or estimate the number of carbohydrates in each meal. In general, you will need 1 unit of insulin to cover 10–15 grams of carbohydrate. It may take a while to figure out the doses that work for you, but once you do, the pump will give you greater flexibility in your schedule.

The pump can be safely taken off during periods of physical activity. Not only is this more convenient, but if you are exercising this will help you avoid hypoglycemia as well. However, if you are using lispro in your pump, do not keep the pump off for more than an hour, because of the risk of hyperglycemia. If you are using regular insulin in your pump, you can probably keep the pump off for 2 to 3 hours.

Insertion Site Problems

■ SYMPTOMS

The needle and catheter should be comfortable at all times, even when you exercise or if someone bumps into you. Any redness or swelling could be a sign of a local allergic reaction or infection. Check your insertion sites for the development of scar tissue. If any of these conditions persist even after you have changed the insertion site, talk to your doctor or health care professional.

■ WHAT TO DO

If you are using a pump, you are subject to many of the same injection site skin problems faced by people who inject insulin with a syringe. The best way to deal with and prevent injection site skin problems is to rotate the insertion site frequently. You should replace the infusion set and move to a new insertion site every 3 days. This will help you to avoid infection and to prevent clogging in the infusion set. Make sure that when you do this, you place the new insertion site at least 1 inch from the old site on the abdomen. Use a regular rotation schedule and avoid inserting into scar tissue or moles. This could interfere with insulin absorption and cause more scarring. If you see any redness or swelling, move your insertion site and replace the infusion set, even if it has been less than 3 days. If the swelling or redness persists, call your doctor. If there are any signs of infection, such as tenderness or the formation or oozing of pus, call your doctor right away. If you have an infection, you will require prompt treatment.

Unexplained Hyperglycemia

■ SYMPTOMS

If you are monitoring your blood glucose, you will notice the first sign of hyperglycemia: a blood glucose reading of more than 250 mg/dl. You may also notice one or more of the following symptoms: dry parched mouth, excessive thirst, warm dry skin with no sweating, frequent urination, and sleepiness or confusion.

■ WHAT TO DO

If you have any symptoms of hyperglycemia, test your blood glucose at once. If it is over 250 mg/dl, you may need to treat it right away. Talk to your doctor about what to do should your blood glucose rise above 250 mg/dl. If you have any of the signs of diabetic ketoacidosis (vomiting, nausea, stomach pain, blurry vision, fever, weakness, or difficulty breathing) you may require emergency treatment (see Chapter 3). You may need to take an extra dose of insulin if your blood glucose is too high, even if you do not show signs of diabetic ketoacidosis. However, if you are using an insulin pump and your pump is clogged, you may be unable to deliver the extra insulin through the pump until you take care of the blockage. If the battery has run out or there is an obstruction in the insulin flow, an alarm will sound. If there is a kink in the line, straighten out the tubing to restore insulin flow. Check for clogs in the line and replace the tubing or infusion set if necessary. Also check that there are no air bubbles in the line, that the battery is working, and the insulin syringe is not empty.

There may be times when blood glucose levels are high and there is no obvious problem with the pump. If this happens, other factors may be contributing. First, check your insulin. If it is not buffered, insulin may crystallize and clog or slow down the flow of liquid through the catheter. Use only buffered insulin preparations. Make sure your insulin has not expired and has not been exposed to extremes in temperature. Check that there are no clumps or floating particles in your insulin preparation. If you have used your vial of insulin for more than a month, replace it with a fresh vial.

If your insulin appears normal, check your insertion site. If the needle is near a scar or mole, move it to another site. Also, move it if it is near your belt line or any other place where there is friction, or if the skin near the site is tender, red, or swollen.

You should also check the infusion set. Make sure the needle is still intact and that insulin is not leaking around the infusion site. Make sure there is no blood or air in the line and that the line did not come loose from the pump. If the infusion set has been in place for more than 2 days, it may be time to change it.

If everything else looks in order, check the pump itself. Make sure that the basal rate is set correctly and the battery has not run down. Check to see if the insulin cartridge has been placed correctly and still contains insulin. Also make sure that the pump is primed with insulin each time a fresh cartridge of insulin is put in. Another possibility is that your pump is just not working correctly. Follow the manufacturer's instructions to see if there is a malfunction of your pump, and call the manufacturer if necessary.

Intensive Therapy

The Diabetes Control and Complications Trial (DCCT), a 10-year study begun in 1983, showed that you can greatly reduce the complications of diabetes by keeping your blood glucose levels under tight control. The study confirmed the suspicion that it is the excess glucose in the blood that leads to eye disease, cardiovascular disease, kidney disease, and nerve disease. By monitoring frequently and taking three to four injections of insulin each day or using an insulin pump, you are more likely to keep your blood glucose levels closer to normal and delay or prevent diabetes complications. The DCCT was conducted using people with type 1 diabetes, but people with type 2 diabetes can also practice tight control through the use of diet, exercise, and oral agents or with the use of insulin.

However, intensive therapy is not without its drawbacks. It requires a great deal of effort and motivation and should not be practiced by patients with cardiovascular disease, severe complications, or a history of drug or alcohol abuse. It is not recommended for young children or the elderly, or anyone with a history of severe hypoglycemia. The chief problems for people adhering to a program of intensive therapy are an increased risk of hypoglycemia and a greater tendency to gain weight. With proper attention and prevention, both problems can be minimized so that you can make intensive therapy work for you.

Hypoglycemia

When you make the switch from traditional management of diabetes to intensive therapy, you are trying to keep your blood glucose levels as close to normal as possible. This means that your overall blood glucose levels are much lower than what you might be used to and you don't have a lot of room for error. A skipped snack, a smaller-than-normal lunch, or an extra lap around the track might be enough to trigger an episode of hypoglycemia. While practicing tight control, you can expect more frequent episodes of all levels of hypoglycemia (mild, moderate, and severe). You might also be more likely to experience hypoglycemia unawareness, a condition in which you are unable to detect the early warning signs of hypoglycemia (see Chapter 2).

■ SYMPTOMS

Symptoms of hypoglycemia include shakiness, nervousness, sweating, irritability, chills and clamminess, rapid heartbeat, dizziness, light-headedness, anxiety, blurred vision, nausea, tingling or numbness in the tongue, confusion, strange behavior, and unconsciousness. (For more information about hypoglycemia and how to distinguish between moderate and severe episodes, see Chapter 2.)

■ RISKS

Anyone practicing tight control is at an increased risk for hypoglycemia. However, if you are male, an adolescent, have had diabetes for a long time, had a high glycated hemoglobin level before intensive therapy and a low glycated hemoglobin level during intensive therapy, and a history of severe hypoglycemia before intensive management, then you are at especially high risk of hypoglycemia while practicing tight control. Hypoglycemia unawareness is also increased for people on tight control.

■ WHAT TO DO

If you think you are having a hypoglycemic reaction, test your blood glucose right away. If it is below 60 mg/dl, you may need to eat a fast-acting carbohydrate snack. Talk to your doctor or health care professional about the level at which you should begin treatment. For some people, hypoglycemia should be treated at a higher blood glucose level. Others may not become hypoglycemic until the blood glucose level is lower than 60 mg/dl. If you are unable to test, but you feel any of the symptoms, treat anyhow. For initial treatment of mild to moderate hypoglycemia, start with 10–15 grams of a fast-acting carbohydrate. Wait 15 minutes, then test and treat again, if necessary. If your hypoglycemia reaction is severe, you may become confused or even unconscious. If this occurs, someone else must take over. If you are unable to eat or drink anything, you may need a glucagon injection. Make sure those around you know the warning signs and know what to do should this situation arise.

■ PREVENTION

If you decide to practice intensive therapy, it is very important to take steps to prevent hypoglycemia from occurring. The most important is to become aware of the symptoms you experience during hypoglycemia. Monitor your blood glucose when in doubt and know the threshold at which your symptoms first appear and when they may change. Be aware that the glucose levels at which symptoms first appear may change during intensive management, compared to what they were on traditional therapy.

Blood glucose monitoring is essential for anyone with diabetes, but if you are practicing intensive therapy it is even more important. You should monitor at least four times a day—before each meal or snack and at bedtime—and you might also consider monitoring 2 hours after each meal. This is especially important during and after a period of increased exercise. If your blood glucose level is low 2 hours after you eat (less than 100 mg/dl), this will tell you that you need to be careful until your next meal. This information will help you to decide whether to increase or decrease any planned activity, whether you need to adjust your next insulin dose, or whether you will need to eat a snack before your meal or increase your food intake in your next meal. Always monitor your blood glucose level before driving.

Also, pay close attention to exercise and physical activity. Even weekend household chores or moderate activity may be enough to trigger an episode of hypoglycemia. Vigorous exercise can trigger hypoglycemia up to 12 to 24 hours following the initial activity.

Finally, to prevent hypoglycemia from occurring frequently, try to figure out what went wrong when you do have an episode. Did you skip a snack or forget to monitor your blood glucose before exercising? Did you oversleep or eat a meal later than usual? Try to figure out what you did out of the ordinary or what signs you may have missed so that you don't repeat any mistakes the next time.

If, despite all your attempts at troubleshooting and preventing hypoglycemia, you still experience repeated episodes, you and your doctor may want to reevaluate your glycemic goals. Maybe you are shooting to keep your blood glucose level between 80 and 120 mg/dl before meals and between 100 and 140 mg/dl at bedtime. If you are attaining these goals but frequently developing hypoglycemia, then maybe you need to shoot for a slightly higher blood glucose level. Maybe a before-meal glucose level of between 100 and 160 mg/dl, for example, will help you keep your blood glucose under control, but prevent the frequent bouts of hypoglycemia. Talk to your doctor about which glycemic goals are suitable for you.

Weight Gain

Many people who switch from a traditional program of diabetes management to intensive therapy experience weight gain. This tendency affects both men and women at any age equally. This may be a result of the tendency to eat more to prevent hypoglycemia. Or it could be due in small part to a more efficient metabolism. Whatever the reason, you may want to take steps to prevent excessive weight gain. This is especially true if you have type 2 diabetes or are already overweight. Excessive weight gain can contribute to further insulin resistance.

■ WHAT TO DO

Even before you begin an intensive management approach, talk to your doctor and nutritionist about changes in your meal plan. Your nutritionist should take a detailed nutritional history that takes into account your daily activities, what you have been eating, and what foods you like as a special treat every now and then. With this information, together you can devise a meal plan that is 200–400 calories per day less than what you have been eating.

You will probably need to reduce between-meal snacks. If you find that you need to take between-meal snacks regularly to prevent hypoglycemia, you may need to reduce your basal dose of insulin instead of eating more snacks. Talk to your doctor about the best way to make these changes.

Instead of treating hypoglycemia with traditional snack items, such as juice or cheese and crackers, treat with pure glucose. If you eat foods that contain many non-glucose ingredients, your calorie intake will increase more than it needs to. These non-glucose ingredients can also slow the treatment of low blood glucose.

Make sure to make exercise a regular part of your daily routine. Talk to your health care team and consult an exercise physiologist to find an exercise program that is right for you. Your best bet is to find an activity you enjoy doing and that is convenient to do. Make it as much a part of your plan as eating and taking insulin. When you exercise more than usual, take less insulin instead of eating more. This may require extra blood testing to figure out the best way to correct an insulin dose for excess exercise.

Don't be afraid to make adjustments in your meals. There may be times when you just don't feel like eating as much or it isn't convenient to eat as much as your plan calls for. At those times, reduce your calorie intake and take less insulin. When you do this, make sure to test your blood glucose more frequently.

Pancreas Transplants

The first pancreas transplant was performed in 1966. Since then, thousands of pancreas transplants have been performed on people with type 1 diabetes. Patients who receive a new pancreas may be effectively cured of diabetes. They no longer need to take insulin and no longer need to test blood glucose levels or adhere to a stringent meal plan. You are probably wondering: if pancreas transplants are such a miracle cure, then why aren't they done more often?

The major problem with a pancreas transplant is that the cure can be worse than the disease. Any kind of surgery poses a risk to patients, and pancreas transplantation surgery is major surgery. Once you receive a new pancreas, your body sees it as foreign matter and will do anything in its power to destroy it. Therefore, any transplant patient must commit to a lifetime of immunosuppressant therapy. Immunosuppressants are drugs that suppress the immune system to prevent organ rejection. The immunosuppressant drugs you must take to prevent organ rejection can cause problems in themselves. Cyclosporine, one of the most commonly used immunosuppressant drugs, can cause kidney damage, high blood pressure, nausea, hearing loss, acne, growth of body hair, and low white blood cell and platelet counts. Prednisone, a steroid drug usually given with cyclosporine, can upset the stomach and cause gastric and duodenal ulcers. It can also cause thinning of the bones, weight gain, cataracts, depression, and other side effects. Imuran, another immunosuppressant, causes nausea, fatigue, and fever.

In addition to the toxic effects of immunosuppressant drugs, patients who take immunosuppressants to prevent organ rejection must live with a suppressed immune system. That makes them less able to fight off a host of bacterial and viral infections. In a person with a suppressed immune system, even common pathogens can be life-threatening. A person on immunosuppressive drugs may also be more susceptible to cancer and other ailments. After all that, 50 percent of all transplanted pancreases are rejected by the patient's immune system and fail within 1 year.

Because the benefits of pancreas transplantation often do not outweigh the risks, pancreas transplants are not usually done alone. However, patients with type 1 diabetes who are having a kidney transplant are often given a pancreas transplant at the same time. Since they have to face the risks of surgery and immunosuppression anyhow, it makes sense to double the benefit: a new kidney and a new pancreas.

■ WHAT TO DO

If you are in line for a kidney transplant and think you might also want to consider a pancreas transplant at the same time, talk to your doctor. At most major hospitals that perform transplants, a double pancreas-kidney transplant is considered routine. The pancreas usually comes from a cadaver and the kidney from a live donor. In some cases a kidney and half of a pancreas can be obtained from a living donor. Half of a pancreas is enough to supply the insulin you need. If pancreas transplants are not offered at your hospital, you might want to locate a medical center that will perform one.

Different medical centers will have different eligibility requirements for a pancreas-only or a pancreas-kidney transplant. In general, you must have type 1 diabetes and be between the ages of 18 and 60. Your health must be good enough to enable you to withstand the stress of surgery and the immunosuppressant drug therapy that follows. You should be of sound mind and emotionally stable. Your chances of having a pancreas transplant are greatly enhanced if you have kidney failure and are undergoing a kidney transplant at the same time. In addition, be aware that organ transplants are costly, ranging from $40,000 to $100,000. You must be able to cover your expenses or have insurance that will.

If you are seeking a pancreas-only transplant, the criteria will be more stringent. Today, only 5 percent of pancreas transplants are single transplants. Pancreas-only transplants are recommended only when you have a very difficult time managing your diabetes on standard therapy and continuing to do so threatens your health. For example, you might be eligible for a pancreas-only transplant if you have brittle diabetes. This means that you are unable to control your blood glucose levels through diet and insulin therapy, frequently experience wide swings in blood glucose levels, have had severe episodes of ketoacidosis, hypoglycemia, and infection, and have hypoglycemia unawareness. You may also have to have two or more complications of diabetes, such as proliferative retinopathy, nephropathy, or neuropathy. In addition, you should understand that pancreas-only transplants are still investigational and have a high risk of failure. You may also be eligible for a pancreas transplant sometime after you have had a kidney transplant, since you are already on immunosuppressant therapy. This type of procedure may require that you have an acceptable creatinine clearance and evidence that your life is threatened by progression in diabetes complications or brittle diabetes.

There are several conditions that may make you ineligible for a pancreas transplant, whether alone or in combination with a kidney transplant. If you have coronary artery disease, cancer, poor lung function, ongoing alcohol or drug abuse, or a history of not taking good care of your health—not taking your medication, for example—you may be ineligible for a pancreas transplant. Talk to your doctor about whether a pancreas transplant would be advisable for you.

Other ways to replace the insulin-producing cells of the pancreas are also being investigated, but none is ready for public use. Researchers are trying to develop ways to transplant the islet cells of the pancreas—the ones that produce insulin. But islet cells are attacked by the immune system more readily than a whole pancreas. For now, islet cell transplants remain in the realm of investigational treatments.

Researchers are also trying to develop an artificial pancreas. This would be no more than an insulin pump that would deliver insulin as the body needs it. Right now, the roadblock is developing the technology for sensing when the body needs insulin. This requires a glucose meter that would work internally and would automatically sense when blood glucose levels are too high or too low, to activate or deactivate the artificial pancreas, much as a living pancreas does automatically. We are not there yet, but many scientists are working hard to solve this problem.

Chapter 5
Solving Oral Medication Problems

Whether you have recently been diagnosed with diabetes or have been dealing with it for some time, your first priority is to start to get your blood glucose levels under control as soon as possible. Fortunately for people with type 2 diabetes, many oral agents are now on the market to help achieve better blood glucose control with or without the aid of insulin. These agents can be taken in pill form on a regular basis. If you cannot control your blood glucose using diet and exercise alone, oral agents can help you get on track. Several choices are available, and not all oral agents will help you. That's because there are many causes of diabetes and you will need to find the drug that helps your specific problem. Some people with diabetes don't make enough insulin and need a drug that helps them make more insulin. Some make enough insulin but their bodies are resistant to insulin. They need a drug that makes cells more sensitive to insulin. And some people are affected by both problems. Your doctor will help find an oral agent that works for you.

Choosing an Oral Agent

If you have type 2 diabetes, your doctor may recommend using an oral agent when diet and exercise alone are no longer working. Oral agents are no substitute for a balanced diet and exercise, but they may provide that added boost to help you get your blood glucose levels under control. Although insulin injections are also an option, you will most likely want to try an oral agent first. Because they come in pill form, oral diabetes agents are easier to deal with. If you are obese, you may be able to avoid the large doses of insulin you would need. Also, with certain oral agents, you are less likely to develop hypoglycemia and less likely to gain weight than you would be using insulin.

■ SYMPTOMS

How do you know you are ready to start using an oral agent? Your doctor may recommend pharmacological intervention if your blood glucose level is over 140 mg/dl before breakfast, if your bedtime blood glucose level is over 160 mg/dl, or if your HbA_{1c} is over 8 percent. Your doctor may also recommend an oral agent if your blood glucose level is above 126 mg/dl but below 140 mg/dl and your HbA_{1c} is between 7 and 8 percent. Doctors and scientists now believe that it is better to begin treatment with oral agents at more modest blood glucose elevations because this may help to better control diabetes, keep it from progressing too quickly, and better prevent diabetes complications.

■ WHAT TO DO

If you are concerned that your blood glucose levels are out of control, monitor them carefully and bring your notes to your next doctor's appointment. If your levels are typically higher than the values listed above, your doctor may test your HbA_{1c} level. This is a measure of how well your blood glucose has been controlled over the long term. If you are having a hard time controlling your blood glucose through diet and exercise, your doctor may recommend an oral agent. There are two basic kinds of oral agents: those that increase the supply of insulin and those that make insulin more effective. You and your doctor will discuss which kind of agent will be better in helping to control your diabetes.

The table on page 151 shows the different drugs available to treat type 2 diabetes. Generally, medications in the same class are not used together because they have the same effect.

Agents that make insulin more effective include metformin, acarbose, and troglitazone. These drugs work differently (this is called their mechanism of action). The table on page 152 shows how these drugs work. Metformin decreases glucose production by the liver. Acarbose and miglitol work in the intestine, where they delay absorption of the carbohydrates you eat, which decreases blood glucose levels after meals. These drugs should always be taken with meals. Troglitazone enhances the effect of insulin on muscle and fat cells by decreasing insulin resistance. This drug should also be taken with food.

MEDICATIONS AVAILABLE TO TREAT DIABETES

Medication Class	Generic Name	Brand Name
Alpha-glucosidase Inhibitors	Acarbose	Precose
	Miglitol	Glyset
Biguanides	Metformin	Glucophage
Meglitinides	Repaglinide	Prandin
Sulfonylureas	Glimepiride	Amaryl
	Glipizide	Glucotrol
	Glyburide	DiaBeta
		Glynase
		Micronase
	Tolbutamide	Orinase
	Tolazamide	Tolinase
	Chlorpropamide	Diabinese
	Acetohexamide	Dymelor
Thiazolidinediones*	Troglitazone	Rezulin

*Pioglitazone (Actos) and Rosiglitazone (Avandia) will be reviewed by the FDA in 1999.

Sulfonylurea drugs and repaglinide increase the supply of insulin and decrease plasma glucose levels. Older, first-generation sulfonylureas require higher doses and often interact with other drugs. They must be used with caution in people with kidney and liver problems and are being used less frequently. More recently developed sulfonylureas, such as glyburide and glipizide, can be used at lower doses.

If your doctor prescribes an oral agent, make sure you understand when and how often to take it, and whether there are any special instructions or precautions you should know about. Discuss how to evaluate whether it is working and under what conditions your doctor should be notified.

Common Side Effects

As with any drug, oral agents all have their side effects. Make sure you and your doctor discuss any possible complications and what to look for.

HOW DIFFERENT DIABETES MEDICATIONS WORK

Medication Class	Site of Action	Action
Alpha-glucosidase Inhibitors (e.g., Acarbose or Miglitol)	Digestive system	Slows the breakdown of starches to glucose. Slows the entry of glucose into the bloodstream after a meal.
Biguanides (e.g., Metformin)	Liver	Decreases glucose production by the liver.
Meglitinides (e.g., Repaglinide)	Pancreas	Stimulates insulin release by the pancreas in response to a meal.
Sulfonylureas (e.g., Glyburide or Glipizide)	Pancreas	Stimulates insulin release by the pancreas.
Thiazolidinediones (e.g., Troglitazone)	Muscle	Enhances glucose uptake by the muscle.

The main side effects of metformin are loss of appetite, nausea, and diarrhea. One rare side effect of metformin is lactic acidosis (see page 154). Metformin may not be recommended if you have a history of lactic acidosis or kidney disease, if you have liver or heart problems, or if you are elderly.

The main side effects of acarbose include flatulence, abdominal distress, and diarrhea. These effects can be minimized by starting at low initial doses and gradually increasing the dose. It may not be recommended if you have inflammatory bowel disease or any other intestinal disorders. The main side effects of troglitazone are fluid retention and weight gain. A rare side effect is liver failure. Your doctor will monitor your liver function for the first year you take it.

The major problem with sulfonylurea drugs is hypoglycemia (see page 153). Because of this, sulfonylureas should be used with caution if you are elderly. The side effects, although uncommon, include gastrointestinal problems such as nausea and vomiting, skin reactions such as rashes, itching, and purpura, and blood problems such as anemia. Sulfonylureas drugs should not be used if you are allergic to sulfa drugs, are pregnant or planning to become pregnant, have heart, liver, or kidney problems, or if your pancreas no longer secretes insulin.

Repaglinide may be an alternative to sulfonylureas for many patients. Its only major side effect appears to be hypoglycemia.

Allergic Reactions

Some oral agents cause allergic reactions. Any type of skin rash—redness, itching, swelling, hives, or discoloration—that develops after you start a new medication could mean that you are allergic to the drug. This is especially true of sulfonylurea drugs. If you suspect that your oral diabetes agent is causing an allergic reaction, call your doctor right away. Sulfonylurea drugs can also make you more sensitive to sunlight. You may burn more easily when in the sun if you are taking a sulfonylurea drug.

Alcohol

You may also experience alcohol intolerance while using oral agents, particularly sulfonylurea drugs. Within 10 to 30 minutes of drinking an alcoholic beverage, or a medicine that contains alcohol, you may experience a headache, a flushing or tingling sensation in the face, nausea, or light-headedness. Even small amounts of alcohol can cause this reaction. If you find that alcohol is causing a problem, discontinue its use. If you have a problem stopping alcohol use, talk to your doctor about the best way to go about this. If you drink alcohol regularly, make sure to tell your doctor before you are prescribed any oral agent.

Hypoglycemia

If you are using a sulfonylurea or repaglinide, you are at a greater risk of hypoglycemia. Both of these drugs increase insulin secretion and thus make it more likely that your blood glucose may fall too low. Oral agents that increase insulin sensitivity, such as metformin, troglitazone, and acarbose, are unlikely to cause hypoglycemia and may be safely used by people with a history of hypoglycemia. If you do require treatment with a sulfonylurea or repaglinide, agents that increase the supply of insulin, there are several steps you can take to minimize the risk.

■ SYMPTOMS

Symptoms of hypoglycemia include shakiness, nervousness, sweating, chills, clamminess, rapid heartbeat, trouble concentrating, headache, dizziness, feeling light-headed, moody, or clumsy, tingling in face, lips, or tongue, and feelings of extreme hunger or irritability.

■ WHAT TO DO

If you have any of the symptoms of hypoglycemia, you should test your blood glucose immediately. If you have a blood glucose level below 60 mg/dl, you will need to eat a fast-acting carbohydrate. If you are having a severe reaction, you will need assistance and may require a glucagon injection or emergency care. Make sure those around you know the warning signs of hypoglycemia and know what to do.

■ PREVENTION

To prevent hypoglycemia while using oral medications, especially sulfonylureas and repaglinide, frequent blood glucose monitoring is essential. This will give you a warning that hypoglycemia is occurring. When beginning therapy with any oral diabetes agent, it is advisable to start with the lowest possible dose and increase the dose gradually, every 4 to 7 days. This will help you decide which dose best helps you control your blood glucose without increasing the incidence of hypoglycemia. If you find that you have more bouts of hypoglycemia as you go from a lower to a higher dose, you may want to cut back to a lower dose.

If you are susceptible to hypoglycemia, you may want to choose an oral agent that has a short duration of action. This is especially true if you have any sort of kidney problems. While taking sulfonylureas and any other oral agent, it is important not to skip meals. Many drugs require that you take them with food, so be sure to check with your doctor or pharmacist to see if this is true of your medication.

Lactic Acidosis

Lactic acidosis is caused by too much lactic acid in your blood. Lactic acid can accumulate when your body doesn't get enough oxygen or when your body's metabolism is disturbed. This can occur with certain diseases and combinations of health problems. Lactic acidosis is more common in people with diabetes who use metformin, but even then it is very rare. Only 1 in 33,000 people who use metformin each year will develop lactic acidosis. Still, in case you are that person, it is important to recognize the symptoms and know how to prevent it from occurring.

■ SYMPTOMS

Symptoms of lactic acidosis include feeling extremely weak or tired, having muscular pain, trouble breathing, or stomach discomfort, feeling cold, dizzy- or light-headed, and having an irregular heartbeat.

■ WHAT TO DO

Lactic acidosis is more likely to occur if you have any sort of kidney, liver, or heart problems, or other serious illness. If you have any of the symptoms of lactic acidosis, are taking metformin, and/or have any of these health problems, you should call your doctor right away. Lactic acidosis is life-threatening if not treated promptly. Usually, an underlying problem is triggering lactic acidosis and you will be treated for that problem first. This may require emergency attention. If there is an underlying problem, lactic acidosis can make it even worse, which is why you need to seek prompt treatment. You may be treated with bicarbonate, dichloroacetate, or other agent to neutralize the excess acid in your blood. However, treatment of the primary problem is most essential. There is no self-treatment of lactic acidosis. You will need to be treated by medical personnel, probably in a hospital setting.

■ PREVENTION

To prevent lactic acidosis from occurring, do not take metformin if you have any serious underlying health problems. Your doctor is unlikely to prescribe it if you have liver, kidney, or heart disease. Make sure you tell your doctor of any other problems you are experiencing so that other complications are not overlooked. Metformin should not be taken by anyone with poor kidney function. If you are taking metformin, you should have your kidney function checked regularly by your doctor. If you have heart failure or liver problems, or if you are hospitalized with a serious illness, you should also avoid metformin. Discuss any concerns about metformin with your doctor.

Common Drug Interactions

Some drug agents interfere with or are affected by other medications. Any time your blood glucose goes out of control for no apparent reason and you have recently changed your medication, think about a drug interaction. Symptoms could include abnormal blood glucose readings or signs of hypoglycemia or hyperglycemia. If you have recently changed the type or dose of a diabetes agent and are taking other medications regularly, or if you are only taking an oral agent but have recently taken any kind of over-the-counter drug, a drug interaction could be responsible. For example, at high doses aspirin can increase the effectiveness of sulfonylurea drugs. Troglitazone can make birth-control pills ineffective.

■ WHAT TO DO

If you suspect that other drugs are interfering with your oral agents, call your doctor right away. Your doctor may advise you to stop taking the medication or may prescribe an alternative therapy. Do not stop taking any medication without first talking to your doctor. If you are taking an over-the-counter medication for a cold, for example, you may want to stop that. But do not stop any medication that could jeopardize your health without first talking to your doctor. Before taking any medication, make sure your doctor and pharmacist know about all the medications you are currently taking.

If you experience any symptoms of hypoglycemia or hyperglycemia, measure your blood glucose level right away and treat appropriately. If you have a blood glucose level below 60 mg/dl, you will need to eat a fast-acting carbohydrate. If you are having a severe reaction, you will need assistance and may require a glucagon injection or emergency care. Make sure those around you know the warning signs of hypoglycemia and know what to do. If your blood glucose level is over 250 mg/dl, you will need to lower your blood glucose. This can be done with a shot of insulin, if you are taking insulin. Do not take any additional oral medication without first talking to your doctor. You may find that delaying your next meal or exercising may bring your blood glucose down to acceptable levels. If your blood glucose is over 300 mg/dl and you experience any of the signs of hyperglycemic hyperosmolar state (see Chapter 3), call for emergency assistance *at once.*

These are life-threatening situations that could result in coma or even death.

Also, be careful of any other drug interactions that might increase the likelihood of hypoglycemia. For example, the following drugs are known to increase the risk of hypoglycemia when taken with sulfonylureas: aspirin, fibrates, trimethoprim, alcohol, beta-blockers, anticoagulants, probenecid, allopurinol, and sympatholytic drugs. Make sure your doctor thoroughly examines prescription drugs that you normally take and any nonprescription drugs you are likely to take or may take on occasion, before you start therapy with any oral agent. If you are on oral therapy, make sure you tell your doctor before taking any other medication. Also, ask your doctor whether there are any other particular medications you should stay away from while you are on your oral diabetes medication.

When Treatment Fails

When you begin to use an oral agent for type 2 diabetes, it is possible, even likely, that at some point the treatment will fail. You may try an oral agent for the first time and find that it never works for you in helping to control your blood glucose. This is called a primary failure. In this case, it is likely that the drug was not the right choice for your kind of diabetes. Maybe your primary problem is insulin resistance, but the drug you tried works by increasing insulin production. Your doctor may now suggest trying a different drug that enhances insulin sensitivity. A primary failure can help your doctor better understand your condition and make a better choice for treating your diabetes.

Sometimes the right class of drug is chosen, but it may not be powerful enough. Your doctor may suggest increasing the dose or switching to a more powerful, but similar, medication. Whenever you start a new drug, be sure to monitor your blood glucose frequently and take notes of your daily activities and meal patterns. This will help you and your doctor decide if your treatment is appropriate for you.

Sometimes a treatment can stop working after it has been helping you for a long time. This is called a secondary failure. This is very likely to happen if you have type 2 diabetes and are taking an oral medication. This can result from changes in lifestyle—maybe you have become less active or have gained weight—or it can result from a progression of the diabetes itself. It is very likely that within 5 years, your oral medication will no longer be effective. This does not mean that you have done something wrong. It just means that your diabetes has progressed to the point where another approach is needed.

■ SYMPTOMS

The first indication that your oral agents are not working is hyperglycemia. If you are monitoring your blood glucose regularly, you will notice that your blood glucose levels are no longer within the target range. If your blood glucose rises dangerously high (over 300 mg/dl) and especially if you have any signs of hyperglycemic hyperosmolar state, you need to be treated right away. If your fasting blood glucose level is typically above 140 mg/dl, talk to your doctor about what changes might be needed. Your doctor will likely measure your HbA_{1c}. Typically, a successful oral agent will reduce your HbA_{1c} by 1 percent when you first start taking it. But when you use the drug continuously, over time, your HbA_{1c} will increase about 0.2 percent per year. This means that after 5 years, your HbA_{1c} will be back to where it was when you started. When this happens, you and your doctor will need to find another approach.

■ TREATMENT

Once you and your doctor have decided that your oral agent is not working, you will have to decide on another treatment. If you have had a primary failure, then you and your doctor will decide upon another drug. Maybe you just need a higher dose or a more powerful drug. Or maybe you will need to try a new class of drug altogether. Your doctor may also suggest you try insulin or a combination of an oral agent and insulin.

If you have secondary failure of an oral agent that has been helping you for several years, it is unlikely that switching to another single drug will be helpful. However, it is possible that a combination of oral agents could help you bring things back under control. Many patients have found that a sulfonylurea with metformin or a sulfonylurea with acarbose can work well. For many patients, diabetes progresses to a point where both insulin deficiency and insulin resistance contribute to the disease. Therefore, a combination of a drug that increases insulin secretion together with one that increases insulin sensitivity has the best chance of success. For example, if you started out with a sulfonylurea, metformin, acarbose, or troglitazone could be added. Three-drug combinations have not been well studied. You should know that eventually, even a combination therapy will fail.

Your doctor may recommend insulin therapy as a first approach when diet and exercise no longer work to control blood glucose levels. Or your doctor may turn to insulin when you have a secondary failure of an oral agent. Alternatively, your doctor may also recommend a combination of insulin and an oral agent. The most likely combination is to use insulin along with an oral agent that increases the effectiveness of insulin, such as metformin, troglitazone, or acarbose.

Chapter 6
Solving Circulation Problems

Circulatory problems—heart disease, vascular disease, and stroke—affect more than 56 million Americans and account for more than 40 percent of all deaths in this country. People with diabetes are three times more likely to die of cardiovascular disease than the general population. And problems with circulation lead to other problems with all parts of the body that depend on a healthy blood supply to function properly.

You are probably tired of hearing your doctor tell you that if you control your blood glucose you are more likely to avoid the complications of diabetes. But it's true. That's because the sugar in your blood makes your blood sticky. And when your blood is thick and sticky, it can't flow well. That's why chronically high levels of blood glucose can increase the risk of cardiovascular disease and other complications of diabetes.

Even if you have controlled your diabetes, you may at some point develop cardiovascular disease or other problems related to circulation. The good news is that new treatments and procedures are emerging all the time. Any time you have a problem related to poor circulation, it is important to seek treatment as soon as possible to keep the problem from getting worse and causing more problems.

Coronary Artery Disease

When your heart muscle doesn't get the blood it needs, you can develop coronary artery disease. This usually happens because something is blocking the blood vessels to the heart. As a result, your heart is deprived of vital oxygen and nutrients carried by the blood. In its mildest form, this could result in angina, a condition signaled by chest pain in which there is partial to near-total blockage of the arteries into the heart. Or it could lead to a heart attack, which occurs when there is a sudden blockage of the arteries leading to the heart. Angina can signal an impending heart attack or a heart attack can come on suddenly without prior warning. At its worst, coronary artery disease can result in sudden death, with or without a history of angina or previous heart attacks.

Coronary artery disease usually begins as the blood vessels in the body begin to clog up. This condition, known as atherosclerosis, or hardening of the arteries, develops over a long period of time. Usually, it begins when something damages the lining of the arteries of the heart. The damage could be caused by smoking, diabetes, high blood pressure, or high cholesterol. When a blood vessel is damaged, the body tries to heal it by sending in macrophages, a class of scavenger cells, to repair the damage. But the macrophages themselves soon become part of the problem. The macrophages and some of the substances they produce begin to stick to the damaged arteries and clog them up further. This adds to the original damage and signals more macrophages to respond, which only makes things worse. Over the years, cholesterol deposits and scar tissue can block the blood vessels further. Eventually, the blood can no longer flow through your blood vessels as it should, and the heart can become damaged.

■ RISKS

Having diabetes is a major risk factor for coronary artery disease. Even if you just have impaired glucose tolerance (see Chapter 3), your risk of developing angina and heart attack are higher than that of the general population. If you have diabetes, and especially if you have problems controlling your blood glucose levels, you are even more likely to develop coronary artery disease. And the longer you have diabetes, the greater the risk. A person who has had diabetes for 15 to 20 years is 10 times as likely to develop coronary artery disease as a person without diabetes.

Other factors also increase the risk of coronary artery disease. These include a family history of coronary artery disease, high blood pressure, a history of smoking, high cholesterol and high triglyceride levels, advancing age, a sedentary lifestyle, and obesity.

Angina

Angina is a form of coronary artery disease in which you experience chest pain. In itself, angina is not a life-threatening condition, but it does signal a reduced flow of blood to the heart and should not be ignored. It serves as a warning sign that something more serious may occur. In its mildest, stable form, the pain occurs sporadically and lasts only a short time. But angina can get worse as the arteries become more clogged and precede a more serious, or even fatal, heart attack.

■ SYMPTOMS

Symptoms of coronary artery disease usually begin to appear when 50 to 75 percent of the blood vessel is blocked and the flow of blood to the heart is slowed. The exact symptoms may depend on which part of the heart is not getting enough blood. Symptoms include pain or pressure in the chest, nausea or pain in the upper abdomen, shortness of breath, weakness, or irregular heartbeat. However, some people with diabetes have neuropathy, or damage to the nerves, and are unable to feel chest pain even though blood flow may be restricted.

The most common symptom of coronary artery disease is chest pain or pressure. It usually comes on gradually, often while exercising and over a period of 30 seconds to several minutes. The pain can intensify, but often it is mild and just goes away. It can also move to the left arm, shoulder, or armpits, or the left side of the neck or jaw. The pain often arises during physical activity and goes away when you stop activity and rest. Emotional stress may also trigger an angina attack. But it can also occur when you are resting and can even awaken you in the middle of the night.

■ WHAT TO DO

If symptoms last only a short time (2 to 15 minutes) and do not occur more often or at low activity levels, you may have stable angina. If this is the case, you should tell your doctor, who will probably conduct a series of tests to assess the condition of your heart. If you do indeed have stable angina, heart tests will show no evidence of permanent damage to the heart.

If the symptoms suddenly get worse or show up when you are not exercising, then you may have unstable angina. This is a sign of more serious heart trouble. When the symptoms of angina get progressively worse, then you may be at risk for a heart attack. Anytime your symptoms get worse, especially if the change is sudden, call your doctor or emergency health care center at once.

Whether you have stable or unstable angina, your doctor will most likely conduct a series of tests to determine the condition of your heart and whether your arteries are significantly blocked. This could involve any of several diagnostic tests.

Your doctor may perform an electrocardiogram, which can detect an abnormal heart rhythm. This will determine whether a heart attack has occurred in the past or is occurring at the time you have your test. Some people, especially people with diabetic neuropathy, can experience a heart attack and not even realize they are having one. As many as one-third of all heart attacks are clinically silent—the symptoms are not recognized or felt by the patient. An electrocardiogram performed at rest will not detect any arterial blockages that have not caused a heart attack, however.

Most likely, your doctor will also recommend a stress test. This is a test that assesses heart activity before, during, and after exercise. You will be asked to walk or jog on a treadmill or peddle an exercise bicycle. You will probably increase the level of exercise in steps until you become fatigued or the electrocardiogram becomes abnormal. Or the test can run until your heart rate reaches a set maximum limit. If you cannot exercise because of some other condition, such as asthma, emphysema, peripheral vascular disease, or other limiting condition, your doctor may perform a chemical stress test. In these tests, an echocardiogram or nuclear imaging technique is done before and after receiving a drug that increases the work of the heart or that expands the arteries of the heart. This test is similar in accuracy to a physical stress test.

Different kinds of stress tests can be performed using different kinds of techniques to look at the heart before and after exercise. A stress test using an electrocardiogram will tell your doctor whether there are parts of your heart muscle that are not getting enough blood. However, an electrocardiogram stress test is not completely accurate. Only 70 percent of people who have a blockage will be detected by this test. And of the people who do test positively, only about 70 percent will actually have a blockage.

Along with the electrocardiogram, your doctor may also perform an echocardiogram before and after you exercise. This is an ultrasonic image of your heart. If you do have a blockage, the echocardiogram will show the area of your heart that is affected, because it will move abnormally when you exercise and immediately after.

Your doctor may also recommend a nuclear imaging test of the heart before and after exercising. With this sort of test, you may be injected with a radioactive tracer that will show the blood flow through your blood vessels and heart. This tells your doctor how many blockages there are and how large they are. The echocardiogram and nuclear imaging stress tests will pick up about 90 percent of the blockages in people tested. About 90 percent of tests that are positive are due to true blockages.

If your stress tests are positive, that is, they indicate that you have blocked arteries, your doctor may also have you undergo a cardiac catheterization and coronary angiography. This is another test that allows a direct view of the arteries and heart. In this test, you will be given a local anaesthetic and a tube, or catheter, will be inserted into one of your arteries. Usually the catheter is inserted into the groin. The catheter is then moved along the major arteries into the chest. The doctor is then able to measure the blood pressures in different chambers of the heart. In addition, a special dye can flow through the tubes and into your heart, so your doctor can see how the different parts of your heart and arteries are functioning, how the blood is flowing, and if there are any blockages in the arteries.

Taken together, the electrocardiogram and imaging stress tests and the catheterization and angiography can give your doctor a good idea of whether or not you have arterial blockages and coronary artery disease. This will help your doctor determine the best way to treat your condition.

■ TREATMENT

Medication

If your doctor determines that you have coronary artery disease, you may be prescribed any of several medications to help your blood flow better and reduce your symptoms. You may be given nitroglycerin or a similar medication. This medicine can be taken under the tongue or through a skin patch or ointment on the skin. It works by lowering the blood pressures of the heart and dilating the arteries to help balance the supply and demand of oxygen throughout the body. Nitroglycerin and similar drugs can only be used 12 to 14 hours a day, however. If they are used continuously, the body stops responding to them. Side effects include headaches and light-headedness. Although nitroglycerin is effective at reducing angina (chest pain), there is no evidence that it actually helps you live longer.

Another type of medication you may be prescribed is known as a beta-blocker. Propanolol (Inderal), atenolol (Tenormin), and metoprolol (Lopressor) are all beta-blockers. These drugs reduce the symptoms of angina by lowering the heart rate and blood pressure, reducing the effect of epinephrine on the heart, and by preventing irregular heartbeats. Beta-blockers have been shown to prolong for 3 to 5 years the lives of people who have already had heart attacks. They also appear to help people with congestive heart failure live longer.

Beta-blockers have some side effects, however. People with type 1 diabetes who have a history of hypoglycemia have to be especially careful. The drugs can interfere with how the body detects and responds to the warning signs of low glucose. If you have frequent bouts of hypoglycemia and are prescribed a beta-blocker, it is essential that you check your blood glucose level often. People with type 1 or type 2 diabetes often find that beta-blockers upset their blood glucose control. Even if you are not prone to hypoglycemia, you will probably need to monitor your blood glucose levels more frequently, especially as you are getting used to the new medication.

Beta-blockers may also raise triglyceride levels and lower high-density lipoprotein (HDL, "good cholesterol") in the blood. If you have peripheral vascular disease, you may find that the symptoms worsen when you are on beta-blockers. If you have asthma or any kind of lung disease, you may be advised not to take a beta-blocker because it can increase the wheezing and make breathing more difficult. If you already have a slow heart rate, you may be advised not to take a beta-blocker, because it may make your heart rate too slow.

Calcium channel blockers work by lowering blood pressure and dilating coronary arteries. Some of these drugs also lower your heart rate. Some types of calcium channel blockers can be used safely by people with diabetes and some cannot. Your doctor will help select the correct medication.

Surgery

There are two types of surgical interventions you and your doctor will want to consider. Angioplasty is a technique that opens up blocked arteries. Cardiac revascularization, or bypass surgery, is a technique using blood vessel grafts that form a detour to move the blood flow around a blocked artery. In the long run, people with diabetes seem to fare better with bypass surgery.

Two types of angioplasty are in common use. With balloon angioplasty, a small balloon is attached to a catheter and inserted into a narrowed artery. Once in the blocked artery, the balloon is inflated, thus compressing the cholesterol plaque and opening up the artery. In many cases, a stent is used in conjunction with a balloon angioplasty. This is a small metal spring or mesh cylinder that is placed at the site of the obstruction to keep cholesterol deposits from closing up the artery again.

Alternatively, a blood vessel can be opened up with a rotoblator, which works much like a small drill to bore through the blocked artery. An atherectomy device can actually remove some of the cholesterol plaque. Stents are often used with both the rotoblator and atherectomy devices.

Angioplasty is not usually recommended for people with diabetes because of the narrow openings in the arteries, which make it technically difficult to perform. Also, it often results in a small tear in the blood vessel lining that can cause a clot to form. This increases the likelihood of the vessel closing up again and provoking a heart attack.

If you have diabetes, you may have better success with a bypass operation. In this procedure, a blood vessel is removed from your leg or chest and used to bypass the arterial blockage. The new blood vessel is first attached to the artery below the blockage and then to the artery above the blockage. This allows the blood an alternate path to flow around the blockage. The surgery typically lasts 4 to 6 hours or even longer. Complications include heart attack, bleeding, infection of the sternum, and infection at the site of the vein removal. Complications are more common in people with diabetes, but most survive with excellent results. The decision of whether to proceed with angioplasty or bypass surgery will be made by you and your doctor based on several factors. Much will depend on the size of the opening in your artery, where the blockage is, whether the blockage contains any calcification, and whether your heart function is otherwise normal.

■ PREVENTION

Your best bet is to take steps to keep coronary artery disease from developing in the first place or to keep it from getting worse. This is especially true if you have diabetes and even more so if you have already had a heart attack. Coronary artery disease, angina, and heart attack occur because there is a buildup of cholesterol-containing plaque along the walls of the arteries that lead to the heart. To avoid coronary artery disease, you need to prevent or minimize this buildup from occurring. If you have cholesterol deposits, then your cholesterol levels are too high and you need to take steps to reduce them. You can do this by changing your diet, reducing your weight, exercising more, and by taking cholesterol-lowering medication.

Other factors also increase the risk of coronary artery disease and heart attack. You can minimize the contribution of these factors by taking steps to lower your blood pressure, lose weight, and stop smoking. Quitting smoking is one of the most effective measures of reducing the risk of heart attack. But it is not easy. If you are having problems quitting smoking, talk to your doctor about medical and psychosocial interventions that may work for you.

Your doctor may also recommend taking aspirin on a daily basis to reduce the risk of coronary artery disease. This has been shown to reduce the risk of heart attack and stroke by thinning the blood and preventing clotting.

Studies have also shown that a diet rich in antioxidants—vitamins A, C, and E—may help prevent coronary artery disease. Consider adding more fruits and vegetables, especially those with deep colors, to your diet. Carrots, sweet potatoes, tomatoes, spinach, broccoli, cantaloupe, pumpkin, apricots, and citrus fruits are all good choices. Vitamin E can also be found in vegetable oils, green and leafy vegetables, wheat germ, whole-grain products, nuts, and seeds.

In addition to all these measures, it is important to control your blood glucose levels, whether you have type 1 or type 2 diabetes. Scientists are continuing to study the connection between blood glucose control and cardiovascular disease.

Heart Attack

A heart attack occurs when the flow of blood to the heart is interrupted abruptly. This can happen when a coronary artery is blocked suddenly. This can come after a long period in which cholesterol plaque gradually builds up in an artery, as occurs in stable coronary artery disease. But then something happens. There may be a crack in a cholesterol plaque that causes a tear in the blood vessel. The vessel hemorrhages and the resulting blood clot now entirely blocks the artery. Or the vessel may become progressively narrower until a small clot or clump of cholesterol plaque completely blocks the narrow opening and the blood supply is cut off. Sometimes something, such as a rapid surge of blood, shears the lining of the blood vessel. This can cause a hemorrhage and a clot in the artery. Or a portion of a cholesterol plaque may shear and form a flap that blocks a coronary artery. Whatever the cause, when a coronary artery is suddenly blocked, a heart attack can ensue.

■ SYMPTOMS

Severe, crushing chest pain under the breast bone that spreads to the left armpit, shoulder, neck, or jaw can signal a heart attack. In the initial stages, the pain may be less severe and may come and go over several hours. You may only experience abdominal discomfort or back pain. But severe pain, often accompanied by nausea, vomiting, sweating, palpitations, feelings of light-headedness, fainting, and shortness of breath, is not unusual. In fact, the pain from a heart attack may be just about the worst pain you have ever experienced.

Unfortunately, people with diabetes sometimes have no symptoms of a heart attack. This is especially true if you have any kind of neuropathy. If you have diabetes and any risk factors for heart disease—obesity, high triglyceride and cholesterol levels, or high blood pressure, for example—talk to your doctor about how to be alert to an impending heart attack. You may experience nausea and abdominal pain with no chest pain. Even a sudden swing in your blood glucose level could be a sign that a heart attack is occurring. If you feel anything out of the ordinary—dizziness, palpitations, sweating, or stomach pain—with or without chest pain, you could be having a heart attack.

■ WHAT TO DO

Any time a heart attack is suspected, you or those around you should call for emergency help at once. If you are having a heart attack, time is of the essence. Don't dismiss the symptoms and wait to see if they get worse, or assume it's just indigestion. Fifty percent of all people who die of a heart attack do so within the first hour. Many of these deaths could be prevented with prompt treatment. Get emergency help right away, if you are even the least bit suspicious.

■ TREATMENT

If you are having a heart attack, emergency treatment will be aimed at getting the blood flowing to your heart. To do this, your medical team will try to open up whatever is blocking the artery. If blood flow is restored quickly, you will have a better chance of avoiding permanent damage to the heart and a better chance of survival with fewer long-term complications.

There are two options at the onset of a heart attack: medical treatment with clot-dissolving drugs, or surgical intervention such as angioplasty to remove the blockage. The decision will be based on your individual circumstances and by logistical factors in the particular treatment setting. For example, if your hospital does not have the means to insert a catheter, angioplasty may be out of the question. On the other hand, medical factors may dictate the course of treatment. If you have a condition that would be made worse by a clot-dissolver—a recent stroke or surgery, for example—then angioplasty may be favored. Your medical team will take into account many factors to determine the treatment that is best for you. If you are unable to communicate, it is important that someone close to you be able to provide your medical team with any critical information. Make sure to tell the hospital or medics that you have diabetes.

If you are given a clot-dissolving medication such as tissue plasminogen activator or streptokinase within 1 hour of the onset of symptoms, your chances of survival will double. This medication works well in people with and without diabetes. You may also be given a blood-thinner such as aspirin. This will not dissolve existing clots, but it will prevent additional clotting from occurring. You may also be given a beta-blocker as part of your initial treatment to slow the heart rate and reduce your blood pressure. Many heart patients will be treated with angioplasty following the administration of a clot-busting drug. However, if you have diabetes, this approach will triple your risk of complications, including death, and is not recommended. If you are able, make sure to discuss the treatment options with your medical team.

■ PREVENTION

Whether you are at risk for a heart attack or have already survived one, it is important to take steps to prevent one from occurring or recurring. The key is to keep your arteries clear and the blood flowing and to keep the arteries from clogging up. If you are a smoker, quitting smoking is the single greatest step you can take to reduce the risk of a heart attack. Reducing fat and cholesterol intake, beginning a modest program of physical activity (if appropriate), losing weight if you are overweight, and eating a balanced diet rich in fruits and vegetables, will all help reduce the risk of a heart attack. In addition, your doctor may recommend taking a low dose of aspirin on a daily basis to prevent stroke and heart attack.

If you have already experienced a heart attack, your doctor may also recommend one of several long-term follow-up therapies to prevent any recurrence of a heart attack. Beta-blockers have been shown to prolong life following a heart attack in people with and without diabetes. Drugs such as angiotensin-converting enzyme (ACE) inhibitors, which prevent the heart from enlarging and also lower blood pressure, lower the risk of death for 3 to 5 years following a heart attack in people with and without diabetes. If you are at risk for a heart attack, and especially if you have already had a heart attack, talk to your doctor about what steps you can take to reduce your risk.

Congestive Heart Failure

When your heart can't pump out enough blood to get to the parts of the body that need it, then congestive heart failure can result. If you have congestive heart failure, you are not having a heart attack, and it does not mean your heart has stopped beating. It just means that the demands of the body are more than it can bear and it just cannot quite keep up with the workload. Several underlying conditions, such as coronary artery disease, high blood pressure, valvular heart disease, and peripheral vascular disease, can all contribute to congestive heart failure.

■ RISKS

Congestive heart failure is a fairly common illness. Nearly 3 million people in this country have congestive heart failure now, and 400,000 new cases will be diagnosed this year. Elderly people are more likely to develop congestive heart failure. With each decade over the age of 45, your risk of developing congestive heart failure doubles. If you have diabetes, you are four to five times more likely to develop congestive heart failure than someone without diabetes. Cardiovascular problems such as angina and coronary artery disease, heart attack, and high blood pressure increase the risk of congestive heart failure. If you have diabetes, you are more likely to develop these cardiovascular problems. But diabetes can also contribute to congestive heart failure, even if you don't have coronary artery disease or high blood pressure. If you have diabetes, the small vessels of your heart cannot dilate well, even with the help of powerful drugs. This makes it hard for your heart to pump and fill properly.

■ SYMPTOMS

Symptoms of congestive heart failure include shortness of breath, difficulty exercising or even walking across the room, difficulty sleeping, fatigue, palpitations, fluid retention, and swollen ankles, feet, and legs.

■ WHAT TO DO

If you are feeling any of the symptoms of congestive heart failure, talk to your doctor as soon as possible. Congestive heart failure is not an emergency situation, but if left untreated it could be life-threatening. Many underlying diseases such as coronary artery disease, high blood pressure, and valvular heart disease can trigger congestive heart failure. In addition, other circumstances, such as too much sodium in the diet, can make it worse. Your doctor will ultimately want to treat the underlying causes of congestive heart failure, but before deciding on a course of treatment, may also want to diminish those conditions that worsen the symptoms of congestive heart failure.

An essential first step in dealing with congestive heart failure is to watch your sodium intake. Ask your doctor what your sodium intake should be. Read the labels of everything and make sure you are not taking in more than you should. If you are retaining too much fluid, your doctor may also want to prescribe a diuretic to help you lose fluid and excess sodium. If you have difficulty sleeping, try propping yourself up with extra pillows.

Treatment of congestive heart failure depends on an accurate diagnosis. Your doctor will probably order a chest X ray and an echocardiogram. This will confirm whether your problem is caused by poor forward heart pump function—your heart has difficulty contracting to pump blood out—or poor relaxation. Your heart needs to be able to contract and relax to pump efficiently. If it can't do one of these functions, it doesn't work properly and congestive heart failure is the result. Often patients with congestive heart failure have problems with both contraction and relaxation.

■ TREATMENT

Your doctor may first want to treat some of the underlying problems that are contributing to congestive heart failure. If you have any form of congestive artery disease, angina, or a history of heart attack, you may be given a beta-blocker or an ACE inhibitor. If you have severe blockages in your arteries, you may need surgical intervention. If you have high blood pressure, you may also be given one of these drugs or another type of drug to reduce blood pressure.

Management of the underlying heart conditions may provide some relief of congestive heart failure. However, if the symptoms do not improve, you may require medications that help the heart pump better. If you have a problem with forward pump function, your doctor will probably suggest a combination of medications. For example, digoxin increases the force of contraction of the heart, and diuretics can help the body get rid of excess fluid. Your doctor may also suggest an ACE inhibitor. These drugs block the production of a hormone called angiotensin II, which causes some arteries to constrict. This is a natural process to help direct the flow of blood to the organs that need it most: the brain, heart, and kidneys. But when the heart is failing, the effects can be detrimental. It places too much of a burden on an already stressed heart. Blocking this hormone with a drug relaxes these arteries and helps the heart pump more efficiently. ACE inhibitors should be used with caution in people with kidney problems. If you have any concerns, talk to your doctor.

■ PREVENTION

Congestive heart failure is a serious condition that can be avoided or minimized with preventive measures. A key first step is to stop smoking if you are a smoker. If you have trouble quitting, talk to your doctor about intervention programs and medical means to help you stop.

If you have diabetes, keep your blood glucose levels under control. Maintain a diet that is low in fat and cholesterol and high in fiber, vitamins, and minerals. This will help reduce the chance that your arteries will clog up. Your doctor may also suggest a long-term aspirin therapy program to reduce the likelihood of atherosclerosis. If you have high blood pressure, reduce your salt intake and excessive alcohol consumption.

Your doctor may also suggest an exercise or activity program you can live with. Even if you can't train for the Boston Marathon, try walking around the block once or twice a day or climbing stairs instead of taking the elevator.

Talk to your health care team about other steps you can take to reduce the risk of congestive heart failure. You may need to make major lifestyle changes and may not be able to take all steps at once. If you find that prospect overwhelming, relax, and take one step at a time. Even if you can't do everything, any preventive measure you take is better than no action at all.

Cholesterol Abnormalities and Atherosclerosis

Cholesterol is a fatty substance the body makes to serve a very important function. Along with other fats, cholesterol helps form the membranes that surround each cell in the body. It also helps form the insulation around the nerves in the body and is needed to make bile, a substance that helps the body digest and absorb fat and fat-soluble vitamins.

The cholesterol in your body does not float around freely in your blood and tissues. Rather, it binds, or attaches, to certain proteins called lipoproteins. Cholesterol binds to both high-density lipoprotein (HDL) and low-density lipoprotein (LDL). Low-density lipoprotein binds a lot of cholesterol and carries cholesterol from the liver throughout the body. It is this form that is responsible for the buildup of cholesterol in blood vessels. Because of that, it is often called "bad cholesterol." You don't want to have high levels of LDL in your blood. High-density lipoprotein, on the other hand, is the form called "good cholesterol." It collects excess cholesterol in the blood and brings it back to the liver where it is broken down. You want to have high levels of HDL.

Too much LDL cholesterol in the blood can be deadly. It can accumulate along the blood vessels that carry blood throughout the body and eventually form blockages that stop the flow of blood. When the blood vessels that supply the heart with blood become blocked, coronary artery disease, including angina, heart attack, and sudden death, can occur. The process that leads to coronary artery disease is called atherosclerosis, also known as hardening of the arteries. It is a slow process that occurs over years, even decades, in which fatty substances in the blood, such as cholesterol, begin to stick to the blood vessel linings. The opening in the arteries gets narrower and narrower. When blood flow to the heart is restricted, it can cause the pain known as angina. When the narrowing finally reaches the point where blood can no longer flow to the heart, a heart attack occurs. This accounts for 30 percent of all heart attacks. Or a piece of a fatty plaque can break off and cause a clot to form instantaneously in the blood vessel. This accounts for 70 percent of all heart attacks. When the arteries to the brain are blocked, the blood flow to the brain may be cut off and a stroke can occur. When the arteries supplying blood to the legs become restricted, you can develop peripheral vascular disease.

Your body needs a good supply of blood to keep all the organs functioning properly. Whenever that blood supply is restricted or blocked, serious consequences can occur. Cholesterol is a major contributor to the slow buildup of plaques that cause arterial blockages. If you have diabetes, have high blood pressure, or smoke, the process of atherosclerosis occurs even faster.

■ SYMPTOMS

Some people with a rare hereditary disease of cholesterol metabolism may develop bumps on the skin and tendons near the elbow and ankle. However, if you are like most people, your body can't tell you when your cholesterol level is too high until it is too late. When your arteries are clogged, you may feel chest pain, or worse, a heart attack or stroke. But you probably want to know well before that point, when you can do something to prevent atherosclerosis and cholesterol buildup.

■ RISKS

If you have high levels of LDL cholesterol, you have an increased risk of developing coronary artery disease, especially if you have diabetes. Researchers have shown that lowering cholesterol can reduce the number of deaths by heart attack and the chance of having a heart attack by 40 percent.

Several different risk factors can contribute to high cholesterol levels. They include heredity, age, sex, diet, weight, exercise level, alcohol intake, cigarette smoking, blood pressure, and diabetes.

Heredity

Researchers don't fully understand which genes cause high cholesterol levels, but one thing is clear. If your parents have high cholesterol levels, the chances are greater that you will too. This is especially true with certain inherited conditions such as familial hypercholesterolemia, which affects 1 in 500 people and leads to early coronary artery disease.

Age and Sex

The older you are, the more likely you are to have high cholesterol. Men over 45, women over 55, and postmenopausal women of any age are at high risk for coronary artery disease, especially among people with diabetes.

Diet

Foods high in saturated fat increase LDL levels. Dietary cholesterol is thought by some to be the major contributor to the high incidence of coronary artery disease in the United States, but others think dietary fat intake plays a much more significant role.

Weight and Exercise

The more excess weight, usually in the form of fat, that you carry around, the greater your risk of high LDL levels. When you lose weight and exercise more, you not only decrease your LDL levels, but you also increase your HDL levels.

Alcohol

Perhaps surprisingly, small amounts of alcohol can raise your level of HDL cholesterol. The key is moderation—a daily glass of wine or beer, for example. Drinking too much alcohol can increase triglyceride levels, affect blood glucose levels, and cause liver damage. Talk to your doctor about the advisability of incorporating small amounts of alcohol into your diet.

Other Factors

Cigarette smoking, high blood pressure, and diabetes can increase the risk of high cholesterol and also increase the risk of coronary artery disease on their own.

■ WHAT TO DO

The only sure way to know whether your cholesterol level is too high is to have your blood tested. If you are over the age of 20, you should have your cholesterol tested every 2 years if it is within normal limits. If it is out of the range of desirable limits, consider being tested on a yearly basis. You will first need to take a test that measures your total cholesterol and your HDL level. This test may not require you to fast.

If your test shows that your total cholesterol level is below 200 mg/dl and you have no other indication of atherosclerosis or coronary artery disease, you can rest assured. If your total cholesterol is above 240 mg/dl or if it is between 200 and 230 mg/dl and you have two or more risk factors listed above, or if you already have been diagnosed with coronary artery disease, then you will have to have another test. This second test measures your lipoprotein profile and will require that you fast before taking it. You will not be able to drink or eat anything except water or black coffee or tea (without milk, cream, or sugar) for 9 to 12 hours before the test. Usually a lipoprotein profile should be scheduled first thing in the morning.

The lipoprotein profile will tell you what your total cholesterol, LDL, and HDL levels are. You should maintain your triglyceride level below 200 mg/dl, HDL above 45 mg/dl, and LDL below 100 mg/dl if you already have diabetes or heart disease. If your cholesterol levels are not within the desirable range, you may need to take steps to bring them within normal limits.

Diet

Depending on your cholesterol profile and LDL and HDL levels, whether or not you have any other risk factors, and whether or not you already have coronary artery disease, you may need to modify or even make drastic changes in your diet. If you do not already have a registered dietitian on your health care team, now is the time to recruit someone to help you devise a meal plan that works for you. Your dietitian may prescribe either a Step I or a Step II plan. Step I and Step II plans are designed to lower cholesterol levels by limiting fat and cholesterol intake.

Under a Step I plan, your dietitian will develop an eating plan for you in which no more than 8 to 10 percent of your calories come from saturated fat and you eat no more than 300 mg of cholesterol per day. In a Step II plan, no more than 7 percent of your total calories come from saturated fat and you eat less than 200 mg of cholesterol per day. A Step II plan should reduce LDL levels by 10 to 15 percent within 6 months.

If you have diabetes or coronary artery disease, your LDL should be less than 100 mg/dl. You may be advised to start a Step II plan right away. If your LDL level does not improve within 6 to 12 weeks, your physician may prescribe a cholesterol-lowering medication.

If your LDL level is under 160 mg/dl and you do not have diabetes, coronary artery disease, or more than two other risk factors, then your dietitian will prescribe a Step I plan. The goal is to decrease your LDL level to less than 160 mg/dl in 3 months. If this does not occur, your dietitian will advise a Step II plan. If there is no reduction in cholesterol levels after following a Step II plan, then your physician may suggest drug therapy.

If you do not have coronary artery disease or diabetes, but you do have more than two risk factors, you should shoot for an LDL level less than 130 mg/dl. To do this, your dietitian will suggest a Step I plan. If there is no improvement after 3 months, then you should proceed to a Step II plan. Drug therapy should be considered if there is no improvement.

Exercise and Weight Loss

You can reduce your cholesterol even further by losing weight. A weight loss of 5 to 10 pounds can lower your blood cholesterol by another 5 to

10 percent. If you reduce your calorie intake by 500 calories a day, you can expect to lose up to a pound a week. However, be sure you do not go below 1,200 calories a day without medical supervison and that you plan your meals to avoid hypoglycemia. Your dietitian should be able to help you with that. You may also consider exercising as another way to lose weight, either with or without a reduction in calories. Make sure your dietitian is aware of any change in your exercise plan and helps you devise a meal plan taking into account your cholesterol goals, weight loss goals, blood glucose control, and physical activity.

Cholesterol-Lowering Medication

Drug treatment should be considered only when diet and exercise fail to lower cholesterol. If you do begin a drug therapy program, you must still maintain a good diet and exercise program. Don't turn to drugs as a substitute for diet and exercise. Your doctor will prescribe one of the following medications to help lower your cholesterol.

Statins

Statins block an enzyme that your body needs to make cholesterol. They also help the liver remove LDL from the blood. This stabilizes the plaque lining the arteries and prevents the ruptures that lead to clots and heart attacks. Statins that are currently available in the U.S. are lovastatin (Mevacore), pravastatin (Pravachol), simvastatin (Zocor), flu-vastatin (Lescol), and atorvastatin (Lipitor). All of these drugs can lower LDL levels by 20 to 60 percent. They are usually given orally as a single dose at bedtime. You can expect to see results within 4 to 6 weeks. Your lipid profile should be reevaluated at that time. You may experience mild gastrointestinal symptoms such as abdominal cramps, gas, and constipation for the first few weeks, but serious complications are unlikely. In rare cases, some people experience soreness and weakness in the muscles. If this happens, stop taking the medication and call your doctor right away.

Bile Acid Resins

Cholestyramine and colestipol are the two major medications of this type. They work by binding cholesterol in the intestines, and they reduce LDL cholesterol by 10 to 20 percent. These drugs can be used in combination with the statins, which limit cholesterol production. They are considered extremely safe, because they are not absorbed into your body. However, they can cause mild gastrointestinal discomfort, such as bloating, constipation, and gas. These effects can be minimized by taking the medication with meals. Do not take these drugs with other medications, because they can interfere with their absorption. If you are on oral diabetes medications, ask your doctor when to take bile acid resins.

Nicotinic Acid

If you have diabetes, you will probably not be prescribed this drug, because it increases blood glucose levels. It has many beneficial effects, however, such as lowering LDL, lowering triglycerides, and raising HDL. If your doctor prescribes this drug, you should take it only under close medical supervision, and pay careful attention to monitoring your blood glucose.

Hormone Replacement Therapy

Postmenopausal women are at greater risk for coronary artery disease because of the loss of estrogen, which protects against high cholesterol. Therefore, many women will want to consider hormone replacement therapy. Estrogen raises HDL, lowers LDL, gets rid of excess fat in the bloodstream, and keeps blood flowing and blood vessels flexible throughout the body. Estrogen comes in three forms: a skin patch, a vaginal cream, and an oral pill. The vaginal cream does not affect cholesterol levels. The patch decreases LDL, but does not affect HDL levels. Your best bet is to take oral estrogen if you want to raise HDL and lower LDL.

Major side effects of estrogen include an increased risk of breast and uterine cancer and an increase in blood clotting, which increases the risk of stroke. Estrogen taken in conjunction with progesterone protects against uterine cancer. Low doses of estrogen (0.625 mg or less) do not increase clotting and do not increase the risk of stroke. The risk of stroke is higher in women who smoke and in those with high blood pressure. Estrogen can also increase triglyceride levels in some women, which could cancel out the benefit to your heart. You and your physician will want to take all these factors into consideration when deciding whether to take estrogen.

Stroke

A stroke occurs when the blood supply to the brain is cut off. This can happen when a blood vessel to the brain ruptures. This is called a hemorrhagic stroke. Or it can occur when a blood vessel that supplies the brain is blocked. This is an ischemic stroke. Eighty percent of all strokes are ischemic. A stroke deprives the brain of the oxygen and nutrients it needs to function. The severity of the stroke depends on how long the brain is deprived of oxygen and what part of the brain is affected. Sometimes a temporary interruption of blood flow, called a transient ischemic attack, can serve as a warning sign that a stroke is imminent or that there is a partial blockage of blood to the brain.

The arteries that supply blood to the brain can become blocked for many reasons, much like the arteries to the heart can clog up. Atherosclerosis, a condition in which the linings of the brain arteries become blocked with deposits of cholesterol and fat, is common. Atherosclerosis is more common in people with diabetes. Atherosclerosis can occur in the large arteries that supply the brain or the smaller arteries within the brain. Ischemic stroke can also be triggered by a blood clot that breaks loose from the heart and lodges within an artery in the brain. Stroke often occurs in people with hematologic or blood abnormalities. In such cases, blood is much more adhesive, or sticky, and much more likely to form clots. This is especially true among people with diabetic kidney disease.

People with diabetes are at an increased risk of experiencing an ischemic stroke compared to those without diabetes, and they tend to fare worse after the stroke. Compared to the general population, people with diabetes are more severely disabled by stroke, are more likely to have another stroke, and are more likely to die from stroke. This is true whether you have type 1 or type 2 diabetes. However, the good news is that you can reduce your risk of stroke by taking steps to keep your blood glucose under control, and by minimizing the effects of other risk factors that also contribute to stroke.

■ SYMPTOMS

Sometimes, but not always, the first warning that a stroke is imminent is a transient ischemic attack. About 20 percent of all people who have a stroke first experience a transient ischemic attack. The symptoms of a transient ischemic attack and stroke are similar, but a transient ischemic attack usually lasts only 5 to 15 minutes. However, it is important to pay attention to the symptoms of a transient ischemic attack, because they mean that a stroke is about to occur.

Symptoms and signs of a transient ischemic attack and stroke include a sudden weakness or numbness in the face, arm, or leg on one side of the body. In rare instances, both sides of the body can be affected. You may feel this weakness as a sort of heaviness or clumsiness in the arm or leg. Or you could feel as though one side of your face is drooping. You might also experience a sudden sense of dimness or loss of vision, especially in one eye. Some people describe this as a haze, fog, or fuzziness over one eye. You may sense a loss of vision from the top to the bottom. If you are having a stroke or transient ischemic attack, you may also notice that your speech is slurred or that you have trouble articulating your words. Others may notice your speech difficulty. You may also have trouble understanding what others are saying to you or you may have trouble reading or writing. You may also feel dizzy, unsteady, or have trouble walking. If you are having a stroke you may feel any combination of these symptoms or only an isolated symptom. Some people are overcome with a sudden violent headache that seems to come out of nowhere. Headaches accompany ischemic stroke about 20 percent of the time.

■ RISKS

Approximately a half million Americans have a stroke each year. People with diabetes are twice as likely to experience a stroke as someone without diabetes. Other factors that increase the risk are advancing age, a family history of stroke (especially if there is also a family history of high blood pressure), diabetes, high cholesterol or blood lipids, sex, and race. Men are more likely than women to have a stroke, but women with diabetes are at higher risk than men with diabetes. African Americans are 60 percent more likely to experience stroke compared to Caucasians.

High blood pressure is the major risk factor for stroke. High blood pressure is defined as any reading greater than 130/85. Smoking can also increase the risk of stroke. Men who smoke are 40 percent more likely to have a stroke, and women who smoke are 60 percent more likely to have a stroke. For women, taking birth control pills increases the risk of stroke, and women who smoke and take birth control pills are 22 times more likely to suffer from stroke. High cholesterol and blood lipids also increase the risk of stroke, although the effect on stroke is not as great a risk factor as it is for heart disease. Heart disease can also increase the likelihood of stroke. Certain drugs that are known to increase blood pressure, such as cocaine, LSD, and amphetamines, can also trigger stroke. Heavy drinking, which also increases blood pressure, makes stroke more likely.

■ WHAT TO DO

If you experience any of the symptoms of stroke, call your doctor right away. If you cannot reach your doctor, call for emergency help at once. If your symptoms disappear, do not dismiss them. They may signal an impending acute stroke. Depending on the severity of your symptoms, you may be admitted immediately to a hospital or advised to see your doctor. It is extremely important to have your situation evaluated as soon as possible. Do not delay!

■ TREATMENT

Whether you are experiencing a stroke or a transient ischemic attack, you will probably be admitted to a hospital. Your doctor can most likely diagnose your stroke based on your symptoms, history, and physical examination. The treatment will depend on what caused the stroke. You may have a computed tomography (CT) scan performed. This provides an image of the brain and can reveal whether the stroke is caused by bleeding (hemorrhagic) or an arterial blockage (ischemic). A magnetic resonance imaging (MRI) scan can help your doctor identify places in the brain affected by stroke that cannot be viewed by a CT scan. Your doctor may also perform a carotid artery duplex scan, which uses ultrasound to look for blockages in the carotid arteries of the neck.

If the stroke or transient ischemic attack is caused by a blood clot that becomes lodged in a narrowed artery, it is very likely that another stroke will follow. Your doctor will try to treat the problem that is causing the blood clots to form. If your heart is beating irregularly, for example, blood clots can form and find their way to the arteries that supply the brain. Your doctor may perform an electrocardiogram to check your heart rhythm or an echocardiogram to see if clots are visible within the chambers of the heart. Your blood may also be tested to rule out the possibility that problems with blood coagulation could be contributing to the problem. Your blood glucose will also be tested to rule out the possibility that low blood glucose may be triggering the symptoms that mimic stroke.

If your stroke is in its early stages and your doctor determines it is due to a blood clot, and not a hemorrhage, you may be given certain drugs that prevent clot formation or dissolve existing clots. Anticoagulants such as heparin and warfarin may help patients who have had a transient ischemic attack or who are in the early stages of a stroke. For example, some strokes begin slowly and progress over several hours or even days. An anticoagulant may prevent further clot formation. However, most strokes happen rapidly with the damage occurring within minutes. Anticoagulant therapy is of little use in this situation. Anticoagulants are also dangerous for people with high blood pressure and for people who have had a hemorrhagic stroke.

Recent studies have shown great promise with new drugs in preventing paralysis and some of the major disabilities of stroke. Drugs such as tissue plasminogen activator and streptokinase work by breaking up or dissolving clots that already exist. They must be given within 3 hours of the onset of symptoms of stroke and cannot be given to patients with hemorraghic stroke.

Your doctor may also suggest a surgical treatment. If your stroke or transient ischemic attack is caused by a blockage in the carotid artery, you may be a candidate for a carotid endarterectomy. In this procedure, the carotid artery in the neck is opened and a layer of cholesterol plaque in the artery is removed. This surgery is helpful to people who have had a narrowing of the artery. If your arteries are less than 30 percent blocked or completely blocked, this surgery is not beneficial. It is not yet known whether carotid endarterectomy can benefit those with a 30 to 70 percent narrowing of the carotid artery. This surgery is not recommended if you have poor heart or lung function, which puts you at high risk for complications from surgery. People with diabetes who have retinopathy, nephropathy, congestive heart failure, heart valve disease, or peripheral vascular disease may be at high risk for complications of surgery.

Surgical and medical treatments for stroke can benefit those in the early stages of stroke and those with a transient ischemic attack, and they may help prevent another, more severe, stroke from occurring. But they will not help a stroke that has already occurred. Once the blood supply to the brain has been shut off, the damage to the brain cannot be reversed. However, rehabilitation can help patients regain function. The brain is a remarkable organ and other parts of the brain can be trained to take over for damaged parts. Many people find that with rehabilitation they can resume normal day-to-day living for years to come. Others are never able to overcome the disabilities of stroke and may have problems eating, speaking, or moving. About 20 percent of those who have a stroke die in the hospital. This is especially true among the elderly.

Rehabilitation can begin as soon as blood pressure, pulse, and breathing are stable. Doctors, nurses, and occupational and physical therapists may work with you in the hospital to keep your muscles strong and maintain flexibility. You may be given specific exercises to do on your own. Once discharged, you may continue with a program of physical therapy on an outpatient basis or you may be transferred to a rehabilitative center for more intensive therapy. Your therapist can help you make the transition from the hospital or rehab center to living at home.

■ PREVENTION

Many of the treatments for stroke are aimed at preventing a second stroke. If you have had a stroke, your doctor may suggest anticoagulant therapy or carotid artery surgery, as discussed above. You may also be treated for any heart problems that are causing clots to form.

Your doctor may also recommend long-term aspirin therapy. Aspirin is a platelet antiaggregant. It thins the blood by preventing blood platelets from sticking to each other. This reduces the likelihood of clot formation. A daily low dose of aspirin has been shown to reduce the risk of stroke by 30 percent. Talk to your doctor about whether this would be advisable for you. Your doctor will recommend a specific dose that suits your needs. In the U.S., recommended doses vary between 81 and 1,300 mg per day. Many people complain of upset stomach when using aspirin and some experience gastrointestinal bleeding. If this is the case, your doctor may suggest an alternative.

If you have been on aspirin therapy but continue to have transient ischemic attacks or even a stroke, your doctor may recommend ticlopidine (Ticlid). Like aspirin, ticlopidine inhibits platelet aggregation, but it does not cause gastrointestinal problems. It is stronger than aspirin and is a potent inhibitor of platelet aggregation. In people with diabetes, it also slows the progression of diabetic retinopathy. However, ticlopidine is more expensive than aspirin and has other side effects. It can cause diarrhea and skin rash. It can also reduce the number of neutrophils, or infection-fighting white blood cells, in the body, a condition known as neutropenia. This is a potentially fatal side effect, but it is reversible if detected early enough. Blood tests should be performed every 2 weeks for at least the first 3 months of therapy.

In addition to surgery and blood-thinning medications, you can also prevent stroke by making lifestyle changes and minimizing the effects of other contributing risk factors. These include quitting smoking, controlling high blood pressure, lowering blood lipid and blood cholesterol levels, and treating heart disease, such as coronary artery disease, congestive heart failure, atrial fibrillation, and other heart-rhythm disturbances. If you drink alcohol to excess, it can also increase blood pressure and increase the risk of stroke. Therefore, try to drink alcohol in moderation. Also, avoid the use of drugs such as cocaine and amphetamines that also increase the risk of stroke.

If you have diabetes, your risk of stroke is two to three times greater than that of someone without diabetes. It is not yet known whether controlling blood glucose levels actually reduces the risk of stroke, but it is a good idea to keep blood glucose under control.

Hypertension (High Blood Pressure)

If you have hypertension, your blood pressure is too high. Your blood travels through a network of arteries from your heart to the parts of your body that need it. If the pressure of the blood flowing through your arteries is too high, it stresses your blood vessels, much like a bicycle tire or balloon is stressed when inflated with too much air. Ideally, your heart pumps with just enough force to move the blood smoothly and swiftly throughout your body. But if your heart pumps with a force that is too great to keep the blood flowing smoothly, the pressure builds up in the artery. Think about what happens when you run water through a tube at a steady, even flow. If you constrict the tube by narrowing the opening or if you turn up the faucet, the water pressure builds and the tube becomes stressed and may even contort. This is what can happen to your arteries. Over time, your whole circulatory system becomes taxed.

There are two types of hypertension: essential and secondary. Essential hypertension has no apparent cause. Secondary hypertension is caused by some specific and recognizable event, such as kidney disease, pregnancy, oral contraceptive use, certain drugs, alcohol abuse, or a hormonal disorder. The vast majority of people with high blood pressure have essential hypertension.

But how much is too much? How do you know you have high blood pressure? Your doctor or health care provider measures your blood pressure in your upper arm with a blood pressure cuff, usually on your regular visit. The pressure of your blood against your arterial wall is measured as your heart contracts to pump out blood (systolic) and as it relaxes to permit the blood to flow (diastolic). The pressure is reported as the systolic pressure over the diastolic pressure. If your doctor tells you your blood pressure is 140/75 or 140 over 75, this means your systolic pressure is 140 and your diastolic pressure is 75. Whether or not you have high blood pressure depends on the values of these readings. In general, when your systolic pressure rises above 130 and your diastolic pressure rises above 85, you have mild hypertension. The higher these values, the more severe your hypertension.

To get an accurate reading, your blood pressure should be measured with a properly fitting cuff. Also, some people experience a rise in blood pressure when they visit a doctor's office. This phenomenon even has a name: white coat hypertension. If you feel tense just from the act of having your blood pressure measured, try taking your own blood pressure measurements with a home blood pressure meter. Keep your own records to show your doctor.

■ SYMPTOMS

There are no symptoms of mild to moderate hypertension. You probably feel fine and may be unaware that anything is wrong. If you have severe to very severe hypertension and you have had it for some time, you may begin to notice headaches, palpitations, dizziness, and an overall feeling of fatigue or just not feeling quite right. However, some of these symptoms are caused by damage to organs and systems in the body a result of high blood pressure, not by the high blood pressure itself. The only way to know for sure whether you have high blood pressure is to have your blood pressure measured on several different occasions, preferably a week apart, by your doctor or member of your health care team. If your blood pressure is over 140/90 on several different occasions, you probably have hypertension.

■ RISKS

If you have high blood pressure, you are at a greatly increased risk for heart failure and heart attack, kidney failure, and, especially, stroke. If you have high blood pressure you are four times more likely to have a stroke than someone without high blood pressure. Even mild hypertension can lower your life expectancy, and severe hypertension can shorten your life dramatically. For example, if you have malignant hypertension, a very severe form of high blood pressure, and it is left untreated, you are at considerable risk of dying within a matter of months. Fewer than 5 percent of people with malignant hypertension survive for a year.

Factors that increase your risk of high blood pressure include a genetic predisposition, increasing age, a sedentary lifestyle, and obesity. African Americans are twice as likely to have high blood pressure as Caucasians, and women are less likely than men. Stress, excessive alcohol consumption, and too much salt in your food can also contribute, especially if you are predisposed to high blood pressure.

■ WHAT TO DO

You should have your blood pressure checked regularly, especially if you have diabetes or any of the risk factors associated with hypertension. If you have any of the symptoms associated with severe or very severe hypertension, see your doctor right away. You could have malignant hypertension, a life-threatening condition that requires immediate treatment. If you are experiencing any symptoms, it means that your organs, especially the kidneys, heart, blood vessels, and brain, may be damaged. You should be treated right away to avoid further damage.

■ TREATMENT

Once your doctor establishes that you have high blood pressure, she will assess whether any of your organs have been damaged. Your retina will be directly examined for retinopathy using an ophthalmoscope. Often a doctor can tell how serious your hypertension is by looking at the condition of your retinas. Your doctor will examine your heart, using an electrocardiogram, echocardiogram, and/or chest X ray. High blood pressure can cause the heart to enlarge. Kidney damage may be assessed by assaying the urine. The presence of protein or blood cells in the urine is an indicator of kidney damage. Your doctor may also check your kidneys in a physical exam and by X ray or ultrasound.

If your high blood pressure is mild to moderately high, your doctor will suggest that you modify certain lifestyle factors. If you are obese, your doctor will suggest you lose weight. Cutting out salt in the diet, reducing alcohol consumption, quitting smoking, and increasing the amount you exercise are some of the steps you can take to lower your blood pressure.

If none of these interventions helps, or if your high blood pressure is severe, your doctor may prescribe a drug to lower blood pressure. Your doctor will prescribe a drug based on many factors, such as your age, sex, and race, as well as lifestyle factors. If you have kidney disease, your choice of drugs may be limited, because certain drugs can cause further kidney damage. And some drugs can upset your blood glucose control and should be avoided if you have diabetes. You may find that you have to try different medications to find the one that works for you.

Your doctor may very well prescribe a thiazide diuretic as a first approach to controlling high blood pressure. These drugs work by helping the body get rid of excess salt and water. This decreases the total volume of fluid in the body and thus lowers blood pressure. However, these drugs can also lower potassium levels. You may be advised to take a potassium supplement while on a thiazide diuretic. These drugs are especially effective in African Americans, the elderly, obese people, and those with kidney or heart failure.

Adrenergic blockers are a class of drugs that blocks the body's response to stress. Normally, your body reacts to stress by causing a rise in blood pressure. But adrenergic blockers prevent this rise in blood pressure. Beta-blockers are the most common adrenergic blockers, and they work well in Caucasians, young people, and people who have had a heart attack, rapid heartbeat, or migraine headaches. Alpha-blockers work by helping blood vessels relax. They do not appear to affect blood glucose levels and may also have a positive effect on blood lipids. However, if you are prescribed an alpha-blocker, your doctor will advise that you use caution. For many people, the first dose can cause blood pressure to drop precipitously. Your doctor may start you on a small dose of this drug.

The ACE inhibitors work by blocking the conversion of an enzyme, angiotensin I, to angiotensin II. Angiotensin II causes arteries to constrict, which increases blood pressure. By blocking the formation of this enzyme, ACE inhibitors work to dilate the arteries. The ACE inhibitors work well in people with kidney disease and protein in the urine. They do not affect blood glucose control and do not increase lipid levels. However, in rare cases, ACE inhibitors can worsen kidney function when both arteries to the kidneys are constricted. Angiotensin II blockers more directly block the action of angiotensin II. The results are similar to those seen with ACE inhibitors—a lowering of blood pressure by dilating the arteries—with fewer side effects.

Calcium channel blockers are also sometimes prescribed for people with high blood pressure. Although they do not appear to affect blood glucose or lipid levels, they should be used with caution. In some people, they can dramatically decrease blood pressure when you stand up, a condition known as orthostatic hypotension. Some calcium channel blockers can worsen the proteinuria found in kidney disease, but others seem to decrease it. For this reason, some doctors do not recommend using some types of calcium channel blockers for people with diabetes.

If you have malignant hypertension, a life-threatening condition in which your blood pressure must be lowered immediately, you may be given one of several drugs intravenously. These drugs include diazoxide, nitroprusside, nitroglycerin, and labetalol. Nifedipine, a calcium channel blocker, is fast acting and can be given orally, but it can cause very low blood pressure and must be used with caution.

■ PREVENTION

The best way to prevent high blood pressure is to maintain a healthy lifestyle. If your blood pressure is already high, modifying certain lifestyle factors can help bring it down. If your blood pressure is in the normal range, keeping fit and eating right can go a long way in preventing high blood pressure from developing.

If you smoke, quit smoking. If you are overweight, losing weight will improve your blood pressure. You may need to reduce the amount of calories you consume, decrease the amount of fat in your diet, and increase the amount you exercise. If you have diabetes, this should be done carefully, with the supervision of your doctor and dietitian. The good news is that modifying these factors will also improve your diabetes control and reduce your risk of stroke and heart attack.

If you drink alcohol, drink only in moderation and talk to your dietitian about how to make this a part of your diabetes control plan. Also, reduce your salt intake and try to reduce the stress in your life as much as possible. Because high blood pressure is a risk factor for other conditions such as heart disease and stroke, preventing it from occurring in the first place will also help reduce the risk of some of these other complications of diabetes.

Peripheral Vascular Disease

When cholesterol plaque builds up in the arteries that supply your legs (and in some cases, your arms) with blood, the arteries can become narrowed and even blocked. This condition is known as peripheral vascular disease. If you have peripheral vascular disease, the flow of blood to your legs is restricted, leading to poor circulation. Without the proper circulation, you can develop foot ulcers, gangrene, and other forms of tissue loss in your feet. If you have even minor foot surgery, or suffer any kind of injury or abrasion to the feet, your feet may be unable to heal properly. Frequently, people with peripheral vascular disease must face limb amputation. Fortunately, with the proper treatment, this can be avoided.

■ SYMPTOMS

The major symptom of peripheral vascular disease is pain in the legs. You may experience pain in the calves while walking or exercising (claudication), or pain while resting or sleeping.

The severity of the symptoms depends on how far peripheral vascular disease has progressed. When the arteries to the leg narrow gradually, you may begin to feel pain, aching, cramping, or tiredness in the leg muscles—especially the calf muscles—while exercising. You may feel the pain while walking, for example. The pain may come on faster and feel more severe when you are walking faster or walking uphill. Many people with peripheral vascular disease feel pain in the calf, but the foot, thigh, hip, or buttocks can also be affected. Usually claudication pain is relieved by resting. If you have neuropathy, or a degeneration of nerves, you may feel no pain, but rather a sensation of numbness or a "dead" feeling in your limb.

As peripheral vascular disease progresses, you may find that the pain kicks in at shorter and shorter distances of walking or amounts of time spent exercising. Eventually you may feel pain while you are resting. You may feel severe, unrelenting pain in the lower leg or foot that gets worse when you try to elevate your leg. You may even feel pain while you are sleeping.

As the blockage in your legs gets worse, your leg may feel cold and numb, with no visible sign of a pulse or a very weak pulse. Your skin may feel dry and scaly and your hair and nails may grow poorly. You may even develop sores, or ulcers, on your toes or heels, or even on your lower leg. At its worst, your leg may shrink, and gangrene, or tissue death, can set in.

When the arteries in the legs become suddenly and completely obstructed, you may feel a severe pain, coldness, and numbness. Your leg may take on a pale or bluish tint and you may feel no pulse below the point at which your artery is blocked.

■ RISKS

If you have diabetes, you are 20 times more likely to develop peripheral vascular disease than someone without diabetes. Your risk is increased further if you smoke, don't eat properly, don't exercise, have high blood levels of cholesterol and other lipids, and have poor blood glucose control. Peripheral vascular disease is prevalent in women as well as men, and is found in both the elderly and younger population.

If you have peripheral vascular disease, you face the risk of developing foot ulcers, gangrene, and amputation. However, if you develop peripheral vascular disease, especially if you catch it in the early stages, it doesn't mean you will eventually face amputation. Only 10 to 15 percent of all patients with peripheral vascular disease go on to face the prospect of losing a limb. Your best bet is to take preventive measures to keep peripheral vascular disease from developing in the first place and to treat it aggressively once it is diagnosed.

■ WHAT TO DO

If you experience any of the symptoms of peripheral vascular disease, contact your doctor right away. Although it is not an emergency situation, you should be diagnosed and treated promptly to avoid permanent damage to your legs and feet and to avoid amputation. The sooner you intervene and treat peripheral vascular disease, the more likely you are to restore circulation to your legs, and the less likely the prospect that you will lose your limbs.

Your doctor will assess the flow of blood to your legs. This can be done by feeling the pulse in the lower leg. If you have a significant obstruction, the pulse will be diminished or even absent below the knee. However, people with diabetes often have calcium deposits in the arterial walls, making the arteries rigid and the pulse difficult to detect. Your doctor may measure the blood pressure in your leg and compare it to that in your arm. Usually the blood pressure in the leg is 90 percent of that in the arm, but with narrowing of the arteries to the leg, the blood pressure can be lower than 50 percent of that in the arm. However, because of the calcification of arteries, it may be more difficult to get an accurate blood pressure reading if you have diabetes. Your doctor may elect to check the blood pressure in your toe instead, because the blood vessels in your toes are not usually calcified even if you have diabetes.

Alternatively, your doctor may measure the amount of oxygen in the skin of your feet. This will tell your doctor whether sufficient blood supply is reaching your feet to keep the tissue supplied with oxygen. Your doctor may also use Doppler ultrasound to detect the amount of blood flowing through your legs. This measures the sound of blood flowing through your arteries. Or you may be given a Doppler color ultrasound, which provides a picture of the artery, with different colors used to illustrate the different flow rates.

In addition to these tests, your doctor may also recommend angiography, an X-ray test that measures blood flow. For this test you will be injected with a substance that appears opaque in an X ray. An X ray is then taken that will provide you and your doctor with a picture of your arteries, showing the extent of obstruction. Your doctor may also recommend magnetic resonance angiography, an imaging technique that can be performed without the use of a dye. This is especially useful in people who have kidney problems.

■ TREATMENT

If your doctor determines that you have blockage in your leg arteries, she may recommend one of several treatments to restore blood flow to your legs. If you are a smoker, you should stop smoking immediately. Ask your doctor for help in finding ways to stop smoking if you find this task daunting. You may also try elevating the head of your bed while sleeping to increase the flow of blood to your legs.

If your peripheral vascular disease is in the early stages and you are experiencing intermittent claudication, your doctor may suggest that you walk 30 minutes each day, if possible, or consider the use of an exercise bicycle. If you feel pain while exercising, stop and rest until the pain subsides, then resume activity. If you do this on a regular basis, you will probably find that you can go longer and longer each time before you feel pain. Exercise increases the circulation to your legs and improves muscle function.

Your doctor may prescribe medication to improve oxygen delivery. Pentoxifylline, for example, can improve oxygen delivery to muscles. Although calcium blockers and aspirin can help some patients, calcium blockers should be used with caution in patients with diabetes. Beta-blockers, which are often used to help people with blockages in the heart arteries, can worsen the condition of people with blockages in the leg arteries.

If your doctor finds a moderate obstruction in your leg arteries, she may perform an angioplasty. This can be done at the same time you are examined by angiography. In an angioplasty, your doctor will insert a catheter equipped with a deflated balloon into your narrowed artery. When the balloon is inflated, it will open up the artery to allow blood to flow. Alternatively, your doctor may recommend another procedure to open the narrowed blood vessel. This could include mechanical cutters, lasers, stents, and rotatory sanders. All of these devices serve to bore through the blockage and open up the blood vessel. Following these procedures you may be given a blood-thinning medication such as heparin or a platelet inhibitor such as aspirin to prevent further blockage or narrowing from occurring.

Angiography is not recommended for people with extensive narrowing, blockages that extend for long distances, or if the artery is severely hardened. If you have significant obstruction in your leg arteries, your doctor may suggest surgery to remove or bypass the obstruction. Surgery is also recommended if there is a blood clot blocking the narrowed blood vessel or if a clot has broken away and blocked a more distant blood vessel.

If the blockage is severe, your doctor may recommend a bypass oper-ation. To do this, a vein from another part of the body or a synthetic tube is grafted to the artery below and above the blockage so that blood can flow around the blocked artery. In some cases, a piece of artery that contains the blockage is surgically removed and replaced with a graft of vein or synthetic tube. Bypasses are only performed when the survival of your limb is threatened. Studies have shown that it can save the limb in 90 percent of cases, even 5 years after surgery.

In severe cases, amputation may be the only way to save a limb. Amputation may be performed to cut out an area of infected tissue, to relieve incessant pain, or to prevent the spread of gangrene. In these cases, the surgeon will do everything to save as much of the leg as possi-ble, especially if you plan to wear an artificial limb.

■ PREVENTION

Like other forms of cardiac and arterial disease, the key to controlling peripheral vascular disease is preventing it from occurring in the first place, or preventing it from progressing as much as possible. For people with diabetes, maintaining good blood glucose control is a key first step. Eating a healthy, low-fat diet will help prevent cholesterol plaque from accumulating in the arteries. And starting or maintaining a moderate exercise or activity program will improve blood circulation and keep blood flowing. Try walking 30 minutes a day or talk to your doctor or exercise physiologist about other activities that will improve blood circu-lation in your legs or arms. Finally, if you are a smoker, quit smoking. Talk to your doctor about programs or medications that can help you stop. This is one of the most important steps you can take to prevent peripheral vascular disease and other types of circulatory problems.

Chapter 7
Solving Neuropathy Problems

Your brain controls virtually everything your body does, from thinking, feeling, and breathing, to eating, sleeping, moving, and making love. It performs this remarkable task by sending messages through your spinal chord and to organs throughout your body through a network of nerve cells. This network of nerves is much like a series of wires that transmits electrical impulses. Like electrical wires, nerves can become damaged or frayed. When this happens, components of the system connected by the wires can malfunction. This type of damage to the nerves is called neuropathy.

No one knows why for certain, but too much glucose in the blood can, over time, damage the nerves of your body. It may be because proteins coated with glucose directly harm the nerve cells. Or it could be that the extra amount of glucose in the blood upsets the chemical balance within nerves. Or it might be that too much glucose interferes with blood circulation and the nerves are unable to get the oxygen they need. Whatever the reason, people with diabetes are more likely to develop nerve problems than people without diabetes. The good news is that keeping tight control over your blood glucose levels can reduce the risk of neuropathy by 60 percent.

Fortunately, the nerves of the central nervous system—the brain and spinal cord—are not usually affected by high blood glucose. But the nerves of the peripheral nervous system, which reach out to muscles, to sensory cells and organs, and to internal organs, can become damaged over time. Sensorimotor neuropathy refers to damage to the sensory nerves, those nerves that send information about how things feel from the skin and from internal organs to the brain. Motor neurons send information from the brain to the muscles of the body about how to move. For instance, if you put your hand down on a hot stove, the sensory neurons send a signal to your brain that you are hurting your hand. Your brain then sends a message through your motor neurons that tells you to move your hand. But when you have neuropathy, these nerve cell transmissions don't work well. You don't always feel pain or things you should be feeling, and your muscles don't always get the message to move the way you want them to move.

There are different types of neuropathies, depending on what nerves are damaged. Neuropathy can affect sensory neurons, motor neurons, or autonomic neurons—those that control internal organs or automatic processes in your body that you don't even need to think about. Nerves are made up of both small fibers and large fibers. Small fibers control sensitivity to heat and cold and to touch. Large fibers control your sense of balance and position. When small fibers are damaged, you may feel pain or a loss of sensitivity to heat and cold. When large fibers are damaged, you may lose your sense of balance or position. Often both small and large fibers are affected by neuropathy.

Neuropathies can also be classified as focal or diffuse. Diffuse neuropathies develop slowly, and over time spread from one set of nerves to another. For example, initially only the sensory and motor nerves may be damaged, but over time, your autonomic system may also become affected. Diffuse neuropathies can affect several different parts of the body at the same time, such as the feet and hands, usually affecting both sides of the body. Focal neuropathies tend to come on suddenly and affect only one nerve or group of nerves. Focal neuropathies can affect very specific parts of the body, such as the wrist in carpal tunnel syndrome. Often diffuse and focal neuropathies can occur together. Fortunately, most types of neuropathies improve with better blood glucose control.

Mononeuropathy (Focal Neuropathy)

Mononeuropathy, or focal neuropathy, is caused by damage to a single nerve or group of nerves. Many mononeuropathies come on quite suddenly and are painful. Nerve damage does not spread from the nerve originally affected and it usually goes away after a while. However, some mononeuropathies have symptoms similar to life-threatening conditions, such as heart attack and stroke, and should not be dismissed without first discussing your symptoms with your doctor. Unlike other mononeuropathies, entrapment syndromes, such as carpal tunnel syndrome, often develop more gradually and persist for long periods of time.

Cranial Neuropathy

Cranial neuropathy is caused by damage to a single nerve from the brain. Cranial neuropathy is rare in younger people, but occurs frequently in elderly people with diabetes.

■ SYMPTOMS

Symptoms of cranial neuropathy include severe headache, drooping of one side of the face, double vision, or difficulty opening one eyelid. Cranial neuropathy is not usually painful.

■ WHAT TO DO

If you experience any of the symptoms listed above, call your doctor. Your doctor will want to rule out the possibility of stroke or other life-threatening conditions. Cranial neuropathy can be frightening, but it usually goes away in a few days or weeks. However, make sure to contact your doctor for an accurate diagnosis and to rule out the possibility of something more serious.

Plexopathy

Plexopathy involves damage to any of the nerve plexi of the peripheral nervous system. A nerve plexus is a sort of electrical junction box that sends out groups of nerves from the spinal cord to various parts of the body. The major plexi include the cervical plexus of the neck, which distributes nerves to the arms, and the lumbosacral plexus of the lower back, which sends out nerves to the pelvis and legs. People with diabetes, especially elderly people, sometimes experience a type of plexopathy known as femoral neuropathy, which affects nerves in the thigh.

■ SYMPTOMS

Symptoms of femoral neuropathy include pain in the thigh and in the calf. The pain is often worse at night. You may also experience weakness in the thigh muscle, which makes it difficult to move your hip and knee.

■ WHAT TO DO

If you experience any leg pain, tell your doctor. Your doctor will want to distinguish it from sciatica. To do this, you will be asked to straighten your leg and raise it. If you have sciatica, this will be very painful, but if you have a plexopathy, you should be able to do this without pain. Usually, this condition is diagnosed by excluding other conditions. Plexopathies, including femoral neuropathy, usually heal spontaneously without treatment. However, it may take several years before you regain muscle strength, and the condition can recur.

Radiculopathy

Radiculopathy is caused by damage to a nerve or group of nerves in the trunk of the body. It affects both men and women with diabetes and is more common in older people.

■ SYMPTOMS

If you have radiculopathy, you may experience pain in the chest or abdomen. The pain usually comes on suddenly and can get worse at night. This could lead you or your doctor to suspect an emergency situation such as a heart attack, ulcer, or appendicitis. The pain of radiculopathy does not usually get worse when you cough or exercise, however.

■ WHAT TO DO

Call your doctor if you experience any chest or abdominal pain. You may need immediate treatment to rule out the possibility of something more serious, such as a heart attack, pneumonia, appendicitis, gastrointestinal disease, or ulcer. Your doctor may need to perform several different tests to correctly diagnose the condition. If you do indeed have radiculopathy, it will go away in a few months on its own. Talk to your doctor if you need help dealing with the pain.

Entrapment Syndromes

Several types of entrapment neuropathies are more common in people with diabetes than in the general population. Researchers do not know for sure why this is true, but they think that diabetes somehow affects nerve transmission. This makes nerves more susceptible to mechanical damage, such as compression. When an already vulnerable nerve is compressed, then damage can occur more readily than in a patient without diabetes. Nerves commonly affected with entrapment include the median nerve in the wrist, which leads to carpal tunnel disorder, the ulnar nerve of the elbow, the radial nerve of the upper arm, the lateral cutaneous nerve of the thigh, and the peroneal nerve of the knee.

Carpal Tunnel Syndrome

Carpal tunnel syndrome is twice as likely to occur in people with diabetes and more likely to affect women than men. It can be caused by repeated motion that compresses the nerve, by changes in metabolism, and by fluid that accumulates within the confined space of the carpal tunnel. People who frequently subject their wrists to forceful repetitive movements such as using a screwdriver or typing at a computer terminal are especially at risk.

■ SYMPTOMS

Symptoms of carpal tunnel syndrome include numbness, tingling, pain, and odd sensations in the thumb, index finger, and middle finger of one hand. Sometimes pain and a tingling or burning sensation also occurs in the arm and shoulder. You may find it more painful while sleeping because of the position of your hand.

■ WHAT TO DO

If you have any of the symptoms of carpal tunnel syndrome, talk to your doctor about what you can do to relieve the pain. You may want to first try to avoid the positions and motions that compress the median nerve. Avoid overextending your wrist or putting extra pressure on your wrist. Using a wrist splint might help. If your problem is a result of overusing your computer keyboard, for example, you might try adjusting the angle or position of the keyboard. Your doctor may prescribe anti-inflammatory drugs to reduce inflammation and help with the pain. In some cases, injection of a corticosteroid can bring temporary relief from pain. You may also be a candidate for physical therapy.

If your pain is severe or your muscles begin to weaken, and none of these measures helps, your doctor may suggest surgery to relieve pressure on the nerve. In this procedure, a surgeon sections a ligament called the volar carpal ligament, which should release the trapped nerve.

Ulnar Nerve Entrapment

The ulnar nerve is also vulnerable and can become entrapped, especially in people with diabetes. This nerve passes through the elbow near the surface of the skin and can become compressed if you repeatedly lean on your elbow or if you have any kind of abnormal bone growth in that area.

■ SYMPTOMS

Symptoms of ulnar nerve entrapment include pain and weakness in the pinkie and ring fingers and the forearm. You may also experience weakness and odd sensations in the hand. If the pain is severe and the nerve compression lasts a long time, then your muscles can atrophy, giving the hand a clawlike deformity.

■ WHAT TO DO

Surgery is generally not successful in relieving ulnar nerve entrapment. Treatment is usually aimed at avoiding pressure on the elbow, and physical therapy can help restore mobility and muscle tone.

Radial Nerve Entrapment

The radial nerve runs beneath the bone of the upper arm. Pressure to this nerve can also cause an entrapment syndrome. This problem is sometimes called "Saturday Night Palsy" because it often occurs in people who drink heavily and fall asleep with an arm draped over the back of a chair or under the head.

■ SYMPTOMS

Symptoms of radial nerve entrapment include weakness and loss of sensation on the back of the hand. Often, the fingers curve and the wrist flops into a bent position (wristdrop) when the wrist is extended.

■ WHAT TO DO

If you suspect radial nerve entrapment, try to avoid any positions or motions that put pressure on the underside of the upper arm. Usually the condition improves once the pressure is relieved. If this does not help, talk to your doctor about possible therapies.

Peroneal Nerve Entrapment

The peroneal nerve runs along the surface of the skin at the top of the calf muscle, in the soft folds of tissue behind the knee. It is often found in people who are thin and bedridden, improperly strapped to a wheelchair, or who tend to cross their legs often and for long periods of time.

■ SYMPTOMS

Symptoms include a weakening of the muscle that lifts the foot. This causes footdrop, an inability to raise or flex the foot, and a loss of sensation at the outer foot.

■ WHAT TO DO

The first thing to do is to identify the cause of the nerve compression. If you cross your legs often, try to avoid doing so. If you are bedridden or wheelchair-bound, talk to your caregivers about finding a position that reduces pressure on the back of your knee. Talk to your doctor about other measures you can take.

Other Conditions

Other nerves are also susceptible to entrapment. Pressure or damage to the lateral cutaneous nerve of the thigh causes pain and sensory loss in the upper thigh. Compression of the sciatic nerve in the buttock can cause sciatica, marked by pain in the lateral thigh, as well as footdrop. And pressure on the medial and lateral plantar nerves in the foot can cause a decrease in sensation on the inside and outside of the foot. Treatments generally include relief of the pressure on the nerve, anti-inflammatory drugs, physical therapy, and in some cases, surgery. Talk to your doctor if you are experiencing any pain or unusual symptoms.

Polyneuropathy (Distal Symmetric Neuropathy)

Polyneuropathy is the most common type of neuropathy found in people with diabetes. It can affect as many as three-quarters of all people with diabetes. You may hear people referring to it by a variety of names: peripheral neuropathy, polyneuropathy, diffuse neuropathy, distal symmetric neuropathy, sensorimotor neuropathy, or painful neuropathy. This kind of neuropathy can affect the nerves in many parts of your body. You might feel numbness, pain, or a loss of sensitivity in your arms, hands, legs, or feet on both sides of your body. Although technically peripheral neuropathy refers to any kind of neuropathy that affects the peripheral nervous system, when people say they have peripheral neuropathy, this is often what they mean.

■ SYMPTOMS

If you have polyneuropathy you may feel one or more of an array of symptoms, depending on what nerves are damaged and the extent of the damage. Nerves are made up of both small and large nerve fibers. If the small nerve fibers are damaged, you may feel symptoms that include a tingling or burning feeling, a sensation of "pins and needles," pain in your arms and/or legs that is usually worse at night, a numbness or loss of feeling in your extremities, cold hands or feet, and swelling, especially in your feet. You may lose the ability to detect temperature. If the large nerve fibers are damaged, you may find that you lose your balance easily, are unable to sense the position of your feet and toes, and develop unusual sensations in your extremities. You could also develop Charcot's joints, a condition marked by redness and swelling in your foot (see page 282). If your motor nerves (the nerves that control your muscles) are damaged, you could lose muscle tone in your hands and feet, develop calluses and open sores on your feet, or develop misshapen or deformed toes and feet.

■ WHAT TO DO

If you are experiencing the pain of neuropathy, tell your doctor. Depending on the symptoms and the extent of the neuropathy, your doctor may suggest exercises that can help reduce the pain, or if the pain is especially severe, your doctor may prescribe a medication to provide some relief. You may also want to take steps to maintain tighter control of your blood glucose levels. If you keep your blood glucose levels as close to normal as possible, you may find that some of your symptoms will disappear. However, some symptoms, even with good glucose control, can persist for 6 to 18 months.

If you do have symptoms of neuropathy, your doctor may want to conduct some tests to accurately diagnose the problem. Neuropathy is often diagnosed by excluding other conditions that could result in the same symptoms. Your doctor will probably test your reflexes. Your doctor may also place a tuning fork against your toe to see whether you can detect vibrations. Your doctor may also place a monofilament wire against the fleshy part of your foot to see if you can detect the sensation of touch. If you have neuropathy, your body may not respond to these stimuli. Your doctor may then send you to a neurologist for a more complete assessment of nerve damage. Your neurologist may elect to conduct an electromyogram to assess nerve function or a neurological exam to determine the severity of your neuropathy.

If you do have neuropathy, it is important that both you and your doctor be aware of it, even if you are not in great pain. This is because the most serious symptom of neuropathy is the loss of sensation, particularly in the feet. Pain signals you that something is hurting you or damaging your body. Without pain, you may not know that you have injured your foot, for example, and may continue to use it and damage it further. This could lead to ulceration, infection, gangrene, and even amputation.

If you have neuropathy or suspect neuropathy, check your feet every day, or have a friend or relative do it for you. Make sure to look at the top of your foot, the bottom of your foot, and between your toes. Any signs of irritation or ulceration should be treated right away. Protect your feet from any sort of injury or damage by wearing the proper shoes, not going barefoot, and inspecting them daily. Your doctor or diabetes educator can show you what to look for and how to examine your feet, as well as how to properly care for them. (For more on foot care, see Chapter 12.)

If you smoke, stop smoking. Talk to your doctor about medical and social interventions if you are having a hard time quitting. Smoking only increases the likelihood of further nerve damage. Avoid alcohol, because it also increases nerve damage. If you have a problem curtailing alcohol intake, talk to your doctor about programs to help you.

Your doctor may also refer you to an exercise physiologist or suggest a program of walking, exercise, or gentle stretching. Some people find yoga especially helpful. Biofeedback techniques and hypnosis have helped some people to deal with neuropathy pain and may be worth a try. If your skin is especially sensitive, you may want to try an elastic body stocking, panty hose, or foot cradles to help keep clothes and bedcovers from irritating your skin. If you have foot problems, lamb's wool or orthotics fitted to your foot can help relieve pressure on your feet.

■ TREATMENT

If you have taken steps to maintain control of blood glucose levels and have quit smoking and drinking but pain and other symptoms persist, your doctor may want to prescribe or suggest certain medications. For example, over-the-counter pain relievers and a capsaicin ointment (0.075%) applied to the skin may help relieve pain. Vitamins, although important as part of a balanced diet, do not usually help alleviate the symptoms of neuropathy. Painkillers that contain narcotics are not recommended for people with diabetes, because of the side effects and potential for addiction.

Other medicines, such as low doses of anticonvulsive agents (phentoin, caramazepine, or gabapentin) or antidepressants (amitriptyline, for example) may also relieve some of the symptoms of neuropathy. Antidepressants may be prescribed alone or along with an anticonvulsive agent. If you do try any of these medicines, give them time to see if they work. It may take as long as 4 to 6 weeks before they take effect, so make sure to give them a fair trial. If you experience any side effects from the drugs, however, make sure to tell your physician right away. Common side effects include sleepiness, dry mouth, constipation, nausea, and dizziness. These are often relieved by taking your dose at bedtime.

Another approach is to use a small battery-operated device known as a transcutaneous electrical nerve stimulation (TENS) unit. This device provides small electrical impulses that block the transmission of pain messages to your brain and provide some relief from pain. This device must be prescribed by your doctor. Some people also find relief from acupuncture and acupressure. Ask your health care team about these methods and any other remedy you may have heard about. Some unorthodox methods actually do have scientific validity, but others may be a waste of your time and money.

■ PREVENTION

The best way to prevent neuropathy is to keep tight control of your blood glucose levels. The Diabetes Control and Complications Trial (DCCT), as well as several other studies in other countries, have shown that keeping blood glucose levels as close to normal as possible can reduce the incidence of neuropathy by as much as 60 percent in people with type 1 or type 2 diabetes. If you have type 2 diabetes and are overweight, losing weight can reduce insulin resistance and in turn reduce the risk of neuropathy. If you smoke, stop smoking, and if you drink alcohol, reduce your alcohol intake. The more preventive steps you can take, the more likely you will reduce the risk of neuropathy now and in the future.

Autonomic Neuropathy

When people say they have neuropathy, they are usually talking about damage to the nerves to the legs, feet, arms, and hands that control the way they walk, move, and feel things in the environment. But nerves to the autonomic nervous system can also be damaged. The autonomic nervous system delivers messages from the brain to control all the internal organs that you don't usually even think about—the heart, lungs, bladder, kidney, stomach, intestines, and reproductive organs, for example. When these nerves are damaged, you may develop autonomic neuropathy. When this occurs, you may experience problems with some of the major organ systems in your body. Autonomic neuropathy can cause problems with bladder control, with the stomach and gastrointestinal tract (see Chapter 10), with sexual function in both men and women (see Chapters 14 and 15), with your heart and blood pressure, with the nerves in the skin that control sweating, and with the way your eyes adjust to lightness and darkness. Autonomic neuropathy can also interfere with the warning signs of hypoglycemia and can contribute to hypoglycemia unawareness.

Neurogenic Bladder

Three different types of nerves control how your bladder functions. Your bladder serves as a sort of vessel to hold the urine that your kidneys make after they have filtered the blood. The kidneys filter the blood and send the blood and blood cells back into circulation. The waste products are collected in the urine, which is sent to the bladder until it is eliminated from the body. The bladder can expand to hold more and more urine until you feel the urge to urinate. One type of nerve sends a message to your brain when your bladder is full and your brain tells you to go to the bathroom. Another type of nerve causes your bladder to contract to push the urine out. A third type of nerve controls the sphincter muscle of the bladder. This muscle opens to allow you to urinate and closes when you are finished. Damage to any of these nerves can cause problems with the way the bladder functions and with the way you urinate. This type of problem is often called bladder neuropathy, bladder dysfunction, or neurogenic bladder.

■ SYMPTOMS

The symptoms of neurogenic bladder depend on which nerves are damaged. You might find that you feel the need to urinate less often, have difficulty completely emptying your bladder, have a weak urinary stream, find it difficult to start urinating and may dribble afterwards, experience urinary incontinence, find it difficult to wait to urinate once you feel the need, or develop frequent urinary tract infections. The symptoms of a urinary tract infection include a frequent need to urinate even though you may not void much urine each time, pain or burning when you urinate, being unable to expel any urine even though you feel the urge, or discolored urine.

■ WHAT TO DO

If you have any of the symptoms of bladder neuropathy, talk to your doctor about what you can do to alleviate the problem. If you have symptoms of a urinary tract infection, talk to your doctor at once. If left untreated, urinary tract infections can cause damage to the kidneys. Urinary tract infections are usually cured rapidly with antibiotics. Even if you have no other signs of neuropathy, frequent urinary tract infections can be an early sign of neurogenic bladder. This happens when the urine is not completely expelled and sits in the bladder for extended periods of time, allowing bacteria to grow. This is especially true for people with diabetes, who may have large amounts of glucose in their urine, providing the bacteria with the nutrients they need to grow.

Your doctor may suggest medications to help with your problem, but there are also several steps you can take yourself to alleviate the symptoms of bladder neuropathy. Because your bladder nerves cannot sense when you need to urinate, you may have to take on the job yourself. Drink plenty of fluids, and instead of waiting until your bladder feels full, try urinating according to a timetable, say every hour or every

2 hours. If you are having problems starting to urinate or completely expelling all your urine, try pushing on your bladder to start the urine flowing and again when you are finished (this is called double voiding). Men may find it easier to urinate sitting down. If you are having problems completely emptying your bladder, try urinating again 5 to 10 minutes after your first attempt.

■ TREATMENT

If timed voiding or double voiding does not alleviate the symptoms of bladder neuropathy, your doctor may want to try a drug therapy, catheterization, or surgery. Your doctor may suggest placing a catheter through your urethra to completely remove the urine from your bladder. A permanent catheter can cause problems, especially in men, including inflammation of the urethra and surrounding tissue. It can also be quite cumbersome. You and your doctor may decide it is preferable to try intermittent self-catherization. In this case, your doctor or nurse educator will show you how to insert a catheter yourself. You can then do this four to six times a day to empty your bladder, removing the catheter after each voiding. This is especially useful if you have a contracted sphincter, which makes it difficult to expel urine.

Drugs such as bethanechol have had limited success in initiating urine flow, but they may nevertheless help some people. However, these drugs do not help if you are having problems fully emptying your bladder. Other medications, such as terazosin or doxazosin, can relax the sphincter to help you empty your bladder. However, these drugs can cause side effects such as dry mouth and constipation and are not generally helpful for people with neurogenic bladder.

Another approach is surgery. Your doctor may suggest bladder neck surgery, which will relieve the spasm of the internal sphincter that prevents emptying of the bladder. The external sphincter is left intact, thus preventing urine leakage.

■ PREVENTION

Your best bet in avoiding bladder problems is to take steps to prevent neuropathy from occurring in the first place or to delay its onset. This includes keeping your blood glucose levels under tight control, avoiding alcohol and smoking, exercising regularly, and keeping your weight under control.

Cardiovascular System

You probably don't even realize it, but as you go about your day, immersed in your various activities—sitting, standing, running, or sleeping—your heart rate and your blood pressure change. This happens automatically because your autonomic nerves control these functions. But if these nerves are damaged, your heart rate and blood pressure may be less responsive to these changing needs. If you have autonomic neuropathy, you may develop orthostatic hypotension, a condition in which your blood pressure drops very low when you stand up. You may also develop an abnormally high heart rate, because of damage to the nerves that control heart rhythm. Another problem with autonomic neuropathy is that you could have a so-called silent heart attack, a heart attack in which you are unable to feel the warning signs due to damage to the nerves that transmit pain signals.

Orthostatic Hypotension

When you stand up suddenly, blood tends to pool in your legs because of gravity. When this happens, less blood returns to your heart and is pumped out by your heart, and your blood pressure falls. Normally, your body rapidly responds to this by signaling the heart to beat faster and stronger, constricting your blood vessels, and blood pressure is quickly restored. However, if you have neuropathy, the signal to change the heart rate and blood pressure is impaired and low blood pressure results.

■ SYMPTOMS

Orthostatic hypotension is marked by a feeling of faintness, light-headedness, dizziness, confusion, blurred vision, or even fainting and convulsions. This is most likely to happen when you get out of bed suddenly or stand up after sitting for a long period of time. The condition is made worse when you are tired, have recently exercised, have eaten a heavy meal, or drunk alcohol.

■ WHAT TO DO

If you frequently feel the symptoms of hypotension when standing suddenly, tell your doctor or health care provider. It is important to first rule out any other condition that may be causing the same problem. If you experience any episode of fainting or convulsions, seek emergency help right away. If you have a history of high blood pressure it is especially important to alert your doctor to this condition.

Your doctor will diagnose orthostatic hypotension by checking your blood pressure in sitting, standing, and reclining positions. If your blood pressure goes down when you stand up but returns to normal when you lie down, you most likely have orthostatic hypotension.

■ TREATMENT

If you are diagnosed with orthostatic hypotension, you can take certain precautions to minimize the symptoms. Avoid standing up suddenly from a sitting or reclining position. If you are lying down, sit up for a minute or two before standing. If you are sitting, stand up slowly. Also avoid sitting or standing still for long periods of time. If you are sitting, get up every now and then and walk around. If your condition occurs because of prolonged bed rest, sitting up in bed from time to time may help. Elevating the head of your bed may also help.

If low blood pressure is occurring because blood is pooling in your legs, then you might find it helpful to wear waist-high support stockings or fitted elastic hose. Make sure to put the stockings on before you get up. In severe cases, your doctor may suggest a total body stocking.

Trying to keep your blood pressure high enough when you stand up must be balanced with not letting it get too high at other times. Make sure that your salt intake is high enough to keep your blood volume large enough. But check with your doctor before you make any changes in your diet, especially if you have high blood pressure.

Your doctor may also suggest one of several medications. Fludrocortisone (Florinef) may help expand your blood volume, which will help prevent your blood pressure from falling too low. However, these drugs can increase the risk of developing high blood pressure or congestive heart failure. Alert your doctor right away if you notice any kind of edema, or swelling. Other medications can work more directly on the blood vessels. These include phenylephrine, ephedrine, Neo-Synephrine nasal spray, beta-blockers, clonidine, octreotide, and Epogen.

Some patients may find some relief with propanolol (Inderal). Some people also experience low blood pressure after eating, especially in the morning. This condition can be helped by octreotide (Sandostatin).

Abnormal Heart Rate

If neuropathy affects the nerves that control your heart rate, you may have an excessively high heart rate, whether you are standing, sitting, exercising, resting, or sleeping. Your heart rate does not change to accommodate the varying needs of your body.

■ SYMPTOMS

You probably won't really feel any pain if neuropathy affects your heart rate. However, you may get the feeling that your heart is racing, even when you are resting. You can check your pulse before and immediately after exercising, as well as an hour after exercising. To do this, find a pulse in your wrist, neck, or other convenient location. Count the beats in a 15-second period and multiply by 4. This gives you your heart rate in beats per minute. Your heart rate should increase during and immediately after exercising (by as much as much as 2- to 3-fold, depending on how strenuous the exercise.) But after an hour's rest, your heart rate should return to preexercise levels. If your heart rate remains high all the time and does not change much (more than 15 percent) in response to various activities and stress, then you may have neuropathy.

■ WHAT TO DO

If you suspect that your heart rate is abnormally high, talk to your doctor. For most people, a normal heart rate is in the range of 60 to 100 beats per minute. It can rise to 120 to 180 beats per minute during exercise. For younger people and those who are physically fit, the resting heart rate can be much lower. If your heart rate is consistently on the high end of this range, or higher, tell your doctor. You will most likely be tested to see if this is a neuropathy-related condition. This condition is potentially serious, for it increases your risk of irregular heartbeat and it may prevent you from feeling the pain of the symptoms of heart attack (see Silent Heart Attack, page 213).

Your doctor may check for changes in your heart rate as you breathe deeply. Or your heart rate may be measured before and during exercise. You may be hooked up to an electrocardiogram or other specialized computer program during this evaluation.

■ TREATMENT

Unfortunately, few satisfactory remedies are available to control the abnormal heart rate due to autonomic neuropathy. Several experimental therapies for neuropathy in general show some promise, and studies are ongoing in this and other countries. These therapies include nutritional factors and dietary supplements, such as vitamins A, B12, and B6, aldose reductase inhibitors, myo-inositol, and evening primrose oil. However, none of these therapies is proven to be effective in widespread studies. Talk to your doctor about the best way to manage cardiac problems resulting from diabetic neuropathy.

■ PREVENTION

Because there are few treatments to alleviate the cardiac problems resulting from autonomic neuropathy, it is especially important to keep blood glucose levels under control. If you have any of the symptoms associated with neuropathy, especially with cardiac complications, you may want to consider maintaining tight control of your blood glucose level. Talk to your doctor or diabetes educator about developing an intensive therapy program.

Silent Heart Attack

A major complication of diabetic neuropathy is the so-called silent heart attack. Often people at risk for heart attack experience warning signs, such as angina, or heart pain. But if your neuropathy is severe, you may not receive any warning that a heart attack is impending. If neuropathy is severe, you may even have a heart attack without experiencing any pain.

■ SYMPTOMS

Unfortunately, with autonomic neuropathy that affects the cardiovascular system, you may not really feel any of the symptoms of a heart attack. Typically, you feel crushing pain in the chest or arms if you are having a heart attack. But with neuropathy, you may not feel this pain at all. The only symptoms you may feel are perspiration, shortness of breath, or fatigue. Another sign that you could be having a heart attack is an unexplained episode of hyperglycemia, or blood glucose levels that go suddenly out of control.

If you have any symptoms of a heart attack, with or without chest pain, call for emergency help at once, especially if you have any history of neuropathy. If you are at risk for a heart attack, talk to your doctor in advance about what to look for and what you should do if you think you are having a heart attack. Do not worry about false alarms. This is a life-threatening situation that should receive immediate attention.

■ TREATMENT

Unfortunately, there are few treatments available to deal with the neuropathy that can lead to a silent heart attack. However, if you are at risk for a heart attack or have had a heart attack, there are several treatments that are mainly aimed at preventing another heart attack from occurring. These include surgery and drug therapy (see Chapter 6).

■ PREVENTION

The best way to prevent a silent heart attack from occurring is to take steps to prevent neuropathy from developing and to prevent heart disease. Have your cholesterol levels checked, and if they are high, take steps to lower your cholesterol level through diet and exercise. If you smoke or drink alcohol, stop. Talk to your doctor about an exercise program that will work for you. Talk to your dietitian about developing a meal plan that will keep your cholesterol and lipid levels low and your blood glucose levels in control. The DCCT showed that you can lower your risk of neuropathy by 60 percent and your risk of cardiovascular disease by 35 percent following a program of intensive therapy. Talk to your doctor about whether this plan would work for you and how to go about implementing it. Even if you don't practice intensive therapy, maintaining your blood glucose levels as close to normal as you can will help control both neuropathy and cardiovascular disease.

Skin and Sweating

Your body regulates your temperature through the skin. Sweating is one way to decrease your body temperature when you get too hot. Your body does this automatically through the sudomotor nerves, which control where and how much you sweat. If you have neuropathy, these nerves may become damaged. Many people with autonomic neuropathy are unable to sweat through the hands and feet, but sweat excessively through the face and trunk. This may be because your body needs to get rid of excess heat. When the peripheral nerves to the arms and legs are damaged, you don't sweat there. Instead, your body sweats more in the face and trunk to make up for the loss of sweating in the arms and legs.

■ SYMPTOMS

When the sudomotor nerves are damaged, you may notice an excessive amount of sweating in your face and on the trunk of your body. You may also notice that you sweat more when you eat certain foods, such as spicy dishes, cheese, chocolate, red sausage, red wine, and even some soft drinks.

You may be less aware that you are not sweating as much in your hands and feet. However, you may notice that the skin on your hands and feet is especially dry and that your hands and feet may be colder than normal. Your skin may also thicken on your feet and hands and be more likely to crack and develop infections.

■ WHAT TO DO

If autonomic neuropathy affects your pattern of sweating, you should talk to your doctor about ways to minimize the symptoms. Avoid extremes of heat and humidity, because your body has a difficult time regulating your body temperature. To treat your dry skin, it is important to use creams and lubricating oils to help retain moisture. Keep on the lookout for any cracks or lesions in the skin. You may need to apply an antibacterial ointment to keep an infection from developing. If your sweating is severe, your doctor may prescribe one of several drugs to help alleviate the problem, such as propantheline hydrobromide, scopolamine patches, or a cholinergic blocker.

Hypoglycemia Unawareness

One serious complication of autonomic neuropathy is hypoglycemia unawareness. When your blood glucose levels get too low, your body releases hormones that cause the liver to release more glucose. Your body also sends out messages that your blood glucose is too low. These signs of hypoglycemia, triggered by the release of the hormone epi-

nephrine, include heart palpitations, irregular heartbeat, anxiety, shakiness, anxiety, and tingling in the mouth.

■ SYMPTOMS

When you have hypoglycemia unawareness, you no longer can detect
the symptoms of hypoglycemia. The only signs that hypoglycemia may
be occurring are the effects of low blood sugar on the brain: irritability,
tiredness, confusion, forgetfulness, and loss of consciousness. Unfortunately, these effects make it even less likely that you will notice that
you have hypoglycemia. The normal warning signs of hypoglycemia—
sweating, palpitations, shakiness, anxiety, and a tingling sensation in
your fingers or toes—are absent or diminished. The longer you have
diabetes, the more likely you are to develop hypoglycemia unawareness.

■ WHAT TO DO

If you suspect you have hypoglycemia unawareness, talk to your doctor
about the best way to treat it. Practicing intensive therapy, for example,
can reduce the risk of neuropathy that triggers hypoglycemia, but it can
also increase the risk of hypoglycemia because you are practicing such
tight control.

The best way to deal with hypoglycemia unawareness is to test your
blood glucose level frequently, especially before meals, before exercising, before bedtime, and before driving a vehicle. If your blood glucose
levels are low, you may need to eat more with your meal or have an
extra snack. Keep a fast-acting carbohydrate snack with you at all times.

Make sure those around you know how to recognize the warning
signs of hypoglycemia. They may be able to notice signals of which you
are unaware, such as irritability, confusion, and forgetfulness. Make sure
your companions know how to administer glucagon and know when to
call for emergency help. Make sure you wear a tag or bracelet that identifies you as having diabetes, so that those around you will know to call
for emergency help.

If your hypoglycemia unawareness is especially frequent, you may
want to consider adjusting your blood glucose goals. Talk to your doctor
about what goals are best for you. (For more information on hypoglycemia, see Chapter 2.)

Chapter 8
Solving Kidney Problems

Your kidneys serve as a collection of tiny filter units that filter out all the toxins and waste products from your blood. Blood enters the kidneys through small blood vessels called capillaries into a complex of tiny blood vessel loops. Through these blood vessels, the blood is filtered. The blood, cleansed of toxins and waste, then reenters the bloodstream, and the waste goes through a series of tubules in the kidneys and is changed into urine. Urine is then sent to the bladder for storage and removal from the body.

If you have diabetic nephropathy, or kidney disease, the capillaries become damaged and are unable to filter the blood properly. They can become blocked, so that not all the wastes and toxins are removed from the blood. They also can become leaky, so that some of the proteins and nutrients that should remain in the blood are excreted into the urine.

It takes a long time for you to feel the effects of kidney damage. Nephropathy progresses through five stages: hyperfiltration, microalbuminuria, nephrotic syndrome, renal insufficiency, and end-stage renal disease. In the early stages, it just means your kidneys have to work over-time to get rid of all the toxic and unwanted products in your blood. But as damage to the kidneys progresses, they cannot keep up with the workload and eventually begin to fail. At this point you may begin to notice the symptoms of kidney damage. Fortunately, there are tests your doctor can perform to detect the early stages of kidney disease. By paying attention to these early signs, you can take steps to prevent or delay serious kidney damage and live a longer and healthier life.

Hyperfiltration

The first sign that your kidneys are damaged is that they are working overtime or hyperfiltering. If you have hyperfiltration, then a higher-than-normal amount of blood is filtered through your kidneys every hour. Hyperfiltration is quite common in the early stages of diabetes. As many as 70 percent of people with type 1 diabetes and 33 percent of people with type 2 diabetes have hyperfiltration early in the course of diabetes. However, less than 50 percent of people with diabetes who have hyperfiltration develop end-stage renal disease, or kidney failure.

■ SYMPTOMS

There are no symptoms for hyperfiltration. The only way to know for sure that you have it is through tests that your doctor can do. Patients with hyperfiltration typically have enlarged kidneys, a high rate of filtration of blood, and an increased rate of clearance of substances from the blood. Your doctor can evaluate whether any of these indicate that you may have hyperfiltration.

■ WHAT TO DO

If you have diabetes, your doctor should be regularly evaluating your kidney function. If any tests indicate that you may have hyperfiltration, you will want to take steps to control your blood glucose levels and your blood pressure. Usually, bringing your blood glucose under control decreases the size of your kidneys and reduces the rate of filtration to within normal levels.

■ PREVENTION

The best way to prevent hyperfiltration from occurring and from progressing to more serious forms of nephropathy is to keep your blood glucose levels under control. If you practice tight control, or intensive therapy, you are 35 to 55 percent less likely to develop kidney disease than is someone who controls diabetes using a standard approach. (For more on intensive therapy, see Chapter 4.)

Microalbuminuria

Microalbuminuria occurs when small amounts of a blood protein known as albumin start to show up in the urine. People without diabetes usually excrete less than 25 mg of albumin in their urine each day. But people with microalbuminuria typically excrete 30 to 300 mg of albumin per day. Microalbuminuria is often present in patients with type 2 diabetes when they are diagnosed with diabetes and usually develops in patients with type 1 diabetes after a year or more. It is important to detect microalbuminuria early to prevent further damage to the kidneys, especially if you have type 1 diabetes. Also, among people with type 2 diabetes, high blood pressure is associated with microalbuminuria. If you have type 2 diabetes and microalbuminuria, you are more likely to have a heart attack or stroke. Therefore, whether you have type 1 or type 2 diabetes, dealing with microalbuminuria early on is a good way to prevent or delay further kidney damage and to reduce the risk of heart attack, stroke, or other serious conditions.

■ SYMPTOMS

If you have microalbuminuria, you will not feel any outward signs or symptoms. The only way to know for sure if you have this condition is through a specific laboratory test conducted by your doctor.

■ WHAT TO DO

If you have had diabetes for a while or even if you are newly diagnosed, your doctor should be testing for microalbuminuria during your routine physical examinations. She will conduct a test that is more sensitive for finding protein in the urine than the routine dipstick tests you may be accustomed to. You will probably be asked to collect a specimen of urine first thing in the morning and bring it to your doctor's office. If this test is positive, you may then be tested for total albumin content. You may be tested on more than one occasion, because the level of albumin in your urine can vary from day to day and throughout the day, depending on your activities. Once you have begun treatment, your doctor may want to retest to see if there is any improvement.

■ TREATMENT

If you do have microalbuminuria, there are changes occurring in the blood vessels in your kidneys that filter out impurities. When these filters in your kidneys are damaged, protein from the blood leaks out. Blood pressure within the kidneys is also elevated and appears to contribute to the problem. Your doctor will probably advise treatment with an angiotensin-converting enzyme (ACE) inhibitor. These drugs lower blood pressure by blocking enzymes that constrict blood vessels. Lowering blood pressure within the kidney's filtering units reduces damage to the kidneys. As a result, less protein will leak into your urine. Your doctor will most likely want to continue testing for microalbuminuria on a routine basis to monitor the condition of your kidneys.

■ PREVENTION

To prevent microalbuminuria and other stages of nephropathy from occurring or to delay their progression, it is important to control high blood pressure, to keep blood glucose levels under control, and to eat a balanced diet. Preventive measures are extremely important at this stage and sooner, because once the disease progresses beyond this point, it is sometimes difficult to prevent end-stage renal failure. If you take action now to lower your blood pressure and control your blood glucose level, it is possible to prevent diabetic nephropathy from progressing.

The single most important step you can take is to control your blood pressure. Early detection is essential. High blood pressure, or hypertension, is defined as anything greater than 130/85 mmHg. If your blood pressure is above this, it is likely to contribute to further damage to the kidneys. If you show signs of hyperfiltration or microalbuminuria, your doctor may want to put you on blood pressure–lowering medications even if your blood pressure is below this value. Your doctor may also recommend controlling the salt in your diet and trying to incorporate a regular exercise program into your daily activities to help control high blood pressure.

Keeping your blood glucose levels under control can also help slow the progression of kidney disease. During the Diabetes Control and Complications Trial, people with type 1 diabetes who maintained tight control decreased their risk of kidney disease by 35 to 56 percent. Even if you do not practice intensive therapy, keeping your blood glucose levels as close to normal as you can will help reduce the risk of damage to the kidneys.

Also talk to your doctor about other things that can harm your kidneys and contribute to kidney disease. In general, you want to avoid anything that could compromise the function of your kidneys. Many over-the-counter drugs can damage kidney tissue. These include ibuprofen (Advil, Motrin, and others) and naproxen (Aleve). Other prescription anti-inflammatory drugs, antibiotics such as cisplatin, and some drugs used to treat psychiatric disorders, such as lithium, can also damage the kidneys. If your kidneys are already damaged, the risk of further injury is even greater. Always talk to your doctor about any prescription or nonprescription medication before you take it. This includes any herbal or so-called natural remedies. You and your doctor should consider both the risks and the benefits of any medication before you decide whether to take it.

If you need to have any X ray or radiographic imaging test done, make sure to talk to your doctor about the possible risks. Coronary angiograms, which evaluate the condition of your blood vessels, and intravenous pyelograms, used to examine the condition of your kidneys, all use a radioactive tracer dye that is injected into your bloodstream. These dyes put you at risk for kidney failure a few days after injection, because they are filtered through your kidneys. Often the condition can be reversed, but it may require kidney dialysis. However, there may be circumstances under which such a procedure is necessary—an emergency coronary artery bypass surgery, for example. If this is the case, your doctors will want to take precautions to minimize the risk. This can be done by giving you extra fluids before and after the procedure to dilute the dye, or by giving you certain drugs, such as theophylline plus allopurinol, that can decrease the risk of acute kidney failure.

If you have any history of neurogenic bladder, or any symptoms of urinary tract infections, incontinence, or an inability to fully empty the bladder, make sure to talk to your doctor right away. Even though it may be embarrassing to discuss some of these issues with your doctor, it is important, especially if there is evidence of kidney disease. When you are unable to fully empty your bladder, urine can back up into your kidneys and cause further damage. There are treatments for neurogenic bladder that can alleviate some of the problems associated with this condition.

Nephrotic Syndrome

As damage to the blood vessels that filter blood in the kidneys progresses, more and more protein from the blood leaks into the urine. In the early stages, the amount of leakage is small and microalbuminuria results. But in later stages, the amount of protein leaking through is substantial. At this point, more than 3.5 grams of albumin pass through to the urine each day. When this happens, you have nephrotic syndrome.

If you have nephrotic syndrome, you are losing measurable amounts of protein from the blood. One of the jobs of the blood protein albumin is to hold the water in blood within the bloodstream. Without sufficient protein, water accumulates in the tissues of the body. In addition, the liver tries to synthesize more albumin to make up for the lost protein. In doing so, it also makes more cholesterol and fats, which create more health problems. At this point, you may begin to notice the symptoms of kidney disease.

Unfortunately, once you show signs of proteinuria—excessively high levels of protein in the urine—it is unlikely that you can prevent progression to end-stage renal disease, especially if you have type 1 diabetes. If you have type 2 diabetes, it is less likely that you will develop end-stage renal failure, but it is important to address the symptoms, because proteinuria is a predictor of stroke and cardiovascular disease. Approximately 80 percent of people with type 2 diabetes who develop nephrotic syndrome die within 10 years from cardiovascular complications and stroke. Therefore, it is extremely important to recognize and treat the problem as soon as possible.

■ SYMPTOMS

If you have nephrotic syndrome, you may feel bloated and heavy and notice swelling in your feet and hands. Fluid may accumulate in your abdomen, chest, and around your heart. You may carry up to 50 pounds in excess fluid retention. This can make you feel tired and short of breath. Your shoes and clothes may feel tight and it may be difficult to carry out even routine activities.

■ WHAT TO DO

If you feel any of the symptoms of nephrotic syndrome, talk to your doctor right away. There are steps you can take to delay the progression of kidney disease and to reduce the risk of complicating conditions such as cardiovascular disease and stroke.

It is also important not to dismiss your symptoms, because there may be other causes that may be contributing to your condition. For example, it is possible that a drug you are taking is contributing to your problem. Make sure your doctor is fully aware of any over-the-counter or prescription medications you are taking. Diabetic nephropathy almost always occurs in conjunction with retinopathy. If you have symptoms of nephropathy without any evidence of retinopathy, make sure you and your physician consider other causes of your kidney problems.

■ TREATMENT

Once nephropathy has progressed to the point of nephrotic syndrome, with protein in the urine, it is less likely that you will be able to prevent progression of the disease. However, you can slow the progression and the worsening of symptoms by controlling your blood pressure and blood glucose levels.

The most important first step is to get your blood pressure under control. To do this, your doctor will most likely prescribe a blood pressure–lowering medication such as an ACE inhibitor. Other drugs that your doctor may prescribe include calcium channel blockers, diuretics, and beta-blockers. Calcium channel blockers may decrease proteinuria and improve renal function and do not seem to impair glucose tolerance. However, you may notice an increase in water retention. Some diuretics can worsen insulin resistance and make it harder for you to control your blood glucose level. They can also increase the likelihood of arrhythmias. Beta-blockers are effective at lowering blood pressure, but they can increase the risk of hypoglycemia. If your doctor does prescribe a beta-blocker, you should monitor your blood glucose levels closely. You and your doctor should discuss the pros and cons of any high blood pressure medication. Your doctor will try to recommend a drug that will provide the maximum benefit to you with the lowest risk for introducing other problems.

If you are overweight, you should try to lose weight. If you are physically inactive, consider incorporating some sort of physical activity into your daily routine, even if it is just going for a walk each day or riding an exercise bike. Also, lower your salt intake, if necessary. You should not be taking in more than 4 to 5 grams of salt each day. Your doctor may suggest that you monitor your blood pressure at home on a daily basis.

■ PREVENTION

Once you develop nephrotic syndrome, it is unlikely you can halt the progression to end-stage renal failure, but you can slow the progression. The best way, of course, is to prevent progression to this stage. You can do this by lowering your blood pressure, keeping your blood glucose levels under control (practicing intensive therapy if possible), exercising regularly, eating a balanced diet low in fat, avoiding alcohol and smoking, and seeing your doctor regularly.

Renal Insufficiency

Sometimes, despite your best efforts, damage to your kidneys worsens. Your condition may progress to the point where your kidneys are no longer able to filter toxins from the blood and cannot keep protein from spilling over into the urine. When this happens, you may have renal insufficiency. This stage of nephropathy is also called clinical nephropathy or kidney failure.

Damage to the kidneys at this stage cannot be reversed by simple preventive measures such as lowering blood pressure and controlling blood glucose. However, paying attention to the same lifestyle factors can slow disease progression. At every stage of kidney disease it is important to control your blood pressure, blood glucose levels, and diet to minimize further damage to your kidneys. You may feel like giving up, but this is the last thing you should do. Even at this stage, treatments are available that can add years to your life.

■ SYMPTOMS

When your kidneys are working at less than 30 percent of their normal capacity, you may begin to feel more of the symptoms of kidney disease. You might feel listless, lose your appetite, find it difficult to concentrate, feel cold, experience bouts of nausea, and your skin may feel unusually itchy. When your kidneys begin to function at less that 15 percent, you may notice that your skin bruises easily and you may lose weight without trying. You may vomit intermittently and experience lethargy and restless legs. You may also feel sleepy or unnaturally drowsy during the day but find it difficult to sleep at night. If you take insulin, you may need less, because less insulin is passing through your kidneys. Clinically, your doctor may also detect anemia, or low iron.

■ WHAT TO DO

If you notice any change in your general state of health or notice any change in your symptoms or new symptoms developing, talk to your doctor. You should be seeing your doctor regularly. Your doctor will routinely examine you and conduct tests to keep tabs on your kidney function. As your kidneys begin to fail, they do a poorer job of filtering impurities and toxins from the blood. Your doctor can get an idea of how your kidneys function by measuring the levels of some of these impurities in the blood. One test, called a BUN, measures the amount of nitrogen in the form of urea that is in the blood. (Urea is a breakdown product of protein degradation.) You probably will also be tested for the amount of creatinine, another metabolic waste product, in your blood or serum. When your serum creatinine levels rise above 2.0 mg/dl, you may be referred to a nephrologist, a doctor who specializes in kidneys. At this point, you, your doctor, and your nephrologist may want to come up with a more aggressive treatment plan.

■ TREATMENT

You and your doctor will want to take several factors into account in developing a treatment or management plan at this stage. In general, you will want to identify and eliminate anything that may be damaging your kidneys, such as a drug or lifestyle factor.

You will also want to continue to keep your blood pressure, blood glucose, metabolic factors, and diet under control to keep your kidneys functioning as efficiently as possible. You may need to reevaluate your blood pressure medication and other drugs you may be taking. Some drugs, including several blood pressure medications, can cause damage to the liver. You and your doctor will want to discuss the pros and cons of any such drug.

Your doctor may also recommend a diet that is low in protein. Several studies have shown that a diet containing no more than 40 to 60 grams of protein each day slows the loss of kidney function.

You and your doctor may also want to reevaluate your blood glucose goals. Once your kidneys have begun to fail, it may not do that much good to maintain an intensive therapy program. If you are practicing tight control, you may face a higher risk of hypoglycemia without the benefit of preventing kidney damage. Therefore, you and your doctor should discuss whether tight control is a prudent goal.

Because the kidney produces many hormones that affect your electrolyte balance, damage to the kidneys can disturb your overall metabolism. For example, potassium and salt levels may become unbalanced.

Some patients may retain excessively high levels of salt and/or potassium, while others may lose large amounts of salt from the body. Your doctor will monitor the levels of salt and other metabolites and may recommend dietary or drug therapy to keep your metabolites in balance. Improper balance of salts and electrolytes can stress the cardiovascular system and can lead to cardiac arrest.

At this point, you and your doctor should also discuss the possibility of future therapy. As kidney damage progresses, you may eventually face the decision of electing a kidney transplant or dialysis. You and your doctor should talk about the pros and cons of these major therapeutic interventions. You may continue for several years in a state of renal insufficiency but should prepare yourself for what to do when you reach end-stage renal disease.

End-Stage Renal Disease

Eventually, your kidneys may become damaged so much that they can no longer function. When this happens, you have end-stage renal disease. If left untreated, your kidneys will be unable to filter your blood adequately. Metabolic wastes, such as urea and creatinine, as well as salts and electrolytes can rise to toxic levels. Fluid can accumulate in all the tissues of your body, including the sack that surrounds your heart. This makes it increasingly difficult for your heart to pump blood. At this point, to continue living, you need to turn to dialysis or kidney transplant.

■ SYMPTOMS

Symptoms of end-stage renal disease include edema, or swelling, in the extremities, particularly the ankles, and in the face, especially around the eyes. Fluid accumulation around the heart and lungs may make you especially tired and short of breath. Even simple tasks may become difficult. You may also have muscle cramps, especially in the digestive tract, which can lead to nausea and vomiting. The bowel can become bloated and sometimes gastrointestinal ulcers develop. Skin can take on an orange-yellow color and muscle and fat may begin to waste away. People with end-stage renal disease often notice blood in their urine. Sleeping patterns may also be disturbed. Neurological symptoms, including convulsions and seizures, can also occur.

■ WHAT TO DO

You should be visiting your doctor regularly. During your visits, your doctor may run some tests to monitor your kidney function. If you experience any worsening of symptoms, any new symptoms, or a general change in how you feel, make sure to tell your doctor right away. Once you develop end-stage renal disease, you need a more aggressive treatment.

■ TREATMENT

If you have end-stage renal disease, you need a treatment that will do the job of filtering impurities from your blood, because your kidneys can no longer perform this function. Currently, three treatment options are available: hemodialysis, peritoneal dialysis, and a kidney transplant.

Dialysis is a way of removing the waste products and toxins from your blood without getting rid of the blood cells that you need. With hemodialysis, your blood flows from your arm, through a machine that purifies your blood, and then back into your arm to your bloodstream. With peritoneal dialysis, a solution is put into your abdominal cavity and drained at regular intervals. This solution, known as a dialysate, removes the impurities from your blood.

Eighty percent of all patients with end-stage renal disease are treated with hemodialysis. If you decide on this treatment, you will most likely visit a dialysis center or clinic three times a week. You will be hooked up to the machine, which functions as an artificial kidney, for 4 to 6 hours during each visit. The disadvantages of hemodialysis are the time commitment and expense, the risk of clotting at the access point (the site at which blood is removed and returned to the body), and the possibility of hemorrhage and infection. Usually, patients undergoing hemodialysis must take an anti-clotting drug, such as heparin. About 80 percent of all patients treated by hemodialysis survive the first year of treatment.

Peritoneal dialysis is another method of cleansing the blood through dialysis. The most common method of peritoneal dialysis is called constant ambulatory peritoneal dialysis. It performs the same function as hemodialysis. But instead of removing blood from the body and cleansing it in a machine, you infuse a solution of dialysate into the peritoneal cavity, your abdominal cavity. There blood from the blood vessels that line the cavity is diluted by the dialysate. The impurities remain in the dialysate in your abdomen while the clean blood moves on to the rest of the body. You then drain the dialysate and remove the impurities from your body. This procedure is repeated every 4 to 6 hours. Your abdomen, in essence, acts as an artificial kidney to clean the blood from your body.

There are several advantages to peritoneal dialysis. You don't have to visit a hospital or clinic as often and are not hooked up to a machine for long periods of time. You can perform the treatment yourself. Also, you don't need to take heparin or another anti-clotting drug. This treatment appears to provide the best hope for rehabilitation and promotes the longest survival rate of any dialysis technique. However, it requires a high degree of patient motivation. The technique also has its disadvantages. You have to pay constant attention to fluid exchange and are at risk for peritonitis, an infection of the lining of the stomach.

By far, the most successful treatment for end-stage renal disease is kidney transplant. During this procedure, your kidney is removed and replaced with a healthy kidney from a living donor, usually a relative or friend, or from someone who has recently died. Usually, people who have kidney transplants are able to completely renew the activities they enjoyed before developing nephropathy.

The biggest disadvantage of a kidney transplant is the threat of rejection of the new kidney by your immune system. Your immune system will see a new kidney as a foreign invader and try to get rid of it. You will be given drugs that suppress the immune system to let your new kidney survive and do its job. Unfortunately, these drugs are toxic and can cause damage to the new kidney.

More than 90 percent of people who get a new kidney survive the first year. This is a greater success rate than dialysis. Twenty percent of people who elect transplants survive more than 10 years. Transplants are highly recommended if you are newly diagnosed with diabetes and end-stage renal disease and if you are under the age of 60.

Many people with type 1 diabetes who decide to have a kidney transplant also elect to have a pancreas transplant done at the same time. This is because the major disadvantage of any transplant is the immunosuppressive drugs that must be taken. But if you are taking them anyway for a kidney transplant, it may make sense to have a pancreas transplant done also. You reap a greater benefit for the same risk. (For more on pancreas transplants, see page 146.)

Make sure to discuss the pros and cons of each treatment with your doctor well before the point at which you need immediate attention. Finding a donor may take time, and it helps to plan ahead, before your condition becomes critical. Often patients awaiting transplant will go on dialysis until an organ becomes available.

Chapter 9
Solving Vision Problems

Whether you have diabetes or not, problems with the eyes are inevitable as you age. But if you have diabetes, you are likely to experience more eye problems and at an earlier age than people without diabetes.

Visual images, or the things you see in the world around you, come into your eye as light. Light enters the eye through your pupil. The cornea and lens that cover your pupil focus the light, which then travels through the posterior segment of your eye. This part of your eye is filled with a gel-like substance known as the vitreous humor. The light passes through the vitreous humor to the back of the eyeball until it hits your retina, the light-sensing part of your eye. Light hitting on the retina transmits signals to your brain through the optic nerve. These signals allow you to see. The brain processes these signals as visual images, or sight. Other nerves also control the way your eyes move, how they focus, and how they adjust pupil size to allow for changes in lightness and darkness.

For your eyes to function properly, you need a good, steady supply of blood to the retinas, to bring them the nutrients they need. Damage to these blood vessels can threaten your vision. Your eyes also depend on healthy nerves to transmit optical signals and to control eye movements. If any of these nerves are damaged, you will experience vision problems. Because diabetes can cause damage to both blood vessels and nerve fibers, the eyes are especially susceptible to problems in people with diabetes.

Some of the eye problems caused by diabetes are mild and easily reversed. Often, maintaining good blood glucose control is enough to make them go away. But other problems can jeopardize your sight and cause blindness if not treated properly. Almost all vision problems triggered by diabetes are treatable if caught early enough. However, most vision problems are not painful and may at first seem like minor nuisances. It is easy to put off doing something about these problems. But that's the worst thing you can do. Anytime you notice a change in how you see things, contact your eye doctor right away. And even if you don't notice any changes, you should see your eye doctor at least once a year. You may even be completely unaware of some of the changes to your eyes caused by diabetes. Therefore, it is extremely important that you see an eye-care specialist on a regular basis.

Retinopathy

The retina is the light-sensing part of your eye, located along the back wall of your eye. It contains the rod and cone cells, which detect light and send a signal to your brain. The retina contains many small blood vessels that supply the retina with the blood, oxygen, and nutrients it needs to function. Unfortunately, these blood vessels can be easily damaged. Poor blood glucose control can change the way your blood flows and can weaken the walls of these blood vessels. When the blood vessels become damaged, retinopathy can occur. Early on, damage to the blood vessels is minimal and can be easily treated. This stage is known as nonproliferative retinopathy. If left untreated, it can progress to proliferative retinopathy, a much more dangerous condition. During either stage of retinopathy, macular edema can occur. This is caused by leakage of fluid into the macula, the region of the retina responsible for color vision and visual acuity. Macular edema can cause loss of vision if not treated.

If you have type 1 diabetes, you will probably not develop retinopathy until you have had diabetes for several years. After 10 years, however, more than half of people with type 1 have retinopathy in one form or another. After 15 years, almost all people with type 1 diabetes have retinopathy. However, only half of all people with type 1 will develop proliferative retinopathy.

On the other hand, if you have type 2 diabetes, you are more likely to have retinopathy at diagnosis and more likely to develop retinopathy early on in the course of diabetes. Twenty percent of all people with type 2 diabetes will have retinopathy at diagnosis. After 15 years, 60 to

85 percent of people with type 2 have retinopathy. At this point, up to 20 percent will also have proliferative retinopathy.

The good news is that retinopathy is preventable. The Diabetes Control and Complications Trial (DCCT) showed that maintaining tight control of blood glucose levels reduced the risk of retinopathy by 76 percent. Early treatment and maintaining good blood glucose control can go a long way in preventing vision loss from retinopathy.

Nonproliferative Retinopathy

If you maintain poor control of blood glucose, the blood vessels that supply your retina can become damaged. When this happens, the blood vessel walls can balloon out, creating tiny aneurysms. This causes the tissue in your retina to swell, a condition known as edema. The blood vessels can also rupture, or hemorrhage, and leak fluid or blood into the retina. When this occurs you have nonproliferative retinopathy. Your retina is cut off from the supply of oxygen and nutrients it needs and doesn't function properly. At this stage, you may experience vision problems or you may be unaware of the problem. If detected early enough, nonproliferative retinopathy can be treated and reversed. However, if left untreated, it can progress to proliferative retinopathy.

■ SYMPTOMS

Unfortunately, nonproliferative retinopathy is often symptomless, especially in the early stages. You may find that parts of your field of vision are distorted, but in the early stages you will probably not experience vision loss, unless macular edema is also present.

Although you may not feel symptoms, your eye doctor can detect nonproliferative retinopathy. The only way to know for sure is through a thorough eye exam conducted by an ophthalmologist.

■ WHAT TO DO

If you have diabetes, you should have a yearly eye exam by an ophthalmologist whether or not you have any symptoms. If you have any symptoms or notice any changes in your vision, tell your doctor or ophthalmologist right away. During your eye exam, your doctor should measure how well you can see (visual acuity), evaluate how you move your eyes, determine whether you need glasses, screen for glaucoma and cataracts, and evaluate changes in both color perception and night vision. Your retina should also be thoroughly examined. This is done by first dilating the pupil, then using one of several techniques to examine the retina. Using an ophthalmoscope, your ophthalmologist can get a magnified view of your retina and look for any changes or irregularities of the optic nerve, the macula, and the blood vessels of the retina. If there is any hemorrhaging, swelling, or new blood vessel formation, your ophthalmologist can detect it.

Your ophthalmologist may also perform a fluorescein angiography test. Using this method, a fluorescent dye is injected into your arm. The flow of dye through the retina is tracked using a special camera. Healthy blood vessels will keep the blood flowing and will not leak, but damaged blood vessels will leak blood and dye. This will help your doctor pinpoint areas in your retina that may require treatment. It will also reveal whether you have any macular swelling that could interfere with vision. After a fluorescein angiogram, you may notice blurred vision, but this condition is temporary. Your normal vision should return rapidly. You may also notice that your skin takes on a tan or yellow appearance for 24 hours and that your urine glows, or takes on an unusual color. This dye is safe, even in people with kidney disease.

Another test your ophthalmologist may perform is ultrasonography. This technique uses sound waves to get a picture of your retina. This is especially helpful for people who have cataracts or hemorrhaging in the vitreous humor. Unlike the angiography, it does not provide a detailed view of blood flow through your retina. Instead, it can tell your doctor whether there is any scarring or retinal detachment.

Other tests may provide additional information. Optical coherence tomography, for example, measures the thickness of the retina and can tell whether you have edema in the retina.

■ TREATMENT

The type of treatment depends on the severity of retinopathy. Nonproliferative retinopathy can be classified as mild, moderate, or severe. If you have mild nonproliferative retinopathy, you may have several microaneurysms, or small areas of ballooning, in your blood vessels. These lesions usually resolve with time or show no change over months and probably require no further treatment. If you have mild nonproliferative retinopathy, you should visit your eye specialist every 9 to 12 months.

If you have moderate nonproliferative retinopathy, you may have more microaneurysms and retinal hemorrhaging. Your doctor may also notice other changes, such as vascular abnormalities and cotton-wool spots—areas of necrosis, or cell death—in the nerve fibers of the retina. If your doctor tells you that you have moderate nonproliferative retinopathy, then you are at greater risk of progressing to proliferative retinopathy and should see your ophthalmologist every 4 to 6 months.

Severe nonproliferative retinopathy involves more extensive hemorrhaging, microaneurysms, and vascular abnormalities. If untreated, half of all cases of severe nonproliferative retinopathy will progress to proliferative retinopathy within 2 years. If you have this condition, you should be treated right away.

If your doctor detects any areas of leakage, she may elect to perform laser surgery to seal off any blood vessels that are leaking. A laser is an instrument that sends out light of a particular wavelength. Laser light can penetrate deep into the retina, where light energy is converted to heat. By selecting specific wavelengths of light, your doctor can zero in on certain kinds of cells or tissues that she may want to destroy without damaging healthy tissues. Laser surgery is usually done in your doctor's office on an outpatient basis. This is performed after fluorescein angiography or a similar test is used to pinpoint specific leaks. Your doctor uses a laser tuned to a specific wavelength of light and aims it at the area requiring treatment. The laser coagulates the blood around the hole in the blood vessel to seal the leak. Laser treatment can also make it easier for the retina to absorb the leakage. However, new zones of leakage could develop over time, which would require additional surgery later on.

If you have any evidence of retinopathy, it is very important to control your blood glucose levels. This is the single most important step you can take to prevent nonproliferative retinopathy from progressing to proliferative retinopathy, a much more serious condition.

■ PREVENTION

If you have diabetes, either type 1 or type 2, you are at risk for developing retinopathy. The best thing you can do is to control your blood glucose levels. At the early stages, this can reverse the effects of nonproliferative retinopathy, and at later stages, it can prevent retinopathy from progressing. The DCCT found that you can reduce the risk of retinopathy by over 75 percent by tightly controlling your blood glucose levels.

Proliferative Retinopathy

As nonproliferative retinopathy gets more severe, the retina receives less oxygen and nutrients than it needs to function. When this occurs, the retina tries to make up for the lack of blood by sending out growth factors that cause new blood vessels to proliferate, or grow. These new blood vessels do more harm than good. They do not supply the retina with the blood it needs and they get in the way. They are fragile and can easily burst. They can get in between the retina and the vitreous humor, cause bleeding, and interfere with the path of light. Scar tissue can form and pull the retina, causing it to detach from the eye. When this happens, the rods and cones stop working and you can no longer see. Because this stage is marked by the proliferation of abnormal blood vessels, it is called proliferative retinopathy. This is a serious condition that, if left untreated, can lead to blindness.

■ SYMPTOMS

Symptoms of proliferative retinopathy include blurred or fluctuating vision, floating spots, distortion or warping of straight lines, and loss of vision. If you see any sort of distortion of straight lines, this could be a sign of macular edema (see below). Floating spots often occur as you age, but they could also be a sign of vitreous hemorrhage. A blockage of vision that looks as if a window shade is being pulled down across your field of view could indicate a detached retina.

■ WHAT TO DO

If you have any symptoms of retinopathy, notify your doctor and get an eye exam right away. Your exam should be performed by an ophthalmologist. The sort of exam you undergo to get a prescription for eyeglasses is not enough. You need to see someone who will exam both the retina and the lens. Your eye doctor will test your vision, test your eye movement, test for cataracts, and test for color and night vision. She will also dilate your pupils and examine your eyes with an ophthalmoscope, which will provide a clear view into the retina. If you have proliferative retinopathy, your eye doctor may be able to detect any scar tissues on the surface of the retina, or hemorrhaging in the vitreous cavity. She will also be able to detect any leakage, swelling, or growth of new blood vessels characteristic of proliferative retinopathy.

Other tests may also be conducted, such as ultrasonography. This technique uses sound waves to construct a picture of the back of the eye. It is particularly useful in people who have obstructions in the eye that make it difficult to directly view the retina, such as cataracts or vitreal bleeding. It can be used to see scar tissue on the surface of the retina or detect a detached retina. However, it does not give information about abnormalities in the circulation. Fluorescein angiography can be used to accurately pinpoint any leaks or blockages in your blood vessels and signs of edema. However, angiography is not routinely used to detect proliferative retinopathy, unless hidden zones of blood vessel growth are suspected.

■ TREATMENT

Proliferative retinopathy can be treated with laser treatment, cryotherapy, or vitrectomy. Your eye doctor will decide on the best treatment depending on what your particular problem is. Retinopathy is typically characterized by the growth of new blood vessels in the retina that don't belong there. But there can be other conditions that coexist with the proliferation of blood vessels. You might have only new vascular growth. Or you could have vascularization along with macular edema, and this would require a different course of treatment. Or you might have hemorrhaging or scar tissue pulling on your retina, in addition to vascular growth. Sometimes, patients will even have new blood vessels growing in the iris as well. Your ophthalmologist will decide on a particular course of treatment depending on your special situation.

Laser Treatment

Laser treatment is useful in treating retinopathy because the light beam can be aimed so exactly at the area needing treatment. A laser can be aimed at a site that is leaking, for example, to seal the surrounding area. It can be aimed at the areas of the retina that are sending out growth factors that trigger abnormal blood vessel growth. When these tissues are targeted, new vessel growth will be prevented.

Laser treatment can also be useful for destroying the abnormal blood vessels that grow during proliferative retinopathy. How this is done depends on where they are growing. If the abnormal vessels are growing on the surface of the retina, away from the macula, they can be directly targeted with the laser and treated in one session. Your doctor will probably want to see you in 2 to 3 months to reevaluate the treatment.

If abnormal blood vessels are growing on the surface of the optic nerve, a different approach may be needed, because focal laser therapy could damage the optic nerve. Instead, your eye specialist may elect to perform panretinal photocoagulation. This technique scatters the laser treatment at different places throughout the retina. By doing this, unhealthy zones are destroyed without damaging the optic nerve directly. It may involve applying 1,200 to 1,800 pulses of a laser beam to the mid-peripheral and peripheral regions of the retina. This type of therapy usually requires two or three sessions. If your doctor were to do it in only one session, it might cause swelling in the retina and macular edema. The net result is to stop the production of the growth factors that trigger abnormal blood vessel growth, increase the amount of oxygen getting to your retina, and to damage the existing abnormal blood vessels.

Laser therapy can be performed in your doctor's office. Usually your eye is anesthetized and a contact lens is placed over it. For scatter laser photocoagulation, the laser is fired in rapid sequence. This is because your doctor does not have to precisely target specific lesions. With focal laser surgery, fewer laser pulses are fired, but more time is required between each laser application. This is because your doctor has to more precisely target specific lesions and more time is required to adjust the direction of the laser beam. Side effects of scatter laser coagulation include some loss of peripheral vision and decreased night vision.

If you have areas of scar tissue in the retina, your doctor may need multiple sessions to treat you. This is because greater care must be taken to avoid the regions of scarring and prevent further contraction. If you have cataracts, they may prevent the laser from reaching the retina. Sometimes your doctor will want to perform cataract surgery first. It might also help to use a laser that emits a red light, since red wavelengths of light may be better transmitted through the cataract. Laser treatment is difficult if you have a vitreous hemorrhage. If this is the case, you may be advised to sleep with your head in an elevated position and avoid exercise or any jarring activity. Once the hemorrhaging has settled to the bottom of the eye, your doctor can examine the eye and treat you with a panretinal therapy.

If you have macular edema along with proliferative retinopathy, your doctor will probably want to treat the edema first. To do this, you will probably be treated with focal therapy to stop any leaking into the macula. Once that has subsided, you may be treated with panretinal therapy to halt the growth of abnormal blood vessels.

Cryotherapy

Cryotherapy is a method that freezes a part of the retina to destroy abnormal blood vessel growth. Cryotherapy can successfully reach areas of the retina that can't be reached by a laser. It is especially useful for patients who have already had laser surgery but still have new blood vessel growth. Cryotherapy is also helpful for people who have hemorrhaging and cannot be treated with laser therapy.

During cryotherapy, you usually will be lying on your back, your eyes will be anesthetized, and your eyelids will be held open with a device called a speculum. Your doctor examines your retina with an ophthalmoscope and applies cryotherapy with a probe that is connected to a cold source. Once the probe is properly located, the freezing can begin. The device freezes specific points in the retina that your doctor can directly target.

Vitrectomy

Vitrectomy can be used to treat patients who have hemorrhaging, or bleeding, in the vitreous humor. Using this technique, your doctor will surgically remove the core of the vitreous gel. This condition, especially if it affects both eyes, can prevent a person from carrying out daily functions. When the blood blocks the macula, it is often difficult to clear up on its own, and it can lead to scar tissue that covers the macula and pulls on the retina.

If you have a vitrectomy performed, you will be given a local or general anesthetic. The surgeon will make small incisions in the wall of your eye. First, your doctor will clear the vitreous cavity, which is often filled with blood. The blood and vitreous gel are removed and the cavity is filled with a clear fluid. Once the vitreous gel is removed, surgery on the retina can be performed. This technique can also be used to remove scar tissue on the retina to help a detached retina to reattach. Tears or holes in the retina can then be treated with laser therapy. A gas bubble can be used to create pressure to hold the retina against the back wall of the eye until the laser treatment creates a secure seal. After surgery, your eye may be filled with a gas to hold your retina in place as it heals. Healing could take a few days or several months. During this period, your vision may be reduced and some of your vision may be completely blocked by the gas bubble. Eventually the gas bubble will break up and be replaced by the natural aqueous fluid made by your body.

Macular Edema

Fluid leaking into the cells of the retina can cause the tissue to swell. One area that is particularly sensitive to this problem is the macula, that area of the retina that allows you to see color and sharp images. When fluid leaks into the macula, you may develop diabetic macular edema. This can occur at any stage of retinopathy—in the early stages of nonproliferative retinopathy or the later stages of proliferative retinopathy. Macular edema accounts for most cases of vision loss, especially in people with type 2 diabetes who do not control blood glucose levels.

■ SYMPTOMS

If you have macular edema, you may notice varying degrees of vision loss, including a blurring of both near and far vision. You may also be less sensitive to blue and yellow colors. You may also notice a distortion of straight lines. This can be evident if you close one eye and look at a pattern of floor tile, for example. If you have symptoms of macular edema, you should have a thorough ophthalmologic exam. Using an ophthalmoscope, your doctor can examine your retina for signs of macular swelling. Your doctor may also conduct a fluorescein angiography exam to locate points in the blood vessels of the retina that may be leaking into the macula, or anything else that may be causing swelling in the macula. Angiography will also tell your doctor whether anything is impairing circulation to the macula, which can also cause loss of vision. You may also be examined using one of several ultrasound techniques, including optical coherence tomography. This gives your doctor an idea of whether there is any swelling in the retina or thickening within the macula, due to macular edema.

■ WHAT TO DO

Any time you notice any change in your vision, tell your doctor right away. If you notice any loss of vision, or any other symptoms of macular edema, contact your physician. You should be examined by an ophthalmologist as soon as possible. Blurred vision is often caused by natural aging or poor glucose control, but if it is indeed due to macular edema, you should be treated as soon as possible.

■ TREATMENT

If fluid is leaking into the macula, your eye doctor will first want to identify the source of the leak. This can be done using angiography or sonography. If a leak or leaks are detected, you may be a candidate for focal laser coagulation. This technique uses a laser to pinpoint specific sites. By aiming a laser at the site of leakage, the tissue coagulates, or closes up, and the leakage is plugged up. The goal is to prevent further leakage and to allow fluid that has already leaked into the macula to be reabsorbed.

If you have macular edema with nonproliferative retinopathy, the goal of treatment may simply be to stop the leaks. If you have macular edema with proliferative retinopathy, you may require several treatment sessions. In the first session, your doctor will want to find sites within the retina that are leaking fluid into the macula. The goal is to fix the leaks and reduce swelling in the macula. Once the swelling has subsided, you can be further treated to get rid of the growth of new blood vessels that are contributing to your problem.

■ PREVENTION

The best thing you can do to prevent any kind of retinopathy is to control your blood glucose and blood pressure levels. This is important to prevent such problems from happening in the first place and to prevent them from recurring.

Cataracts

Over time, the lenses of your eyes can develop areas of cloudiness. When this happens, you have a cataract. Often, cataracts have no effect on how you see things. But some cataracts interfere with your vision. If this occurs, you may need surgery.

Cataracts happen naturally as you age. But if you have diabetes, they may occur earlier than normal. Often people with diabetes develop cataracts in their 30s or 40s. Early cataract formation is thought to be due to poor blood glucose control over time. Fortunately, new surgical techniques are available to effectively treat cataracts. The best way to reduce your risk of early cataract development is to control your blood glucose levels.

■ SYMPTOMS

Dulling of vision, decreased reading vision, a need for more light when you are reading, or difficulty seeing when you are driving are all signs that you may have cataracts. If you have cataracts, an oncoming headlight while you are driving at night may look like a bursting star or sparkler.

■ WHAT TO DO

If you notice any of the symptoms of cataracts, contact your doctor or ophthalmologist. Your eye doctor will examine you to determine whether you have any cataracts that are causing your vision problems.

■ TREATMENT

Cataracts that interfere with your vision and prevent you from carrying out your normal day-to-day routines require surgery. Usually cataract surgery is performed in your doctor's office on an outpatient basis. Before you have surgery, your doctor will evaluate your eyes and take measurements for an artificial lens that is prepared before your surgery. During the actual surgery, your eye doctor will remove the lens from your eye and replace it with a plastic, artificial lens. Usually, the lens capsule, or posterior membrane, is left in place.

Sometimes, cataracts will develop in the lens capsule and also interfere with vision. These are called aftercataracts. Your doctor may treat aftercataracts with laser surgery. In this procedure, a laser is used to burn a clear hole in your membrane to remove the cataract that is clouding your vision. Lasers are not used to remove cataracts in your actual lens.

After you have cataract surgery, you will probably still need glasses for reading, distance, or both. Your lens naturally focuses your vision. When you have an artificial lens implanted, your vision is focused for only one distance. Glasses will allow you to focus at different distances. You will need to have your eyeglass prescription reevaluated after cataract surgery.

Glaucoma

If you have glaucoma, then the pressure exerted by the fluid inside your eye is too high. If this pressure, known as the ocular pressure, remains too high, over time it can damage the optic nerve. Normally, your eyes produce a fluid known as the aqueous humor. The aqueous humor fills the front part of your eye, circulating from behind the iris, through the pupil, and into a chamber between the iris and the cornea. This fluid is normally drained at the same rate it is produced. If something happens to interfere with the drainage of the aqueous humor, glaucoma can result. The draining of the aqueous humor can be blocked for several reasons; thus, glaucoma can have several different causes. Not all causes of glaucoma are related to diabetes.

Open-angle glaucoma, or chronic glaucoma, is the most common type of glaucoma. It can be affected by diabetes. It occurs when the drainage network (also known as the filtration angle) that drains the fluid from the eye is blocked. When circulation is poor and the eye doesn't receive the oxygen and nutrients it needs, extra blood vessels can grow where they don't belong. When these unwanted blood vessels grow across the drainage network, fluid can't leave the eye and pressure within the eye builds up.

Angle-closure glaucoma, also known as acute glaucoma, is caused by a filtration angle that is too narrow, which prevents the drainage of fluid. Angle-closure glaucoma is not affected by diabetes. Your doctor can tell from a complete eye exam whether or not you are prone to angle-closure glaucoma and can treat it before it becomes a problem.

Neovascular glaucoma is also caused by the growth of new, unwanted blood vessels. In this case, the blood vessels grow on the surface of the iris and eventually reach a point where they block the filtration angle. Diabetes can increase the risk of neovascular glaucoma, especially if you have proliferative retinopathy.

■ SYMPTOMS

The symptoms of glaucoma depend on what type of glaucoma you have. If you have open-angle glaucoma, you probably will not notice any symptoms. The only early sign of open-angle glaucoma is a slight loss of small areas of peripheral vision. This loss of vision usually occurs in one eye, on the side near the nose. You may not notice this because the peripheral vision of the other eye makes up for it. Gradually, the extent of loss of peripheral vision increases and the second eye will also be affected. By the time you notice the loss of vision some damage has been done.

The symptoms of angle-closure glaucoma are more noticeable. You may experience an acute glaucoma attack, characterized by blurry vision, the appearance of halos around lights, and pain and redness in the eye. Your cornea may also begin to look hazy. Usually preliminary attacks precede a fully developed attack. If you have a fully developed attack, you may also experience excruciating pain in the head as well as the eye. Sometimes the pain is so great that you will vomit. The cornea may look gray and granular and your eyeball may be painful to the touch.

Symptoms of neovascular glaucoma may vary. You may feel no symptoms at all or you may feel symptoms similar to those found in angle-closure glaucoma.

■ RISKS

Acute glaucoma is relatively rare and tends to run in families. Chronic glaucoma, however, is more common. About 1 to 2 percent of the population over 40 will develop this type of glaucoma, and if you have diabetes, you are twice as likely to develop it. The risk continues to rise with age. If the condition is not caught early, your peripheral vision in both eyes will be lost. If not treated, it can also affect your ability to see straight ahead, and eventually both eyes may become totally blind.

■ WHAT TO DO

If you feel the symptoms of an acute glaucoma attack, call your doctor right away. If you are unable to contact your regular doctor or eye care specialist, or a physician on call, go to the emergency room of your nearest hospital.

If you have any symptoms of open-angle, or chronic, glaucoma, notify your doctor as soon as you notice any vision loss. Unfortunately, you cannot regain the vision lost through this disorder, but you can prevent further vision loss. Because the symptom itself is vision loss, it is important to have your ophthalmologist test you on a regular basis. This is especially true for people with diabetes.

■ TREATMENT

Treatment for glaucoma depends on the kind of glaucoma you have. If you have open-angle glaucoma, your doctor will first treat you with eye drops to reduce the pressure in the eye. You may be given eye drops or medication that opens up the drainage vessels or that decreases the rate of production of aqueous humor. Most of these medications must be taken for life. If your condition does not respond to this treatment, you may require laser surgery. In this procedure, your doctor will use a laser to create an artificial drainage channel in the angle.

If you have angle-closure, or acute, glaucoma, you need emergency attention. In the emergency room, you will be given eye drops to encourage the iris, which may be blocking the drainage channel, to withdraw. You may also be given an injection of a drug to block the production of the aqueous humor. You may also be treated with a procedure known as a laser iridotomy. Using a laser, your doctor will create a small hole in your iris that allows the aqueous humor to pass through the drainage angle. You will need careful follow-up evaluations after this type of surgery.

Neovascular glaucoma is usually treated with laser surgery to the retina. This is because the blood vessel growth in the iris is the result of problems in the retina. If the problem does not respond to laser treatment of the retina, you may need to take eye drops or have laser surgery performed directly on the abnormal blood vessels in the iris.

With any treatment of glaucoma, it is important to schedule follow-up visits with your ophthalmologist, to make sure that the treatment has succeeded in improving your condition.

■ PREVENTION

The best way to prevent the type of glaucoma triggered by diabetes is to control your blood glucose levels. Also schedule visits with your ophthalmologist on a regular basis to be tested for glaucoma. By catching glaucoma in the early stages, you can prevent the loss of vision that may occur if detected too late.

Blurry Vision

Not every vision problem is a sign of retinopathy. Sometimes you may develop temporary problems with your vision, such as blurring. This often can happen when your blood glucose levels are out of control. See your ophthalmologist when you notice any change in vision to make sure you don't have a serious condition that could get progressively worse.

■ SYMPTOMS

You will notice blurry vision and changes in how well you see throughout the day. You may notice that your vision is especially blurry when you look in the distance, but your near-range vision may actually improve. If you normally wear reading glasses, you may even find that you don't need them.

■ WHAT TO DO

Notify your doctor or your ophthalmologist if you notice any change in your vision. Blurry vision could be a sign of retinopathy, a serious condition that could lead to blindness if left untreated.

However, your vision could also get blurry when your blood glucose levels get out of control. Blurry vision is a symptom of both hypoglycemia and hyperglycemia. If you have an episode of blurry vision that comes on suddenly, especially if you also have other symptoms of hypoglycemia or hyperglycemia, test your blood glucose level at once. If it is dangerously low or high, take treatment steps right away. If left untreated, hypoglycemia could lead to convulsions and unconsciousness. Hyperglycemia can lead to a life-threatening condition such as diabetic ketoacidosis, which is more common in people with type 1 diabetes, or hyperglycemic hyperosmolar state, which is more common in people with type 2 diabetes.

Blurry vision in itself may not necessarily be a sign that you have a sight-threatening condition such as retinopathy. It could be a temporary situation that will go away on its own. But it could signal a low or high blood glucose reaction, situations that require immediate attention.

If you have recently switched from an oral medication to insulin, have changed the dose or timing of any medication, or have started intensive therapy, you may also experience blurry vision. These effects are often only temporary and are likely to go away in 3 to 6 months. However, if you are tightening your control of diabetes or switching medications, it is a good idea to schedule regular eye examinations to make sure you don't develop any serious eye problems.

The bottom line is that any time you experience a change in the way you see things, including blurry vision, notify your doctor. It could signal an emergency situation, such as hypoglycemia or hyperglycemia. Or it could signal a potentially serious eye condition, such as retinopathy, that should be treated at once to preserve your eyesight.

Double Vision

Diabetes can also cause a condition that makes you see double. This condition, called diplopia, is caused by damage to the nerves and blood vessels that control the muscles that move the eyes. Your eyes are surrounded by six muscles that control their movements. The movement of these muscles is coordinated by nerves so that they maintain simultaneous focus on whatever you may be looking at. If your nerves are damaged by a poor blood supply, the muscles may not coordinate the movement of the eyes. When this happens you have double vision. This is a type of mononeuropathy (see Chapter 7).

■ SYMPTOMS

Symptoms of diplopia include double vision, drooping of the eyelid, and sometimes pain over the affected eye.

■ WHAT TO DO

Notify your physician if you have any of the symptoms listed above. Usually, the nerves regain function over several months and the eyes regain their coordinate vision. In the meantime, you may be treated with a eye patch to eliminate one of the two images. Or you may be given an optical device called a prism, in a spectacle lens that attempts to align the two visual images. In rare cases, surgery on the muscle of one eye may be performed.

Double vision can sometimes signal a potentially life-threatening situation. Therefore, it is important to tell your doctor right away if you are seeing double. Although it could be due to a neuropathy that clears itself up, you want to rule out something more serious. Tell your physician about any abnormality or change in your vision right away.

■ PREVENTION

The best way to prevent diplopia is to keep your blood glucose levels as close to normal as possible.

Chapter 10
Solving Gastrointestinal Problems

Your gastrointestinal (GI) tract carries out an important job. It processes all the food your body takes in, directs all the energy and nutrients to where they are needed, decides what your body doesn't need, and eliminates the waste. Food enters your mouth and travels down your esophagus to your stomach where it is digested. A powerful system of muscles propels the food and waste from your stomach, through your large and small intestines, and to your rectum for elimination. As your food moves along, specialized cells along the GI tract absorb the needed nutrients and shuttle them off to where they are needed.

The muscles that propel food along your GI tract are controlled by a network of nerve fibers. These nerves are part of the autonomic nervous system. They carry out their job without you even being aware that they are working. But when these nerves become damaged, you can develop autonomic neuropathy. When this happens, your GI tract can't do its job as efficiently. Food stays in your stomach longer and moves more slowly through the tract. You can often feel the effects as gastrointestinal discomfort. If you have diabetes, you are more likely to have neuropathy, or nerve damage, and are more likely to experience problems with the gastrointestinal tract, from the mouth to the rectum.

Gastroparesis

Your stomach is a big, hollow, muscular organ. Through strong, regular contractions, it grinds up the food that you eat, breaking down big pieces into tiny particles. At the same time, gastric juices chemically digest your food to break it down further. Once pieces of food are small enough, they can pass through the pyloric sphincter, a kind of valve between the stomach and small intestine. Larger pieces are propelled back to the stomach for further processing. In between meals, when your stomach is not actively digesting food, larger, undigested particles are pushed through to the intestines.

If you have diabetes, you are more likely to have autonomic neuropathy. If this happens, damage to the nerves that control the stomach muscles can prevent or slow down their action. As a result, your stomach can't efficiently break down your food into smaller pieces, and food remains in your stomach too long. In a person who does not have autonomic neuropathy, liquids empty out of the stomach in 10 to 30 minutes and solids remain for 1 to 2 1/2 hours. But if you have neuropathy, both liquids and solids can remain for much longer. The mechanism that allows undigested matter to pass through is also disturbed. Sometimes food particles can remain in your stomach for days.

■ SYMPTOMS

If you have gastroparesis, or delayed stomach emptying, you may experience frequent bouts of nausea and vomiting. This often occurs along with weight loss. Episodes of nausea and vomiting may last for days, or, less frequently, for months. Or you may experience these symptoms in cycles. You may feel bloated in your abdomen and have an uncomfortable feeling of fullness after a meal. Often, you feel full before you have eaten very much. If you vomit, you may notice food that you ate several days ago.

Blood glucose levels may be difficult to control, because glucose is delivered to your bloodstream erratically. You might have frequent bouts of hypoglycemia because it is more difficult to match your insulin doses to your meals, because your meals are not being processed in a timely manner.

Gastroparesis often occurs when you have other complications of diabetes, especially those caused by neuropathy. These include retinopathy, nephropathy, and peripheral neuropathy. You may also experience the symptoms of other autonomic neuropathies. These include a sluggish pupil response to changing light conditions, lack of sweating, facial sweating while eating certain foods, dizziness when you stand up, impotence or diminished ejaculation if you are male, and poor bladder function with frequent bladder infections. If you experience any of these other problems related to neuropathy, it is likely that your stomach discomfort may also be due to neuropathy.

■ WHAT TO DO

If you have any recurrent bouts of nausea and vomiting, notify your physician. You will want to rule out other causes that could be contributing. If you do have gastroparesis, your doctor may need to conduct several tests to correctly diagnose the problem and to come up with the proper treatment.

Any time you have nausea and/or vomiting, check your blood glucose level. If you have any signs of dehydration, diabetic ketoacidosis, or hyperglycemic hyperosmolar state, you may need emergency help. If your blood glucose level is above 250 mg/dl, call a member of your health care team at once. You may need to treat the hyperglycemia. If your blood glucose level is over 500 mg/dl, call for emergency help or have someone take you to a hospital immediately. (For more on diabetic ketoacidosis, hyperglycemic hyperosmolar state, and treating hyperglycemia, see Chapter 3.)

If your blood glucose level is below 60 mg/dl, you have hypoglycemia. You should take a fast-acting carbohydrate right away. However, delivering glucose to your bloodstream can be difficult if you have gastroparesis, especially if you are vomiting. Try taking a fast-acting carbohydrate that contains 10 to 15 grams of carbohydrate (2 tablespoons of raisins, 4 ounces of orange juice, 6 jelly beans, 2 teaspoons of sugar, 10 gumdrops, or 2 to 5 glucose tablets, for example.) Wait 15 minutes and then retest your blood glucose level. If it is still below 60 mg/dl, take another dose of carbohydrate. If your blood glucose level remains low and your vomiting makes you unable to keep down any food, call your doctor immediately. If you show any signs of severe hypoglycemia, seek emergency help at once. (For more on hypoglycemia, see Chapter 2.)

If you have frequent bouts of nausea and vomiting, talk to your doctor about what to do in an emergency situation, should your blood glucose level rise too high or fall too low. Know what signs to look for and make sure you and those around you know what to do.

■ TREATMENT

If you have severe nausea and vomiting and are at risk for dehydration, you will need emergency treatment. If your dehydration becomes severe, you will require hospitalization. In the hospital, your stomach will be pumped to quickly remove the contents and relieve the symptoms. You will be given intravenous fluids containing the appropriate nutrients and metabolites to rehydrate you and restore any metabolic imbalance due to hypoglycemia, hyperglycemia, low potassium, or ketoacidosis. If you are malnourished, you may be given a feeding tube that bypasses the stomach.

Once you are stable, your physician will want to first rule out any conditions that have symptoms similar to gastroparesis. These include chronic peptic ulcer, cancer, uremia, pregnancy, or the side effects of any medications you may be taking. Medications used to treat high blood pressure and depression frequently cause a delay in stomach emptying.

Once your doctor has ruled out other factors, she may want to conduct a stomach-emptying test. To do this, you will be asked to eat a meal containing a radioactive tracer. After eating the meal, the level of radioactivity will be measured at different times to determine the rate of stomach emptying. You will be given specific instructions about what to eat before the test. It will be important that your blood glucose level remains below 240 mg/dl throughout the test. This is because hyperglycemia itself slows the emptying of the stomach. If your glucose levels are too high, it will be difficult to know whether your gastroparesis is due to a true neuropathic condition or simply a reflection of hyperglycemia at the time of the test.

Your doctor may also conduct a gastroscopy test. This is a method used to look inside your stomach. Your doctor will insert a probe that contains a tiny camera. This will provide a view of the inside of your stomach and will alert your doctor to any abnormalities.

Once diagnosed, treatment for gastroparesis may include a combination of diet and drug therapy. Your doctor or dietitian may suggest that you eat small meals more frequently rather than a few large meals each day. Avoid eating high-fat and high-fiber foods, including uncooked vegetables. You do not want to eat foods that are difficult to digest, such as legumes, lentils, and citrus fruits. This can aggravate the symptoms of gastroparesis. In addition, undigested food can form hard lumps, known as bezoars, that remain in the stomach. These bezoars will further worsen your symptoms of gastroparesis, contributing to feelings of bloating, nausea, and abdominal discomfort. They can be very difficult for your doctor to remove.

You may also be given medication that stimulates your stomach to contract and empty its contents. If one drug doesn't work for you, you may be given a different drug or a combination of drugs. Sometimes a particular medication works for a while, then stops working. If this happens, make sure to tell your doctor so she can switch you to a different drug. Also notify your doctor if you experience any side effects of medication. Some people have symptoms of gastroparesis for years and then they mysteriously disappear. Others deal with gastroparesis for years, managing it through diet and drug therapy. But if you find that your symptoms make your life unpleasant and uncomfortable, keep talking to your doctor until you find a suitable way to manage your condition. This may require referral to a specialist.

Also, if you have gastroparesis, especially if it is accompanied by bouts of vomiting, you need to keep close tabs on your blood glucose levels. This means testing more frequently and treating hypoglycemia and hyperglycemia when they occur.

■ PREVENTION

The best way to prevent gastroparesis from occurring is to keep your blood glucose levels under control. Over the long term, if you keep your blood glucose levels as close to normal as possible, you can delay or prevent any neuropathy from occurring in the first place.

Gastroesophageal Reflux

Your GI tract has the job of moving food through your body from your mouth to your rectum. Fortunately, your GI tract has a built-in mechanism for preventing food from backing up along the way. Your GI tract is compartmentalized, and at each juncture specialized valves operate to keep your food from backing up. This is especially important at the junction of the stomach and esophagus, because the environment of the stomach is extremely acidic and can damage the tissues of the esophagus. At this junction, a special muscle called a sphincter muscle closes once food makes it into your stomach. This keeps food and stomach acid from backing up into the esophagus. If the sphincter muscle does not close as it should, you can develop a condition called gastroesophageal reflux.

■ SYMPTOMS

Gastroesophageal reflux is marked by heartburn, a burning pain behind the breastbone, or any burning sensation in the chest or throat. This can occur after eating a meal, when lying down, or when bending over. These feelings can even awaken you from sleep. You could simply feel that you have a sour taste in your mouth and throat. You may also experience chest pain during a meal or after eating or drinking. You may also have a physical sensation that liquid or solid food stops or passes with great difficulty through your throat and into your stomach.

People with type 1 diabetes may have a lower incidence of heartburn than people with type 2 diabetes or people without diabetes. This appears to be due to a decrease in stomach acid production in people with type 1 diabetes, because of neuropathy that affects the acid-producing cells of the stomach.

■ WHAT TO DO

If you experience heartburn or any of the symptoms of gastroesophageal reflux, talk to your doctor. It is not an emergency situation, but it can be very uncomfortable. Over time, the excess stomach acid can damage the lining of the esophagus and make you more prone to esophageal problems, such as esophageal cancer.

If you are experiencing chest pain, call your doctor right away. Do not dismiss any sort of chest pain as indigestion, since it may be something more serious, such as a heart attack.

■ TREATMENT

If you experience heartburn or pain in the throat and chest, your doctor will probably conduct a series of tests to rule out other conditions and properly diagnose your condition. If you have chest pain, you may require a series of tests to rule out poor circulation to the heart. Your doctor will probably also conduct an upper-GI X ray or an examination of the upper GI with an endoscope. This will rule out esophagitis (inflammation of the esophagus) or other conditions, such as a yeast infection or cancer of the esophagus.

Your doctor may first suggest changes in lifestyle to minimize the symptoms of gastroesophageal reflux. These include losing weight, stopping smoking, and avoiding foods that trigger acid reflux, such as caffeine, chocolate, tomato sauce, and high-fat foods. Avoid lying down for 2 hours after a meal. Also, elevate your head 6 inches when you do lie down to prevent stomach contents from traveling up the esophagus.

If these measures provide little relief or if your condition is more serious than feelings of mild discomfort, your doctor may prescribe a medication to help relieve symptoms. The choice of drug will depend on the severity and frequency of your particular symptoms, and whether your esophagus shows signs of inflammation. Your doctor could prescribe an antacid or other medication to decrease the production of stomach acid. Antacids can be taken an hour after meals and before bedtime to reduce stomach acidity. Or you could be given a drug that acts as a proton pump inhibitor. These are the most effective drugs for healing ulcers in the esophagus that may be caused by excess stomach acid.

If your symptoms are mild, and you have heartburn less than once a week, you may find that altering lifestyle patterns and taking antacids will provide the relief you need. However, if you have heartburn more than once a week, you may need stronger treatment.

■ PREVENTION

To prevent gastroesophageal reflux, you should first consider a long-term approach to prevent neuropathy from occurring in the first place. Try to keep your blood glucose levels as close to normal as possible. Also, avoid lifestyle habits that may encourage acid reflux. Stop smoking and avoid drinking alcohol to excess. Avoid chocolate, caffeine, high-fat containing foods and certain drugs, such as anticholinergics.

Diarrhea

About 5 percent of people with diabetes experience frequent bouts of diarrhea. Diarrhea is especially common among people who have had diabetes for a long time and among those who use insulin. The causes of diabetic diarrhea are not completely clear. It may be a result of neuropathy. The nerves that control movement of food through the bowel and the absorption of fluid from food don't function properly. You can also be affected by fecal incontinence, when the nerves that control the anal sphincter muscles are damaged and interfere with the normal way you sense the need to defecate.

Diarrhea may also be triggered by ingestion of artificial sweeteners, particularly sorbitol, a practice common among people with diabetes. Diarrhea may also be caused by the overgrowth of bacteria in the colon, because the muscles that move food along naturally do not function properly. This causes food to sit longer in the digestive tract, allowing bacteria to flourish.

Diarrhea could also be triggered by a problem with the production of bile acid, which helps you digest fat. Whatever the cause, the symptoms can be severe enough to keep you from wanting to go out of your home.

■ SYMPTOMS

The main symptom of diarrhea is a loose, watery bowel movement. It can occur at any time, often with little warning. Often, people with diabetic diarrhea experience fecal incontinence, an inability to control bowel movements. You may find that you leak stool, but don't feel the urge to defecate. Episodes of diarrhea often, but not always, occur at night.

Diarrhea can last from a few hours to a few weeks. You may have periods of remission, in which you have no diarrhea. You may even have periods in which you are constipated. During episodes of diarrhea, you will probably notice an increase in the frequency and the amount of your bowel movements.

■ WHAT TO DO

If you have any episode of diarrhea that lasts more than a day, contact your doctor. If diarrhea is severe, you need to watch out for dehydration, especially if you also have any kind of nausea or vomiting. Make sure to test your blood glucose levels more frequently. If there is any evidence of hypoglycemia or hyperglycemia, treat right away and call your doctor.

If your diarrhea occurs without the threat of dehydration, it is less of an emergency, but it nevertheless may be distressing enough to require prompt treatment. This is especially true if you have frequent episodes. Talk your doctor about your problem, in order to begin treatment as soon as possible.

■ TREATMENT

Diarrhea can have several causes, so you and your doctor may have to try several different approaches to find the one that works for you. If neuropathy is causing your diarrhea, then you probably have reduced sensation around your anus. Your doctor can detect this with a pin. If you have neuropathy, you may be unable to sense a pin prick. Your doctor may also give you a rectal exam. If you have neuropathy, you may have a lax anal sphincter muscle. When a finger is inserted, the sphincter muscle will fail to contract. You may also show a loss of the anal wink reflex. This is a contraction of the anus in a "wink" when the skin around the anus is stroked. There may also be a loss of the bulbocavernosus reflex in men. This occurs when the anus contracts as the glans penis is squeezed between the fingers. Your doctor may test all or some of these reflexes to see if neuropathy is the cause of your diarrhea.

Before conducting any further tests, you and your doctor may want to go over all the food in your diet to see if anything you are eating or drinking could be causing the problem. For example, many foods contain sorbitol, which can trigger diarrhea in some people. Check the labels of everything you eat, including any diet drinks, sugar-free candies, or even gum. Excessive amounts of caffeine, found in coffee, tea, chocolate and cocoa, and many soft drinks, can also trigger diarrhea. Many people with diabetes take magnesium-based antacids, which can contribute to diarrhea. Go over all the medications you are taking, including over-the-counter drugs. Some medications, such as metformin, can cause diarrhea.

If you fail to find an obvious dietary cause of diarrhea, your doctor may suggest a wheat gluten–free diet. This is because the gluten in wheat can cause an allergic reaction in some people that triggers diarrhea. Other food allergies may also be the culprit. A visit to an allergy specialist may be in order.

Your doctor may suggest that you take a course of antibiotics to control the possible overgrowth of bacteria in your bowel. Your doctor may first want to test your bowel to see if you have too many bacteria growing there. If the test reveals that you have more than 100,000 micro-

organisms per milliliter, then you may need an antibiotic. You will probably be prescribed an oral antibiotic for 10 days. Make sure to take the
entire dose of drug for the whole 10 days, even if your diarrhea goes
away before then.

If antibiotics fail to improve your condition, you may be given an
anti-diarrheal drug, such as diphenoxylate (Lomotil). If your condition
shows no improvement, your doctor may then conduct an upper-GI
endoscopy exam. This test allows a look at the lining of your small intestine. Your doctor may also collect a sample of bacteria to see if a bacterial infection in the small intestine could be causing the problem.

In rare cases, diarrhea is caused by poor action of pancreatic
enzymes. This can be tested by collecting a 72-hour stool sample. If you
have pancreatic enzyme insufficiency, you may be given supplementary
pancreatic enzymes for treatment.

Problems with the absorption of the bile acids produced by your
gallbladder have also been implicated as a cause of diarrhea. However,
this is fairly rare. Your doctor may suggest taking a medication such as
cholestyramine, which binds bile acids, or loperamide (Imodium),
which slows the amount of time food spends in the small intestine.

Once your diarrhea is under control, your doctor can then help you
control fecal incontinence. Often fecal incontinence is confused with
diarrhea, but they are two different conditions. Fecal incontinence
refers to the inability to detect or control bowel movements and often
coexists with diarrhea. One way you can control fecal incontinence is by
using biofeedback techniques. Another is to do specific exercises called
Kegel exercises to train your anal sphincter muscle. A nurse educator or
physical therapist can show you how to do these exercises. Basically, they
work by squeezing your lower abdomen and pelvis as though you are
trying to prevent urine or stool from coming out. You can try doing
these exercises several times a day, whenever you have free time. Try it
when you are sitting at a stoplight or standing in line at the grocery
store. In people with good rectal sensation, these exercises, along with
biofeedback techniques, reduce fecal incontinence 70 percent of the
time. Your doctor may also suggest the drug octreotide acetate
(Sandostatin), which frequently works with great success.

Diarrhea can be an embarrassing condition, and you may feel
uncomfortable discussing it with your physician. However, the sooner

you talk to your doctor about it, the sooner you can begin treatment to alleviate the problem.

■ PREVENTION

Diarrhea may be prevented by avoiding foods and medications that may trigger the condition. Over the long term, controlling your blood glucose levels may also reduce or prevent the neuropathy that can lead to diarrhea and rectal incontinence.

Constipation

Any time you have fewer than three bowel movements a week, you have constipation. Constipation is probably the most common GI complication of diabetes. It affects 25 percent of all people with diabetes and more than half of people with neuropathy.

Constipation can have many causes. Most commonly, people with neuropathy develop constipation because the fecal waste moves so slowly through the GI tract that too much water is absorbed. This makes the feces hard and difficult to pass. It can also be caused by some sort of obstruction at the rectum, such as a rectal sphincter muscle that is not functioning properly. This may be due to damage to the nerves that control the sphincter. Also, poorly functioning pelvic muscles can also contribute to constipation, because you need to contract your pelvic muscles in order to have a bowel movement. Fortunately, there are many noninvasive treatments available that can alleviate the symptoms of this sometimes painful condition.

■ SYMPTOMS

The primary symptom of constipation is the inability to have regular bowel movements. If you have fewer than three movements a week, or every other day, you are probably constipated. Not everyone keeps track of the timing of their bowel movements, but if you infrequently pass a stool and find that the stool is hard and that you have to strain to pass it, you probably have constipation. Sometimes you may even have to bend over or assume a contorted position to eliminate the stool. You may also have rectal discomfort and have a sense that you have not completely eliminated your feces. Bouts of constipation may alternate with episodes of diarrhea.

Constipation is not necessarily an emergency situation, although it can become quite uncomfortable and the symptoms can worsen the longer it goes on. The longer you wait to defecate, the more difficult it can be. If you are constipated, talk to your physician about how best to treat it. In the meantime, you can try several self-help measures to see if they alleviate the problem.

Try drinking plenty of water during the course of the day, particularly during hot weather. Eight glasses a day is a good rule of thumb. Also, regular exercise can stimulate the bowels into action. Go for a walk or jog, or take a bike ride, or try any other activity that you like to do. Just keep moving. If you sweat excessively, drink plenty of water before and after you exercise. Eating also helps intestinal movement, so be aware of any urges, no matter how slight, after a meal.

You should try to eat 20 to 35 grams of fiber each day. If you are not doing so already, try increasing your fiber intake. However, this may not be advised if you have gastroparesis. You can incorporate fiber into your diet by eating more fruits, vegetables, legumes such as beans, peas, and lentils, and whole grains. You are better off trying to change your diet before trying medications to loosen your stools.

If dietary changes do not help, ask your doctor about over-the-counter medications. Stool softeners or psyllium (a fiber supplement) may be effective, especially in combination with other self-help methods such as diet and exercise. However, be careful about doing too much too soon. If you eat too much fiber (more than 35 grams a day), you may find that your symptoms of constipation worsen and that you are plagued with flatulence (intestinal gas). Try increasing the fiber in your diet gradually. Talk to your doctor before using any laxative, especially if you have diabetes. Your body may start to depend on laxatives and you may lose the ability to eliminate waste on your own.

■ TREATMENT

If your constipation persists, even when you change your diet and increase your activity level, talk to your doctor. She may want to conduct an examination of your rectum. This can be done using proctosigmoidoscopy. This device consists of a long tube with a light on the end that allows your doctor to look into your rectum and intestines. You may also be given a barium enema. This is an X ray of your intestines after you have been given an enema that contains barium, a soft metal that is opaque to an X ray. The barium will show up any blockages. Your doctor may also want to conduct a colonoscopy to examine the lining of your colon.

Your doctor will also check to see if the mucous membranes of your colon and rectum look normal. She will also evaluate your muscles to see how efficient they are at eliminating stool during a simple rectal exam. You may also be evaluated to see if your pelvic muscles and the nerves supplying the muscles of the anus and rectum are functioning properly. If pelvic nerves and muscles are normal, then your doctor may use an X ray or gamma camera to measure how fast solid matter moves through your colon.

Depending on the results of these tests, your doctor may prescribe one of several medications to improve your bowel movements. Your doctor may suggest including fiber or laxatives, such as milk of magnesia, as part of your diet. Regular enemas may also be in order. Your doctor may also recommend a drug that increases colonic motility, such as bisacodyl (Dulcolax), a drug called cisapride, or a glycerin suppository.

■ PREVENTION

To prevent constipation, eat a balanced diet with plenty of fruits, vegetables, and fiber, exercise regularly, and drink plenty of water. Avoid the overuse of anti-diarrheal medications. For long-term prevention of the neuropathy that may cause constipation, do your best to keep your blood glucose levels as close to normal as possible.

Abdominal Pain

Almost everyone develops some sort of abdominal pain from time to time. And people with diabetes may suffer from the same problems as the rest of the population. But if you do have diabetes, you may be more likely to develop gallbladder disease, and this can contribute to abdominal pain. This may be because neuropathy affects the way the gallbladder functions. The gallbladder stores bile from the liver and releases bile to aid digestion. But if you have neuropathy, the gallbladder may have a difficult time contracting efficiently. As a result, bile pools in the gallbladder and forms a sort of sludge. Ultimately, the sludge forms stones. When the gallbladder attempts to push bile out, the stones get in the way and can cause pain.

Abdominal pain can also be caused by impaired circulation to the intestines, caused by atherosclerosis of the blood vessels that supply the abdomen. Damage to the nerves of the midsection can also cause abdominal pain.

■ SYMPTOMS

Symptoms of gallstones include pain in the upper abdomen. It may come in waves and be particularly acute in the upper abdomen. Pain may get worse after a meal or in the middle of the night. You may also experience nausea or vomiting.

You may also feel pain in the girdle area if you have diabetic radiculopathy (see page 200). This is caused by damage to the nerves that conduct impulses to the chest and abdomen. Gastroparesis and circulatory problems may also result in abdominal pain.

■ WHAT TO DO

Talk to your doctor if you experience any kind of abdominal pain. Abdominal pain can have many causes, which may or may not be related to your diabetes. If your pain is severe or debilitating, call your doctor or seek emergency help. If your doctor suspects gallstones, she will probably examine you by an X ray called a cholecystogram. Your doctor may also take blood for a blood analysis. Sometimes an ultrasound or computed tomography (CT) scan will also reveal gallstones.

■ TREATMENT

If your tests show that your pain is due to gallstones, your doctor may recommend surgery. In the past, this operation was performed under general anesthesia in a hospital or clinic. The surgeon made a small incision in the upper abdomen and removed the gallbladder and any stones in the bile duct. The procedure usually took about 1 1/2 hours. Ask your doctor about newer techniques for gallbladder and stone removal involving a laparoscope.

■ PREVENTION

To prevent gallstones, eat a balanced diet. Avoid foods that are high in fat or bring on pain or indigestion. To avoid neuropathy that may trigger gallstone development, keep your blood glucose levels as close to normal as possible over the long term.

Chapter 11
Solving Infection Problems

Everywhere you go, everything you do, microorganisms are on the prowl, trying to get into your body. They would like nothing better than to use you as a cheap hotel, complete with free food and drink. Fortunately, your body has a sophisticated security system of sorts—your immune system. Your immune system has both surveillance and search-and-destroy units that work together to keep unwanted invaders out and to destroy those that make it in.

Your primary defense against invaders is your skin and the mucous membranes of your intestinal and genitourinary tracts. Your skin and mucous membranes serve as natural barriers to unwanted microorganisms such as viruses, bacteria, and fungi. Some microorganisms are allowed to live in your body and may actually help you. Your intestinal tract, for example, contains millions of *E. coli* bacteria that actually help break down waste products. Some helpful microorganisms also protect against infection by other, more harmful, pathogens.

When microorganisms that can do you harm enter your body, your immune system springs into action. White blood cells produced in your bone marrow are dispatched to your bloodstream where they seek out and destroy foreign matter. For most people the immune system does a fairly good job of keeping harmful microorganisms at bay. But every now and then, a disease-causing microorganism, or pathogen, makes it past your body's defenses and proliferates out of control. When this happens, you have an infection.

Unfortunately, if you have diabetes, you are more likely to develop infections than the general population. The reasons aren't exactly clear, but people with diabetes do have more glucose in their blood. This provides an excellent food source for microorganisms and encourages their growth in your body. Also, if you have diabetes, there are defects in how your body produces and dispatches infection-fighting cells. The ability of the immune system cells to target and move toward the site of an infection is impaired. Also, people with diabetes are more likely to have problems with circulation. This means that as your immune cells travel through the bloodstream to their targets, they have a harder time getting to where they need to be. A further complication in people with diabetes occurs because of neuropathy. If you have damage to your nerves, you may be less likely to sense the pain that accompanies an infection. By the time you sense there is a problem, the infection may be out of control and more difficult to treat.

Infections can be especially dangerous to someone with diabetes. That is because your blood glucose levels can rise unexpectedly and be difficult to control when you have an infection. When your body is trying to fight off an infection, it becomes stressed. To deal with stress, your body releases an array of stress hormones, including cortisol and glucagon, which trigger the release of glucose from the liver and can cause insulin resistance. This causes your blood glucose level to go up.

The good news is that most infections are treatable. You can help your body fight infection by taking steps to prevent infections from occurring, being on the lookout for any signs of infection, and taking prompt action when they occur.

Urinary Tract Infections

People with diabetes are at increased risk for developing urinary tract infections compared to the general population. This is partly because the urinary tract serves as a rich glucose-containing medium for the growth of microorganisms in people with diabetes. The risk is even greater if you are a woman, if you are elderly, if you have any abnormalities in your genital or urinary structures, or if you have had diabetes for a long time. The most common urinary tract infections are bacteriuria, cystitis, and pyelonephritis.

Bacteriuria

Normally, urine is sterile. That means there are no bacteria or other microorganisms growing in it. Bacteria typically enter the urinary tract from the intestinal tract and from the vagina in women. Usually these microbes are washed out by the flushing action of urine when you urinate. But sometimes bacteria grow in urine. When you have more than 100,000 bacteria per milliliter growing in your urine, you have a condition known as bacteriuria.

■ SYMPTOMS

Bacteriuria itself is symptomless. It causes no symptoms, pain, or discomfort. The only way to know for sure that you have a high concentration of bacteria is to have a urine culture performed.

■ RISKS

Bacteriuria often develops in women following sexual intercourse. It is also quite common in people with diabetes because of the high glucose content of urine, especially in people with neurogenic bladder. If you have neurogenic bladder, you may have a problem emptying your bladder. This allows bacteria to spend more time in your urine and increases the chance of infection. Bacteriuria commonly occurs in people with neurogenic bladder who have to use a catheter to empty the bladder.

Bacteriuria has no symptoms and is not problematic in itself. The danger of bacteriuria is that it can progress to cystitis, infection of the bladder, and to pyelonephritis, infection of the kidneys.

■ TREATMENT

Most bacterial infections can be treated with antibiotics, drugs that kill bacteria. If you have bacteriuria and no symptoms of pain or discomfort, there is little benefit to be gained in taking antibiotics. That is because the overuse of antibiotics can lead to drug-resistant strains of microorganisms that can be more dangerous and more difficult to get rid of. However, if you have any sort of obstruction to urinary flow or bladder dysfunction, are pregnant, have immune system problems, or are having a bladder catheterization or other sort of invasive procedure of the urinary tract, your doctor may suggest that you take a course of antibiotics.

If you do use a catheter for emptying the bladder and develop bacteriuria, the catheter should be removed before treating with antibiotics, if at all possible. If the catheter is kept in, you or your caregiver should remove it frequently. Your doctor will probably prescribe an antibiotic only if you are experiencing symptoms of infection. Bacteriuria itself does not usually produce symptoms unless it has progressed to cystitis.

Cystitis

Bacteriuria can often progress to the point where the tissue of your bladder becomes inflamed. When this happens, you have cystitis. Most bladder infections are caused by an overgrowth of bacteria. However, sometimes people with diabetes develop fungal infections of the bladder, which require a different drug therapy.

■ SYMPTOMS

Symptoms of bladder infection include a feeling that you always have to urinate and a burning, painful sensation when you do urinate. You may feel pain over the bladder, which lies above the pubic area. Occasionally you may also develop a fever. Your urine may be cloudy and have a foul odor. You may even notice blood in your urine.

■ WHAT TO DO

If you have frequent, painful urination, contact your doctor. You may need to have a urinalysis performed to confirm the infection and identify the organism responsible. This will dictate the course of treatment.

In the meantime, you can start some self-help steps to begin to clear up the infection. Drink plenty of fluids. The more liquid that moves through your bladder, the greater the chance that your urine will flush out your bladder. Some people find that drinking cranberry juice helps, but check with your dietitian and make sure to make allowances for the sugar from the juice in your meal plan.

■ TREATMENT

If your infection is bacterial, your doctor will prescribe one of several antibiotic drugs, depending on what type of bacteria are responsible. Usually the condition clears up within a few days. However, if you are prescribed an antibiotic, it is important that you take the drug for the entire course of treatment (usually 10 days) to prevent reinfection.

If your infection is due to a fungus, your doctor will prescribe a different type of drug, an antifungal agent. Sometimes fungi form a large mass called a fungus ball in the bladder or anywhere else in the urinary tract. If this occurs, you may have to have it surgically removed.

Pyelonephritis

Sometimes infected urine can travel from the bladder and up the ureters (the tubes that connect the bladder to the kidneys) to the kidneys. When this happens, one or both of your kidneys can become infected. If you have neurogenic bladder, you are at a greatly increased risk of developing pyelonephritis.

■ SYMPTOMS

Pyelonephritis can be quite painful. You may experience fever, chills, nausea, vomiting, and severe pain in your side or upper back. If you have pyelonephritis, these symptoms can occur along with the symptoms of cystitis (see above) or shortly thereafter. You may also find that your blood glucose levels are very high.

■ WHAT TO DO

If you have recently had a bladder infection or suspect that you have one and develop any of the symptoms of pyelonephritis, contact your doctor or health care professional right away. If you are vomiting, have a high fever, have blood glucose levels over 400 mg/dl, or have positive urine ketones (with type 1 diabetes), you may require hospitalization.

■ TREATMENT

If your symptoms are severe, you will be treated in a hospital setting where you will probably receive intravenous therapy for several days. If your symptoms are less severe, you may be treated on an outpatient basis. You will probably need to take antibiotics for 2 full weeks.

If your symptoms have persisted for several days, your doctor may take an X ray of your abdomen. This is to determine whether you have a condition known as emphysematous pyelonephritis. This is a complication that is characterized by the presence of gas in your kidneys. Although rare, most cases of emphysematous pyelonephritis occur in patients with diabetes. It may be that the bacteria or fungi that are causing the infection feed on the glucose in the urine to produce gas. If you have emphysematous pyelonephritis, you will require immediate hospitalization. If you have a kidney infection and do not treat it promptly, you risk the death not only of kidney tissue, but also of the tissues surrounding the kidney.

■ PREVENTION

It is not always easy to prevent infection, especially if you have diabetes. Try to keep your blood glucose levels as close to normal as possible for both the short and long term. In the short term, the lower your glucose levels, the less hospitable a climate you provide for invading pathogens. In the long term, good glucose control can go a long way in preventing neuropathy. This can help minimize the possibility of developing neurogenic bladder, which puts you at risk for urinary tract infections.

Keep your genital region clean, especially if you are a woman. Try to avoid any contact between your vagina and fecal waste. Also, drink plenty of fluids to promote the flushing out of any bacteria by the urine flow. You are more susceptible to infection when you are overtired, overstressed, and eating poorly, so try to get enough rest, avoid or reduce stress as much as possible, and eat a balanced diet.

If you have frequent urinary tract infections that occur with pain and discomfort, your doctor may suggest a low-level daily dose of antibiotics to prevent bacteriuria from occurring. However, when you do this, reinfection often occurs when you stop taking the antibiotics, and the resultant infection may be harder to cure.

If you do develop a kidney infection, you should be thoroughly evaluated by your doctor to identify any factors that may predispose you to urinary tract infections. This exam will probably include an ultrasound examination of the kidneys, measurement of urinary flow, excretory urogram using an injected dye, or cytoscopy, a method of looking into the bladder with a special instrument.

Ear Infections

People with diabetes are at high risk for a serious form of ear infection called malignant external otitis. In fact, malignant external otitis occurs almost exclusively in people with diabetes. The term "malignant" here means only that the condition is serious. It does not mean you have cancer. This condition is caused by the *Pseudomonas aeruginosa* bacteria. The infection starts in the soft tissue and cartilage around the external auditory, or outer ear, canal. As the infection progresses, it can spread to the bones of the ear canal. If untreated, the infection can sometimes reach the cranial nerves, which extend into the brain, or into the compartments of the brain itself. In some cases, malignant external otitis can abscess or rupture into the meningeal space—the space between the brain and its membrane—and cause death. The best defense against this serious infection is early, aggressive intervention.

■ SYMPTOMS

Symptoms of malignant external otitis include a severe, persistent headache. Often you may notice a foul-smelling discharge of pus from the outer ear. You may also experience a loss of hearing in the affected ear. If the infection progresses, you may also notice a drooping of facial muscles due to infection of the cranial nerves. You may also show signs of a systemic infection, such as high fever and chills. Your blood glucose levels may rise significantly. In clinical tests, your doctor may also find that you have a high white blood cell count.

■ RISKS

Malignant external otitis occurs almost exclusively in people with diabetes. It typically occurs in people over the age of 65 who are male and have had diabetes for a long time.

■ WHAT TO DO

If you experience any of the symptoms of malignant external otitis, call your doctor *at once!* The earlier you seek treatment, the greater the chance that you can prevent the spread of infection.

As with any sign of infection, make sure to monitor your blood glucose levels frequently. If you show signs of hyperglycemia, you will need to bring down your blood glucose levels. This may involve taking an extra dose of insulin or altering the timing of your meals. Ask your doctor about the best way for you to deal with hyperglycemia.

■ TREATMENT

The treatment of malignant external otitis will depend on an accurate diagnosis and an assessment of how far the infection has progressed. Your doctor may take an X ray or use magnetic resonance imaging or another scanning technique to see whether the infection has spread to soft tissue, bone, or beyond.

Once it is known how far the infection has spread, your doctor will surgically remove any infected tissue or bone and then wash out the site with antibiotic solution. You will then begin an intensive course of therapy with antibiotics. Most likely you will have to take the drug for 6 weeks or more, either orally or intravenously. It is important to schedule follow-up appointments with your doctor, because this type of infection can recur.

■ PREVENTION

Serious *Pseudomonas* infections tend to affect people with weakened immune systems. Your best bet to avoid this infection is to follow a healthy lifestyle. Eat balanced meals and keep your blood glucose levels under control. Exercise to whatever extent is possible and keep your weight under control. Try to get plenty of rest and avoid stress. Also practice good hygiene and keep your ears clean and dry. Make sure your doctor checks your ears at your routine examinations.

Sinus Infections

Whether you have diabetes or not, you are likely to develop sinus infections on occasion. Most sinus infections can be easily treated with antibiotics. But if you have diabetes, especially if you are prone to diabetic ketoacidosis, you need to be on guard against rhinocerebral mucormycosis. This is a rare infection, caused by the fungus *Zygomycetes*, that can infect your nasal sinuses and the palate of your mouth.

The zygomycetes fungus can exist in your blood without causing much harm, and normal blood stops its growth. However, these organisms can grow rapidly in the presence of high concentrations of glucose and in an acid environment. Both of these conditions occur if you develop diabetic ketoacidosis. When this occurs, the infection can progress rapidly with a potentially fatal outcome.

The infection may begin in the nostrils or sinuses and spreads at an amazingly rapid rate. Within days, the zygomycetes fungus can eat through to the deep recesses of the sinuses, infecting nerves and blood vessels, until it reaches the brain.

■ SYMPTOMS

The earliest symptom of a rhinocerebral mucormycosis infection is often pain in your eyes or face. This is followed by a yellowish-white nasal discharge that may be tinged with blood. You may also experience swelling around the eyes, increased tearing, visual blurring, and tenderness in the sinus and nasal passages.

■ WHAT TO DO

If you have any of these symptoms, especially if you have had a recent episode of diabetic ketoacidosis, hyperglycemia, or ketones in the blood, call your doctor *at once.* This is a life-threatening condition that could cause death within days. If you cannot contact your doctor immediately, seek emergency help.

■ TREATMENT

A rhinocerebral mucormycosis infection must be treated quickly and aggressively. Your doctor will examine you physically to determine whether you have rhinocerebral mucormycosis. If you do, your doctor will notice a darkening or ulceration in the nasal passages or palate of your mouth. You will also be examined by X ray or other imaging technique to confirm the diagnosis and evaluate the extent of disease.

If you have rhinocerebral mucormycosis, you will require immediate surgery. Your doctor or surgeon will remove all dead and infected tissue and surrounding tissue. This procedure may have to be repeated. This will be followed by an aggressive course of antifungal medication to kill the fungus that is causing the infection.

If your condition is accompanied by diabetic ketoacidosis and/or hyperglycemia, these conditions will have to be brought under immediate control.

■ PREVENTION

The greatest risk factor for rhinocerebral mucormycosis is diabetic ketoacidosis. To prevent rhinocerebral mucormycosis and diabetic ketoacidosis, it is essential to keep your blood glucose levels under control. You, your doctor, and your dietitian should together develop an eating and insulin schedule you can follow. Never skip a dose of insulin, even if you are not feeling well. Monitor your blood glucose level frequently, especially if you are feeling sick, are under stress, have an infection, or have changed your daily routine.

Mouth Infections

Oral hygiene may seem like no big deal, or maybe even a nuisance. There are so many other things to worry about if you have diabetes. But the truth is, if you have diabetes, it is critical to take good care of your mouth, teeth, and gums. People with diabetes are more prone to gum disease and infections. Infections can undermine your efforts to control your blood glucose levels and lead to emergency situations. And, pain in your mouth could have a hidden consequence. Any time you have pain or discomfort in your mouth, you may not be able to eat. That is one of the worst things that could happen to someone with diabetes, because maintaining good blood glucose control depends on carefully balancing your food intake with available insulin. Therefore, it is critical to maintain good oral health by taking preventive measures to keep your mouth, teeth, and gums in top form.

Diabetes can affect your oral health in several ways. If you have diabetes you are more likely to have high blood glucose levels, and this can affect your circulation. This means that the small blood vessels that supply your mouth with oxygen and nutrients are easily damaged. As a result, you are more likely to develop gum disease, and gum problems in someone with diabetes are slower to heal than in someone without diabetes.

If you have diabetes you are more likely to develop infections and also have a harder time fighting off infections. If you have a deep cavity, for example, your white blood cells are less capable of fighting off invading bacteria than are those of people without diabetes. As a result, you are more likely to develop abscesses and other infections. This may be because you probably have higher levels of glucose in your saliva. This glucose feeds the bacteria in your mouth that can cause infection and damage your gums.

If you have diabetes, you are at high risk for autonomic neuropathy. When the nerves that control the production of saliva in your mouth are damaged, you could develop a condition known as "dry mouth," or xerostomia. Without a good supply of saliva, you are at an increased risk for cavities and infections of the mouth.

Fortunately, you can minimize the risk of infection, gum disease, and other problems of the mouth by practicing good oral hygiene and keeping your blood glucose levels under control.

Periodontal Disease

Periodontal disease is also known as gum disease. Your teeth are anchored in your mouth by bone, and your gums provide a soft covering of the juncture between tooth and bone. Bacteria can grow in the space between your gums and teeth. When this gets out of control, you have gum disease.

In its earliest stage, referred to as gingivitis, your teeth become covered by a thin film known as plaque, which is rich in bacteria. As the disease progresses to periodontitis, a harder material known as tartar also adheres to the teeth and gathers between the teeth and gums. Tartar, also known as calculus, is equally rich in bacteria. As gum disease progresses, the gums recede and the underlying bone erodes away. Without treatment, the loss of your teeth and further erosion of the gums and bone is inevitable. Fortunately, the process can be stopped at any stage with proper treatment.

■ SYMPTOMS

Symptoms of gingivitis, the earliest stage of gum disease, include redness and swelling of the gums. You may find that your gums bleed easily, especially when you are flossing or even brushing your teeth. Plaque and tartar are visible along the surface of the teeth and below the gum line. As gum disease progresses, the gum line recedes, exposing the roots of your teeth. As the gum line recedes further, the bone holding your teeth in place also begins to erode, further exposing the roots. Eventually the bone loss will be so great that your teeth will become loose and may fall out.

■ WHAT TO DO

Gum disease in itself is not life-threatening and does not require emergency attention. However, as soon as you see any signs of gum disease, including redness of the gums, or if you notice that your gums bleed easily, schedule an appointment with your dentist right away. The earlier you seek treatment, the less likely you are to lose your teeth. Once your gums and bones recede, they will not grow back again. However, you can prevent further loss of gum and bone by proper treatment.

■ TREATMENT

If you haven't seen a dentist in a while, you will be given a thorough examination on your first visit. Your dentist will first examine your gums and teeth to look for signs of gum disease. Your dentist may also take X rays of your teeth. This will reveal whether any bone loss has taken place. Your dentist may also measure the depth of the pocket that surrounds each tooth to further evaluate the extent of gum disease. Your teeth will also be examined for any signs of decay, broken, chipped, or cracked teeth, defective crowns, or missing or misfit fillings.

If your gum disease is in its early stages, the treatment can be as simple as routine dental cleanings every 3 to 6 months. During these visits, your dentist or dental hygienist will remove the plaque and tartar with dental instruments. If the plaque and tartar buildup is more substantial, your dentist may recommend a scaling and root planing treatment. This deep-cleaning treatment will probably involve several trips to the dentist and will require a local anesthetic. Once you have this procedure performed, your dentist may recommend more frequent follow-up visits than the standard 6-month interval.

When gum disease is more severe, it may be more difficult to conduct a deep cleaning of the gums and teeth. This is because there is not enough bone to support the teeth. In this case your dentist may refer you to a gum specialist, a periodontist. Depending on the state of your gums, the periodontist may perform gum surgery. The goal of this type of surgery is to reshape the bone and reposition the gums to make your teeth and gums easier to clean. Without this sort of reshaping, the pockets between your teeth and gums can become so deep and accumulate so much plaque and tartar that they are impossible to clean. This leads to further gum recession and bone loss that inevitably leads to tooth loss. The goal here is to stop the cycle and allow you to preserve your gums, bone, and teeth.

■ PREVENTION

The simplest way to prevent gum disease is to keep plaque and tartar from accumulating on your teeth. Although maintaining good oral health is more difficult for people with diabetes, it is not impossible.

Once you have an initial, thorough cleaning, your dentist may recommend that you brush your teeth after every meal and before bedtime, and floss daily. If you have bridgework that makes it difficult to get between your teeth, your dentist may be able to give you an instrument to aid cleaning. Electric toothbrushes may help if you have a hard time moving your hands to brush your teeth manually. You may also consider using dental care products at home aimed to kill plaque and bacteria and prevent tartar buildup. And don't forget to visit your dentist on a regular basis: every 3 to 6 months for a thorough cleaning.

Dry Mouth

As its name suggests, dry mouth is a condition characterized by a lack of saliva. It is thought to be caused by autonomic neuropathy. Saliva performs several functions in your mouth. It helps you digest your food, keeps your mouth lubricated, and helps keep your mouth clean. When you don't have enough saliva, the condition can be more than annoying. It can become more difficult to speak and eat and it can give your mouth a bad taste and odor. Also, if you have dry mouth, you are more likely to get dental cavities.

■ SYMPTOMS

Symptoms of dry mouth include a lack of saliva, a bad taste and odor in the mouth, and difficulty swallowing, eating, and talking.

■ WHAT TO DO

If you have symptoms of dry mouth, talk to your dentist. She can prescribe gels or rinses that have a high fluoride content. These will help to remineralize or fill in holes or small cavities. However, these products should only be used under the advice of your dentist. Your dentist may also recommend artificial saliva. This can be sipped and swished around your mouth to help you eat or speak better.

There are other techniques you can use yourself. Try chewing gum or sucking on candies or mints (sugarless, of course). Chewing gum and candy will stimulate the flow of saliva. A bonus of chewing sugarless gum is that it decreases cavity formation. Water will also help keep your mouth moist. Taking frequent small sips throughout the day or sucking on ice chips may work well.

Because dry mouth is caused by neuropathy, the best way to prevent it is to control your blood glucose levels over the long term, which reduces your risk of neuropathy.

Thrush

Thrush is type of infection in the mouth caused by a yeast-like fungus known scientifically as *Candida albicans*. If left unchecked, thrush can cause your blood glucose levels to swing. It occurs more frequently in people with diabetes, because the *Candida* microorganism thrives on the extra glucose found in the saliva of people with diabetes.

■ SYMPTOMS

Symptoms of thrush include the appearance of creamy white patches or red areas of irritation in the mouth. These patches can be scraped off easily with a finger or a spoon. Your mouth may feel sore or you may feel a burning sensation. If you wear dentures, they may become impossible to wear.

■ WHAT TO DO

Notify your doctor or dentist right away if you experience any of these symptoms. Like any infection, thrush can upset your blood glucose control. Thrush can be easily treated, but the sooner you begin treatment the easier it is to get rid of.

■ TREATMENT

Thrush can be treated by prescription antifungal drugs available in several forms. You can take a pill that kills the fungus systemically. Or you can use a medicated rinse that you swish around in your mouth and spit out. A lozenge that dissolves slowly in your mouth is also available.

Dental Treatment

A trip to the dentist can make anyone anxious and uncomfortable. But if you have diabetes, you may have special concerns when you visit the dentist, whether for extensive treatment or routine care. If your diabetes is well controlled, routine care should pose no more problems for you than for a person without diabetes. But if your diabetes is not well controlled, your dental visits may be more challenging.

If your diabetes is well controlled, you may only have to follow a few extra precautions for routine dental visits. These include your routine exam, cleaning, X rays, and simple fillings. If you require a local anesthetic, you may need to avoid the use of anything with epinephrine. This is especially true if you have had diabetes for a long time, have any evidence of neuropathy, or have any history of heart problems. Epinephrine can cause your heart to beat rapidly, a condition known as tachycardia, and should be avoided in many patients.

After you go to the dentist, depending on what procedures you have performed, you may find it difficult to eat or chew. This may interfere with your blood glucose control if you cannot follow your regular eating plan. If you take insulin or an oral medication, try to schedule your visits for the mid-morning. This will make it easier for you to take your morning medication and eat a normal breakfast. Try to schedule it so that there will be ample time for any anesthetic to wear off before your next meal is due. Monitor your blood glucose level before your visit, and tell your dentist what your blood glucose level is. You may want to ask your dentist to use a shorter-acting anesthetic so you don't have to skip or postpone a meal. You may want to try taking a liquid meal while you are recovering from the anesthetic or the procedure itself.

If your diabetes is well controlled, you can probably undergo more extensive treatments without much adjustment. Make sure your dentist consults with your doctor to see if any special precautions should be followed. For example, your doctor may want you to take an antibiotic before and after surgery, to prevent any bacterial infection from developing. Also, monitor your blood glucose levels before and after any dental work. Stress, anxiety, pain, and infection can all affect your blood glucose level.

If your diabetes is not well controlled, you may need to take extra precautions. Make sure your dentist consults with your doctor, even for the most routine visits. If you are not under the care of a physician, you should not have any major dental work done without first having an overall assessment of your health.

Report any heart problems or other complications of diabetes to your dentist before having anything done. People with heart valve abnormalities, for example, should take a preventive dose of antibiotic before even the most routine care, including cleaning.

■ PREVENTION

The best way to prevent any problems with your dental visits is to make sure your dentist knows you have diabetes, ask your dentist to consult with your doctor before any dental treatment, and try to time your visits so they will not interfere with your blood glucose control. Realize that even the mildest amount of stress or anxiety can affect blood glucose levels, so monitor your blood glucose both before and after your visit.

Chapter 12
Solving Foot Problems

Your feet are triply cursed when it comes to diabetes. They can be affected by poor circulation and neuropathy, and they are susceptible to infection. To make matters worse, these problems can feed on each other. If you have nerve damage to your feet, you can't feel pain and you may not realize that something is irritating your feet. This can lead to ulceration, or the formation of an open sore. A foot ulcer can easily become infected, and without proper circulation, the infection can be slow to heal. Some people with diabetes develop foot infections that can ultimately lead to amputation.

Of the 16 million people with diabetes in the United States, 15 percent will develop a serious foot problem at one time or another that can threaten their limbs or even their life. More than 50,000 people with diabetes lose a limb to diabetes each year. This can be disturbing news if you have diabetes, and particularly if you have any symptoms of neuropathy or circulatory problems. But the good news is that most of these problems can be prevented or minimized. By keeping your blood glucose levels under control, taking care of your feet with daily foot inspections, visiting your doctor and podiatrist regularly, wearing properly fitting shoes, being alert to early warning signs of neuropathy or circulation problems, and treating any problems that arise, you can prevent ulcers and infections from occurring.

If you have sensorimotor neuropathy, you can't feel pain or sensation in your feet and legs the way someone without neuropathy would. You could develop a blister or step on a thumbtack and not even realize it. Even a minor irritation, if left untreated, can develop into something major. If you have a small sore or abrasion and you continue walking on it and don't treat it, you can injure it further. Eventually an ulcer can develop and that can become easily infected. Neuropathy can cause further problems, because it can result in muscle weakness and the loss of muscle tone. When this happens, your feet and legs can become easily deformed and more prone to trauma and injury.

Once a lesion develops, your body calls on its immune system to prevent and combat any infection that develops. But your immune system needs a good circulatory system in order to do its job. Unfortunately, if you have diabetes, you are likely to have impairments in your circulation, particularly in the legs. This means that any lesion that develops can be slow to heal and may be easily infected.

This chapter deals with three other factors that contribute to foot problems: foot deformities, foot ulcers, and infections of the foot. For more information about how neuropathy can lead to the formation of ulcers on your feet, see Chapter 7. To learn more about circulatory problems, such as peripheral vascular disease, and how they can contribute to infection, see Chapter 6.

Foot Deformities

Foot deformities are not unique to people with diabetes. Hammertoes, bunions, and metatarsal disorders are not uncommon in the general population, especially among older citizens. But foot deformities can have more serious consequences if you have diabetes. If you have a problem in the way your foot is structured, it can cause pressure on certain points of the foot just from walking, especially when you wear poorly fitting shoes. If you have neuropathy, any calluses, corns, blisters, and/or ulcers that develop can go unnoticed. They can worsen or be slow to heal if your circulation is poor. If left untreated, these lesions can develop into serious infections. The key to dealing with foot deformities is to have your shoes properly fitted and to inspect your feet daily for any signs of irritation or abrasion. This can prevent serious lesions and infections from developing.

There are several common types of foot deformities among people with diabetes: hammertoes, claw toes, prominent metatarsal heads, bunions, limited joint mobility, partial foot amputations, and Charcot's joints.

Hammertoes

Hammertoes are caused by a buckling of the toes, such that the structure of the toe resembles the neck of a swan. Hammertoes are often caused by a weakness of the small muscles of the foot. These muscles can't stabilize the toes on the ground. This causes the toe to bend back and sit up on the metatarsal head. If you have hammertoes, you place extra pressure on the ball of your foot. This position causes irritation at the tip and top of the toe. If you have hammertoes, you probably have a difficult time getting shoes to fit properly. If your shoes don't fit right, you may find that your foot rubs at the top of the toe and can easily develop an ulcer.

Claw Toes

Claw toes are similar to hammertoes. However, there is more buckling and the toes are more deformed. The toe is bent quite a bit at the first and second joint. If you have claw toes, your toes sit on top of their metatarsal heads and push down on the ball of the foot. You are more likely to have claw toes if you have high arches. Like hammertoes, claw toes are difficult to fit properly. You will need to find a shoe with a large toe box.

Prominent Metatarsal Heads

Prominent metatarsal heads can occur if you have one metatarsal bone that is longer or lower than its neighboring bones. The metatarsal bones are the five long bones located in the mid- and forefoot, just behind the toes. The metatarsal heads are similar to the knuckles of the hand. They are found in the ball of the foot and support your body's weight. Normally your weight is distributed evenly across these heads. But sometimes, one metatarsal head can carry a disproportionate amount of weight. This can cause pain, callus formation, and ulceration of the foot.

Bunions

Bunions are caused by an enlargement of bone at the base of the big toe joint. They are often blamed on tight-fitting shoes, but more often than not, bunions are inherited. If you have a bunion, then your big toe points toward the second toe. When this happens, your big toe may sit over or under the second toe. If you have a bunion and wear a tight or ill-fitting shoe, especially high heels, you put pressure on the metatarsal head of your big toe. This can cause an ulcer to form. Arthritis may occur along with bunions and this can cause pain and stiffness in the joint. You can also develop a callus or ulcer under the big toe.

Limited Joint Mobility

Limited joint mobility of your foot and ankle can put an abnormal amount of pressure on the bottom of the foot. This can lead to skin damage and ulcer formation. Arthritis is one disorder that can limit the range of motion of many of the joints in your foot. When it affects one of your big toe joints, specifically the first metatarsal phalangeal joint, your toe can't bend normally when you walk. To compensate, your weight shifts to the ball of your foot as your heel lifts off the ground. As a result you have extra pressure under the big toe (called the hallux). Calluses tend to form here and lead to ulceration. This condition is called hallux limitus.

Partial Foot Amputation

Sometimes, in order to save the foot, doctors recommend partial foot amputation. However, if you have one or more toes removed from your foot, this creates a foot deformity and can create further problems. If you have toes missing, the pressure you exert on the bones of the foot is uneven as you walk. This can cause ulcers to form and can increase the chances of further amputation down the road. Many patients have avoided this dilemma by having a transmetatarsal amputation performed. In this procedure, all the toes up to part of the metatarsal bones are removed so that, in effect, the forefoot is amputated. This type of surgery results in greater balance, flexibility, and mobility and reduces the risk of developing pressure points, ulcerations, and future amputation. If you have this operation, you will not have to wear a prosthesis, but you will need extra padding in your shoes.

Charcot's Joints

Charcot's joints is a somewhat rare but debilitating foot injury that results from sensorimotor neuropathy. When the nerves of your feet are damaged, you lose the ability to sense pain. Over the years, minor injuries and fractures hurt the joints in your feet, but you probably didn't even notice. Ultimately, the damage becomes so great that the joint is permanently destroyed. You probably won't notice anything until your foot is red and swollen. Once this occurs, the joint can become completely destroyed in a matter of months. Once the middle of the foot collapses, the foot may take on a rocker-bottom configuration, which increases the pressure on the bottom of the foot. Walking can become difficult and ulcers are likely to develop.

■ SYMPTOMS

Symptoms of foot deformities may vary depending on the exact condition. However, several signs may indicate that you have a potentially serious foot problem. Any redness, swelling, or increased skin temperature of the foot or ankle, or a change in the size or shape of the foot or ankle could mean you have a foot deformity. Any pain in your legs while at rest or while walking could indicate a circulation problem that can contribute to foot problems. Any open sores with or without drainage, no matter how small, or any nonhealing wounds, ingrown toenails, corns or calluses, or skin discoloration could be due to a foot deformity and require immediate attention. If you have Charcot's joints, you may not feel pain in your foot, but you may notice a coarse, grating sound when you move your foot.

■ WHAT TO DO

If you notice any of the symptoms associated with foot problems, contact your doctor or foot specialist right away. Although it is not an emergency situation, you should be examined as soon as possible. Foot ulcerations can be extremely slow to heal, so the earlier you seek treatment, the better. Some foot deformities, such as Charcot's joints, can rapidly progress to a point where damage is irreversible. Any change in the shape of your foot, especially if there is any redness, swelling, or pain, should be taken seriously. If you continue to use your foot, you could permanently disable it. If you notice these signs, you need to stop bearing weight on your foot immediately and see your foot care specialist at once. Any foot problems should be evaluated and treated as soon as possible.

■ TREATMENT

Your exact treatment will depend on the nature of your problem. Certain conditions, such as Charcot's joints, may require a specially fitted cast or splint to prevent further damage to the joint and to allow any existing fractures to heal. In some situations, and depending on your general state of health, foot surgery may be recommended to correct a deformity. For example, surgery might be advised to correct a hammertoe to relieve the pressure beneath a metatarsal head or over a prominent toe. Your doctor may also suggest surgery to treat hallux limitus, especially if it leads to ulcers under the big toe. This type of surgery increases the range of motion of the big toe and relieves the pressure on the toe to help the ulcer heal. However, surgery can only be performed if you have good circulation to the legs and feet.

If you have diabetes, properly fitting footwear is essential. For many patients, a good-fitting pair of athletic shoes with plenty of cushioning may do the job. But if you have any sort of recognizable foot deformity or loss of feeling in your feet, you may need therapeutic shoes. These shoes differ from normal shoes in that they are prescribed by a foot specialist and specially designed to accommodate your particular foot problem. Your therapeutic shoes should offer relief of pressure, should accommodate any deformities you have, should provide support for your foot, and should limit joint motion (if needed).

You should first see a podiatrist who is specially trained in the treatment of diabetic foot disorders. Your podiatrist will measure your feet and evaluate your foot structure and your particular problem. Your podiatrist can write a prescription for therapeutic shoes if you need them. You can then take the prescription to a place that sells this type of shoe. Most likely, you will visit a special therapeutic shoe store, or you may be referred to a special foot clinic or orthotic-prosthetic facility to have your shoes fitted. There, you will probably see a pedorthist, who is specially trained in fitting therapeutic shoes. You may also need to see an orthotist, who is trained to fit prostheses. It is usually necessary to make an appointment to have your shoes fitted.

There are several things to keep in mind in fitting any shoes, but these are especially true if you are buying therapeutic shoes. Have your feet measured for size every time you buy a new pair of shoes. The length, width, and shape of your foot may change. Also make sure to have both feet measured. Don't be surprised if they are different sizes. Try to schedule your appointment in the afternoon or near the end of the day. Your feet have a tendency to swell as the day goes on. If you have your shoes fitted in the morning, they may be too tight for you in the afternoon. By having them fitted in the afternoon you can be assured that they will fit all day long.

Don't pay attention to the size of shoe marked on the box. Sizes of shoes, even therapeutic shoes, can vary according to the manufacturer. Make your decision by how the shoe feels on your foot. When you put the shoes on, you should have 3/8 to 1/2 inch of space between your longest toe and the tip of the shoe while you are standing. Also, make sure that the ball of the foot fits well into the widest part of the shoe. Finally, walk around in your shoes to make sure they feel comfortable. They should not be too tight. Don't count on them stretching out as you wear them. Make sure they fit you at the time you buy them. Also make sure the heels don't slip too much. If they don't feel 100% comfortable, don't buy them.

Most likely, your pedorthist will have shoes on hand that will suit your needs. About 85 percent of people seeking therapeutic shoes can be properly fitted with off-the-shelf shoes. However, your pedorthist may need to make adjustments in your shoes to ensure that they fit right. You may need to have the uppers stretched, you may require additional padding or lifts, or you may need to have wedges and flares added to the soles for greater stability. Rocker soles or metatarsal bars can also be added to reduce pressure on certain areas of the foot. You may also need to have special inserts called orthotics placed inside your shoes to accommodate any special foot problems. You are better off with a softer orthotic to avoid any sort of rubbing or damage to your feet. If your pedorthist cannot find a pair of shoes in stock to suit you, you may need to be fitted for a pair of custom-made shoes. These can take 3 to 6 weeks to be made and delivered.

If you do need therapeutic shoes or inserts for your regular shoes, you may be able to get reimbursed for part of the cost by Medicare or your insurance company. Check with your specific plan to see if you are covered. Your primary doctor will need to fill out a form that certifies you are in a comprehensive plan of diabetes care, have evidence of diabetic foot disease, and need therapeutic footwear or orthotic devices.

■ PREVENTION

Foot deformities can be difficult to prevent. Your best bet for the long term is to keep your blood glucose levels under control. This will help prevent the neuropathy that underlies diabetic foot disease. Also take steps to keep your circulatory system healthy. This means eating a balanced diet that is low in fat and stopping smoking. Foot problems can be exacerbated when your feet must support excess weight. If you are overweight, try taking steps to reduce your weight now.

You will also need to see a foot care specialist on a regular basis. You should have an annual exam to assess the degree of physical sensation in your feet, evaluate blood circulation to your feet, and check for any foot deformities or other problems that may put you at risk for ulcers and infections of the foot. If you have any particular foot problems, or are at risk for developing a foot problem, you should see your podiatrist more often.

Foot Ulcers

An ulcer is open sore. In people with diabetes, especially those with sensorimotor neuropathy, ulcers commonly develop on the bottom of the foot or the top or tip of a toe. An ulcer can develop from any source of irritation to the skin: a corn or callus that grows too thick, excessive pressure or abrasion of one part of the foot, or a splinter or other type of trauma that injures the surface of the foot. If you have neuropathy, you may not even notice that you have hurt yourself or that your skin is irritated, because you can't feel the pain. But the wound could still be doing you harm, even if it doesn't hurt. If you continue to walk on your injured foot, you can make the ulcer worse. It may be slow to heal and is likely to become infected. An infection can be even harder to cure and may eventually penetrate the bone, a condition that could require amputation.

■ SYMPTOMS

The most obvious sign of a foot ulcer is an open sore on the bottom of your foot or toe. However, it is very likely that you will feel no pain. If you notice any open sore, bleeding, or irritation, no matter how small, you may have an ulcer or be at risk for developing one. Even if you don't have a visible ulcer, any sort of callus, corn, or area of redness requires prompt attention. If there is any redness, swelling, warmth, or drainage around the ulcer, you may have an infection (see below).

■ RISKS

Untreated ulcers put you at great risk for infection and foot amputation. The risk is greatest among people with diabetes who maintain poor blood glucose control and among those who smoke. Among people with diabetes, 90 percent of all foot amputations occur in people who smoke. If you have any signs of neuropathy or peripheral vascular disease, your risk of developing foot ulcers and infection is greatly increased.

■ WHAT TO DO

If you notice any sort of cut, abrasion, or open sore on your foot, call your physician right away. The sooner you begin treatment, the greater you decrease the risk of infection. Do not put off seeking treatment because it doesn't hurt or the sore is not too big. You need to be seen by your doctor or foot care specialist right away.

In the meantime, if you have any ulceration, do not walk on your injured foot and do not exert any pressure on the ulcer. This will only make it worse and increase the risk of infection.

Also make sure to keep your blood glucose levels under control. If you have an ulcer, you are at risk for developing an infection. You need a healthy immune system to fight off infection, and high levels of glucose in your blood impair the ability of your white blood cells to fight infection.

■ TREATMENT

Your doctor will evaluate the depth and size of the ulcer. Your foot will also be X-rayed to determine whether there is any foreign matter in your foot, whether there are signs of infection in the bone, and whether there is any gas or air deep in the wound. Gas or air in a wound is a sign of infection. Your foot may also be examined using a more sophisticated imaging technique, such as magnetic resonance imaging. Your doctor may also choose to biopsy your ulceration, especially if it is in an unusual place. Most foot ulcers develop on the toes or the ball of the foot. If you find an ulcer somewhere else, your doctor will want to find out what caused it. A biopsy may also be in order if the ulcer is not responding to treatment.

Your doctor will probably remove or debride any dead tissue present in your ulcer. Dead tissue makes it more difficult to heal and increases the chances of infection. Your doctor will also culture material from the ulcer to make sure there are no bacteria or other microorganisms present, which indicate infection.

While your ulcer is healing, you will need to keep it clean and dry. Your doctor will give you instructions on daily care, including how to clean it and what dressings to apply. You may be given an over-the-counter or prescription antibiotic solution or ointment to apply to the wound to prevent infection. Your doctor may suggest applying a wad of plain gauze that has been soaked in an antiseptic solution. This can be applied to the open ulcer once or twice a day. If there is any sign of a fissure or crack in the skin, treat it with an antibiotic ointment daily and cover with plain gauze.

A foot ulcer can take months to heal. It is important during this period to keep your blood glucose levels under control and to stay off your foot. Peripheral vascular disease can impair the healing of a foot ulcer. If you have significant blockages that are preventing blood flow to your legs, your doctor may suggest bypass surgery. Any evidence of infection could also be hindering the healing of your ulcer.

■ PREVENTION

You can take several steps to minimize the risk of developing foot ulcers and infections. Make sure to visit a foot specialist on a regular basis. You need to see a podiatrist who is trained in the care of the diabetic foot. Your podiatrist should examine your feet and check for signs of neuropathy, circulatory problems, and any potential trouble spots. Your podiatrist will also trim your toenails and calluses before they become a problem. You should see your foot care specialist several times each year. If you have any signs of neuropathy, foot deformities, peripheral vascular disease, or previous foot ulcers, you should schedule your appointments more frequently.

Your podiatrist should also determine whether you need any special therapeutic footwear or any orthotic devices to keep your feet well protected. You may find that a good pair of athletic shoes work just fine. Make sure to bring your regular shoes to your appointments so that your podiatrist can tell whether any changes are needed. Your podiatrist will also determine whether you need any special accommodations to reduce pressure points in your feet. You may need extra padding, insoles, orthotics, or special therapeutic shoes. Your podiatrist will also evaluate whether you need any sort of prophylactic surgery to correct any existing or developing foot deformities, such as hammertoes.

In addition to regular visits to your doctor and podiatrist, there are several steps you can take to prevent ulcers from developing or getting worse. You can start by inspecting your feet daily for signs of blistering, bleeding, abrasion, ulceration, or lesions on the bottom of the feet and between the toes. Use a mirror to see the bottom of your feet and toes. Ask a family member to help if necessary to ensure a thorough inspection. Make this a part of your daily routine, much like brushing your teeth.

Wash your feet daily with warm, soapy water. Dry them well, especially between the toes. When you are done, put on clean socks. Use a moisturizing lotion on your feet each day, preferably after they are clean and dry. Make sure to avoid any lotions that list alcohol as the first ingredient. Keep your toenails trimmed, following the curve of your toe. If you have a difficult time doing this, schedule regular, frequent appointments with your podiatrist, who will do it for you.

Don't soak your feet. Also avoid the use of acids or chemical corn removers. If you have corns or calluses, schedule an appointment with your podiatrist as soon as possible. Do not try any "bathroom surgery" or try to remove corns, calluses, or treat ingrown toenails on your own.

Avoid any extremes in temperature. Don't use any hot water bottles or heating pads, ice packs, or electric blankets on your feet. Before you get in a bathtub, test the water with your elbow.

Don't walk barefoot, ever. Make sure you have a pair of well-fitting shoes that have been approved by your podiatrist. Before you put on your shoes, check inside for any tacks, rough linings, bumps, stones, or foreign objects. Call your doctor immediately if you notice any redness, pain, or swelling in your foot, or if there is any sign of ulceration or infection.

Also, over the long haul, develop good lifestyle habits to prevent neuropathy and circulatory problems. Eat sensible, well-balanced meals and avoid too much dietary fat. Keep your blood glucose levels as close to normal as possible, and don't smoke. By following these guidelines, you can avoid the likelihood of developing foot ulcers that could lead to infection and amputation.

Foot Infections

Any time a break in the skin occurs, bacteria, fungi, and other pathogens can enter and cause an infection. The foot is an especially rich source of bacteria and invading microorganisms, because your shoes provide them a perfect environment in which to live. Therefore, any time you notice a lesion, ulcer, cut, or sore on your feet, you need to take prompt action to prevent infection. A foot ulcer is the most likely source of infection in the foot. When an ulcer becomes infected, microorganisms can eat through layers of skin and bone tissue to create a deep hole. When the infection spreads or becomes too deep, amputation may be needed.

■ SYMPTOMS

Symptoms of an infected ulcer include fever, redness, swelling, warmth around the wound, and any sort of drainage or oozing of pus-like material.

■ RISKS

An infected ulcer can eat away at your soft tissue and make its way into the bone. If the infection is deep, a part of the foot or even the entire foot or leg may have to be removed to save your life.

■ WHAT TO DO

If you notice any signs of infection in a foot ulcer, notify your doctor or podiatrist right away. You need to be seen at once before the infection spreads further. You may notice signs of infection even if you don't have an open sore or ulcer. If you notice any redness, swelling, or oozing around your toenail, for example, or at the site of a cut or splinter, you also need to call your doctor right away.

■ TREATMENT

Your doctor will probably first culture material from the sight of infection. You will probably be treated with an antibiotic depending on what sort of organism is causing the infection. This could be an antibiotic or an antifungal agent that can be taken orally, one that is applied topically, or both.

Your doctor will also conduct blood tests to check your blood glucose level and your white cell count. You may also be examined by X ray to make sure there is no sign of bone infection. If the infection is not severe, you will be treated on an outpatient basis, but you should be seen every 2 or 3 days for the first week or so. Most infections will show some improvement in a few days. If you have a soft-tissue infection, you will probably need to take antibiotics for 2 weeks. If the infection has reached the bone, you may need antibiotic therapy for 6 weeks or longer. Make sure to take the prescribed antibiotics for the entire time, even if you think it is getting better. If the infection gets worse, contact your provider immediately, even if you are scheduled for an appointment soon. Signs of a worsening infection include fever or an elevation in an existing fever, increased pain, redness, warmth, or pus formation.

Besides antibiotics, your doctor takes other steps to encourage the healing of your infected ulcer. For an ulcer to heal, it has to be covered with a healthy layer of tissue, with no dead cells in the way. To ensure this, your doctor may perform a surgical debridement. This means all dead tissue will be removed from the wound. This needs to be done frequently as the wound is healing. *Do not attempt to do this yourself!*

Your doctor may give you instructions for dressing the wound. You may be given an antibiotic solution or ointment. After cleaning the site of infection, you can either apply the ointment directly or soak a piece of clean gauze in antibiotic solution and apply it to the wound. You will probably want to cover the wound with clean sterile gauze in between dressings.

Also make sure not to walk on your infected foot. If you need to get around, consider using a pair of crutches or even a wheelchair. If you notice any swelling, keep your leg elevated.

While your infection is healing it is important to keep your blood glucose levels under control. This may be a bit of a catch-22 situation. Infection can upset your blood glucose levels, but too much glucose in the blood can impair healing and promote infection. Therefore, test your blood glucose levels frequently and treat hyperglycemia or hypoglycemia if necessary.

To prevent ulcers or other areas of the foot from becoming infected, make sure to keep any open sore clean and dry. Your doctor may suggest treating any ulcer with antibiotic ointment or solution to prevent infection.

Make sure you avoid walking or further irritating the ulcer. Keep a close eye on the wound for any further changes in its appearance. Also, while your ulcer is healing, keep your blood glucose levels as close to normal as possible.

Nail Infections

The most common nail infection among people with diabetes is onychomycosis. This infection is caused by a fungus and most frequently affects the nail of the big toe. If you can tolerate the unsightly appearance of the toe, it may not seem like that big of a deal. But if left untreated, a fungal toenail can lead to ulceration and infection of the toe itself, which can have serious consequences for someone with diabetes.

■ SYMPTOMS

The primary symptom of onychomycosis is an unsightly toe. Your toenail may become thick, rough, and yellow. Debris from the infection may collect under the top edge of the nail. After awhile, the entire nail may become soft and crumbly and may even fall off.

■ WHAT TO DO

Talk to your doctor or podiatrist if you notice any of the symptoms of onychomycosis. Before treating, your doctor will need to accurately diagnose the problem and identify the fungus responsible. This can be done by taking a sample of debris from the nail edge, examining it under a microscope, and culturing it.

■ TREATMENT

Fungal infections are traditionally difficult to cure. Your doctor may prescribe an oral medication such as terbinafine (Lamisil) or itraconazole (Sporanox). However, these and some other antifungal drugs have side effects. Make sure to discuss these potential side effects with your doctor before taking any new medication. These drugs are newer and have a higher success rate than traditional therapies. You will probably have to take the drug for up to 12 weeks. Following this regimen, 80 percent of nails are successfully treated. However, the condition may reoccur, especially if you discontinue treatment early. Don't be surprised if it takes your new toenail up to 2 years to grow out normally once the fungus has been destroyed.

■ PREVENTION

To prevent fungal infections, make sure you keep your feet clean and dry. Keep your toenails well trimmed and wear correctly fitted shoes. Visit your podiatrist regularly for a routine foot examination. Also, keep your blood glucose levels under control and eat a well-balanced diet.

Chapter 13
Solving Skin Problems

People with diabetes experience a wide array of skin problems. The exact cause of many of these conditions remains unknown, and it is not even clear whether diabetes is to blame. However, it is known that many skin conditions are more common in people with diabetes. Some skin problems seem to be associated with metabolic imbalances. Others are caused by infection. And some skin problems may be triggered by your diabetes medications. Fortunately, most of the skin problems associated with diabetes are not harmful, but they can be unsightly and uncomfortable. On the other hand, other conditions, such as infections, can be life-threatening. It is important not only to learn how to manage the nonthreatening conditions and make your life more comfortable, but also to recognize the warning signs of those conditions that could be more serious.

Digital Sclerosis

If you have type 1 diabetes, you may have a tendency to develop stiffness in the small and large joints. More than a third of people with joint problems also develop thick, waxy skin. This combination of symptoms is called digital sclerosis. The exact cause of this condition, which affects up to 30 percent of people with type 1 diabetes, is not known. Scientists do know that glucose molecules attach to collagen, the underlying connective tissue of the skin. This may disrupt the collagen, which provides elasticity to your skin and structure to your tendons and ligaments. When your collagen structure is disrupted, your joints don't work right, and your skin takes on a thick and waxy appearance. Fortunately, the condition is not usually painful, but it can limit mobility. Patients who have this kind of joint immobility also seem to experience more microvascular problems.

■ SYMPTOMS

Symptoms include a thickening of your skin, which takes on a waxy feel. You may find it difficult to move your joints because they are stiff, but not painful. If you try to place your hand flat on a tabletop or press the palms of your hands together in a praying position, you may find it difficult to straighten your fingers completely.

■ WHAT TO DO

There is no known treatment for this condition. However, some studies have shown that maintaining good blood glucose control can improve and even reverse the symptoms.

■ PREVENTION

The best way to prevent digital sclerosis is by maintaining good control of your blood glucose levels.

Dupuytren's Contracture

For unknown reasons, some people with diabetes develop a thickening and shrinkage of the tissue that lies under the skin on the palm of their hand. The tendons seem to contract and their fingers may become permanently bent.

■ SYMPTOMS

Signs of Dupuytren's contracture include a thickening of the tissue on the palm of your hand. Eventually you may be unable to bend your pinkie and ring fingers. One or both hands may be affected. There is no pain associated with the condition, but it can render your hand useless. Sometimes you may also notice thickened skin pads on the balls of your feet.

■ WHAT TO DO

The only known treatment for Dupuytren's contracture is surgery. The earlier it is detected, the greater the success of the surgery. If you notice any of the symptoms of this condition, tell your doctor as soon as possible.

Yellow Skin

Several different conditions can make your skin or fingernails look yellow. Some of these conditions, although not unique to people with diabetes, are fairly common in people with diabetes. For example, both carotenoderma and xanthochromia seem to occur in people with diabetes and in those who eat a lot of yellow and orange vegetables. Yellow nails can be caused by fungal infection or peripheral vascular disease, but for many people with this symptom, there is no apparent cause. Fortunately, none of these conditions is painful or life-threatening.

■ SYMPTOMS

If you have carotenoderma, you may notice that your skin has a slight yellowish color. This is due to deposits of carotene, found in yellow and orange vegetables, in the skin. Carotenoderma can be distinguished from jaundice in that there is no yellowing in the whites of the eyes. Xanthochromia is a fairly rare condition characterized by yellowing of the skin on the soles of the feet.

Some people with diabetes have yellow fingernails and toenails. The first sign can be a brown or yellow color on the nail. Later, all the nails can turn bright yellow.

■ WHAT TO DO

If you notice a yellow tinge to your skin, look in the mirror at the whites of your eyes. If they are clear, you probably have nothing to worry about. You may have carotenoderma, which is a harmless condition. However, if you notice any yellowing in the whites of your eyes, you could have jaundice due to liver or gallbladder disease. If this is the case, call your doctor right away.

If you notice that only the soles of your feet are yellow, you could have xanthochromia. This is thought to be caused by the liver's reduced ability to convert carotene in certain foods to vitamin A. The condition is not harmful, but you might want to talk to your doctor or dietitian about whether or not vitamin supplements are in order.

If your toenails and fingernails are yellow, talk to your doctor. Half of all cases of yellow nails have no known cause. However, yellow nails could signal a fungal infection that should be treated as soon as possible to avoid further infection. Your doctor will probably prescribe a topical or oral antifungal agent. Yellow nails could also be a sign of peripheral vascular disease. This is a serious complication of diabetes that can sometimes lead to foot disease and amputation. Talk to your doctor about it, especially if you notice any leg pain.

Diabetic Dermopathy

Diabetic dermopathy is characterized by the appearance of small, round, colored spots on the lower part of your legs. This condition is more common in men with diabetes, although people without diabetes sometimes develop it. Seventy percent of all men with diabetes over the age of 60 develop diabetic dermopathy.

■ SYMPTOMS

If you have diabetic dermopathy, you may first notice small pink spots on your shin or lower leg that eventually turn brown. The lesions usually range in size from 0.5 to 2 cm. Sometimes the skin can become scaly. The cause is not known, but it seems to be more common in those with neuropathy. The spots often disappear spontaneously, but new spots tend to develop nearby.

■ WHAT TO DO

Diabetic dermopathy does not produce any symptoms other than the appearance of the spots themselves and requires no treatment. If they do produce any kind of discomfort, talk to your doctor.

Necrobiosis Lipoidica Diabeticorum

Necrobiosis lipoidica diabeticorum is another skin condition that affects the shins and lower legs. It is associated with a breakdown of collagen under the skin. Necrobiosis lipoidica diabeticorum is a fairly rare condition that usually affects people with type 1 diabetes. It can occur in young adults and is more common in women than in men. Sometimes the symptoms may appear before diabetes has even been diagnosed.

■ SYMPTOMS

Early signs of necrobiosis lipoidica diabeticorum are the appearance of red bumps on the shin. These lesions can also appear on the scalp, face, arms, and body, but they are more common on the lower leg. Sometimes the bumps are reddish brown to purple. They eventually grow together and enlarge. These larger lesions usually develop a thin yellow center and the skin takes on a shiny, almost transparent, appearance. Often you can see small blood vessels under the surface of the skin. These lesions frequently form ulcers, or open sores.

■ WHAT TO DO

Tell your doctor if you notice any unusual bumps or lesions. Necrobiosis lipoidica diabeticorum often goes away by itself in 10 to 20 percent of the cases. If you develop an ulceration, or open sore, contact your doctor right away. You will want to take steps to make sure the sore does not become infected. Any infection can have serious consequences.

There is no effective treatment for necrobiosis lipoidica diabeticorum. Your doctor may suggest that you apply a steroid cream and cover the area with a light bandage. Steroid cream and injected steroids may prevent new areas from appearing. Some experimental treatments, including low doses of aspirin and the antiplatelet drug dipyridamole, have been encouraging.

You may want a cosmetic treatment to cover up these lesions. Some women have found that a green-based waterproof cosmetic cream may cover areas of discoloration. Consult with an experienced cosmetologist to help you select the appropriate cosmetic treatment. Before applying any topical creams or cosmetics, check with your doctor first to make sure it will not further aggravate your condition.

Granuloma Annulare

Granuloma annulare is an inflammatory disorder of the skin. It most commonly affects the hands or feet of children and young adults with type 1 diabetes, but it can spread across the arms, neck, and trunk. The cause of granuloma annulare is unknown.

Granuloma annulare first appears as flesh-colored, red or red-brown bumps. These begin to grow together to form ring-shaped patches. You may even mistake it for ringworm. The skin in the middle of these rings is flat and may be red or flesh-colored. It usually appears on the hands and feet. If it spreads across the trunk of the body, it is called generalized granuloma annulare. There are no other symptoms other than the appearance of the spots themselves.

■ WHAT TO DO

Granuloma annulare usually goes away on its own. In the meantime, it can be treated with injected steroids, steroid creams, or niacinamide.

Scleredema

This condition can be a little confusing. It sounds like a more serious autoimmune disease, scleroderma, but it is quite different. Scleredema can occur in people with diabetes, usually men who are overweight. It can also occur in people without diabetes, usually children, following a streptococcal or viral infection.

■ SYMPTOMS

Scleredema is characterized by the appearance of a patchy thickening of the skin, usually on the back, shoulders, and neck. If you have scleredema, your skin almost looks like the skin of an orange. Less often, it affects the face, upper arms, abdomen, lower back, and tongue. In people with diabetes, the condition is usually painless, although you may have a decreased sensitivity to pain or touch in the affected areas. You may also notice a redness associated with it.

■ WHAT TO DO

When scleredema occurs in children following an infection, it usually goes away on it own. But if you have diabetes, scleredema is less likely to disappear spontaneously. Unfortunately, there is no known treatment for this condition.

Bullosis Diabeticorum

Bullosis diabeticorum is a blister that develops for no apparent reason in people with diabetes. The condition is rare and tends to occur in people who have had diabetes for a long time, especially those with neuropathy.

■ SYMPTOMS

If you have bullosis diabeticorum, you may notice blisters on the skin of your forearms, fingers, feet, and toes that contain clear fluid. The blisters range in size from a few millimeters to a few centimeters and appear on normal (uninjured) skin.

■ WHAT TO DO

Bullosis diabeticorum heals on its own with no treatment and usually goes away in 2 to 4 weeks. Do not attempt to break the blisters. Let them dry up on their own. As the blisters heal, they may darken or even turn black. If you do break the blister, tell your physician and be on the lookout for signs of infection.

Xanthomas

If you have poor control of your blood glucose and triglyceride levels, you may develop bumps on the skin called xanthomas. There are several types of xanthomas, including eruptive xanthomas, which usually appear suddenly, and a type of xanthoma found on the eyelid, called a xanthelasma. Xanthelasmas are more common in women than men. The bumps are frequently filled with lipids, or fats. They usually don't cause any trouble on their own, but they could serve as a warning sign that your fat and cholesterol levels are too high.

■ SYMPTOMS

Eruptive xanthomas are small red bumps with yellow heads, about 4 to 6 mm in diameter that appear suddenly and are not easily broken. They usually appear on the elbows, knees, buttocks, or at the site of an injury.

Xanthelasmas first appear as small yellow-orange bumps on the eyelid, then thicken and can eventually cover the entire eyelid.

■ WHAT TO DO

Xanthomas rarely break or cause ulcers and do not lead to any more serious complications. If they occur, talk to your doctor and try to control your blood glucose, cholesterol, and triglyceride levels. This may require a visit to your dietitian. They may disappear if you lower your blood cholesterol and triglyceride levels. More importantly, they serve as an indicator that you need to control your fat intake and blood glucose levels. Failure to do so could lead to more serious complications, such as cardiovascular disease.

Acanthus Nigricans

Acanthus nigricans is a skin discoloration often found in people with type 2 diabetes who are obese and have insulin resistance.

■ SYMPTOMS

The only symptom of acanthus nigricans is a darkening of the skin from velvety tan to dark brown on the sides of the neck, sides of the body, armpits, and groin. It sometimes also occurs in the joints of the hand, fingers, elbows, and knees.

■ WHAT TO DO

Acanthus nigricans itself is not harmful, but it can be a sign of high insulin resistance. Usually losing weight and bringing your blood glucose levels under control will improve the condition. If you want to improve the way it looks, you can try topical agents such as urea and retinoic acid, but check with your doctor first. Retinoic acid can cause birth defects, so do not use it without the advice of your physician if you are pregnant.

Vitiligo

Vitiligo is a skin condition found more commonly in people with type 1 diabetes. Its exact cause is not known, but some evidence suggests that it may be caused by an immune disorder.

■ SYMPTOMS

Vitiligo appears as patches of discolored skin. Usually these patches have lost pigment and have no color. If you are exposed to sunlight, these areas will not tan. It usually affects the trunk of the body but can also be found near the nostrils, eyes, mouth, and other openings.

■ WHAT TO DO

Talk to your doctor if you notice any sort of pigment discoloration. Certain fungal infections can have a similar appearance. There is no treatment for vitiligo, but it can be covered with makeup.

Pruritus

Pruritus is a general name for itchy skin. Itchy skin in someone with diabetes can have several causes. It can be due to the irritation of your sensory nerve endings, for example. Itchy skin can also be a symptom of kidney complications, which are common in people with diabetes. High levels of urea in the blood, a condition known as uremia, can also cause itching. Shingles, a condition caused by the same virus that causes chicken pox, can also cause intense itching. Shingles is common in people with diabetes.

■ SYMPTOMS

The primary symptom of pruritus is itchy skin. When it affects the feet and legs it can become very uncomfortable and difficult to control. This may make you want to scratch a great deal. The itchiness associated with shingles can be especially painful.

■ WHAT TO DO

If you have painful itching and find it difficult to resist the urge to scratch, talk to your doctor. Excessive scratching can damage the skin, and depending on the condition that is causing it, can lead to ulcer formation. Your doctor can prescribe a steroid cream that may provide some relief. If your condition is due to a kidney problem, maintaining good control of blood glucose levels could improve your condition. Often the itchiness may go away on its own.

Necrolytic Migratory Erythema

A rather uncommon skin condition can be caused by a tumor of the pancreas. This type of tumor, called a glucagonoma, can cause a meta-

bolic imbalance that triggers a skin rash called necrolytic migratory erythema.

■ SYMPTOMS

Necrolytic migratory erythema appears as a bright red to brownish red
skin rash on the abdomen, buttocks, hands, feet, or legs. If you have a
tumor, you will probably notice the rash well before the tumor is discov-
ered. If you have necrolytic migratory erythema, you might also have
anemia and diarrhea. Your tongue may be smooth and bright red, and
you may experience weight loss.

■ WHAT TO DO

If you notice any of these symptoms, contact your doctor right away. If
you are found to have a glucagonoma, the tumor should be removed
promptly. Usually the symptoms disappear immediately. Without tumor
removal, the rash resists treatment, although the symptoms may come
and go.

Yeast Infections

Yeast are a type of microscopic fungus. The type of yeast that most commonly causes infections in humans is called *Candida*. Yeast like to find
moist places to grow that can provide a source of nutrients. If you have
diabetes you are at greater risk for yeast infections because of the high
glucose content in your body. Yeast often grow in warm moist places,
such as skin crevices in the armpit and groin or under the breasts, and
in mucous membranes such as the mouth, rectum, and vagina. Yeast
infections can be very uncomfortable, but they are easily treated.

■ SYMPTOMS

The symptoms of a yeast infection will vary depending on what part of
the body is infected. In the mouth, a yeast infection is called thrush.
The tongue and cheeks may be covered with a thick, white, cheesy substance. Near the corners of the mouth, yeast infections are usually red
and moist. If *Candida* infects skin folds around the breasts, groin, or
anus, you may notice a bright red spot surrounded by smaller dotted
spots. These smaller dots often have central yellow pustules. Vaginal

yeast infections are common in women with diabetes. If you have a vaginal yeast infection, you might notice a white curd-like discharge. Yeast infections of the vagina and skin are often very itchy. If you have a vaginal yeast infection, you may also notice a burning sensation when you urinate.

■ WHAT TO DO

The first step in combating any kind of yeast infection is to control your blood glucose levels. You should also try to avoid or reduce stress and get plenty of rest. Also keep areas of infected skin clean and dry. Try to keep moisture from accumulating around the corners of your mouth.

You should also contact your doctor, who may prescribe an antifungal medication to kill the yeast. You may use an antifungal rinse in your mouth—swish it around and spit it out. Or, you may choose an oral lozenge that dissolves slowly to kill yeast. Yeast that are resistant to these topical agents may respond to a drug that is swallowed, such a fluconazole. Topical antifungal agents such as nystatin or terbinafine seem to work well on infections at the corners of the mouth.

To treat yeast infections in the folds of skin on the body, it is important to keep the skin clean and dry. This is to prevent a bacterial infection from also developing, which can lead to the destruction of skin tissue. After cleaning and drying the area, apply a topical antifungal cream.

Vaginal yeast infections can be treated with over-the-counter or prescription antifungal creams or suppositories. Make sure to use a cream that is designed for use in the vagina. If your infection is difficult to clear up, you may need an oral antifungal agent. You may need to be examined by your physician, since vaginal infections often have symptoms similar to bladder infections. If you have a yeast infection in the rectal area, cleanse the area with water, then apply an antifungal cream.

If your yeast infections tend to recur, as they often do in people with diabetes, your doctor may suggest a preventive program. This could include using antifungal powders on your skin and regularly applying topical antifungal creams to infected sites to prevent reinfection.

Fungal Infections

In addition to yeast, other types of fungi can infect your body. Fungal infections can occur between your toes, in your groin, on the bottoms of your feet, on the palms of your hands, or under your nails. Fungal infections can be dangerous if you have diabetes, because they can create an area of irritation that can provide an opening for a more serious bacterial infection.

■ SYMPTOMS

Symptoms of fungal infections depend on the sites at which they occur. If your feet become infected, you will probably first notice white and softened skin between your toes. This often occurs between the fourth and fifth toes, but it can quickly spread to the other toes.

Fungal infections of the groin are more common in men than in women. The infection often starts as an irritation of the inner thighs. You may notice a red, scaly rash. Usually the scrotum is not affected.

You can experience a dry, powdery scaling that often starts in a small area on the soles of your feet and the palms of your hands. It then spread to the sides of the feet in what is sometimes called a "moccasin-type" of infection.

Fungal infections of the nail are difficult to cure and perhaps the most unsightly of all fungal infections. The nails tend to become thick and yellow. They are most common in the toenails, but can spread to other nails of the feet and hands. You may also notice dark streaks in infected nails. The nail can become dull and eventually the entire nail can become soft and crumbly and may fall off.

■ WHAT TO DO

Talk to your doctor if you develop any of the symptoms of a fungal infection. She may prescribe or recommend a topical antifungal cream. To treat your feet and toes, dry well between your toes after bathing and apply an antifungal cream, such as clotimazole or miconazole, twice a day. Once the infection clears, use an antifungal powder on a daily basis. Also wear shoes and socks that breathe well and minimize excess sweating of your feet.

For infections of the groin, keep the area clean and dry and apply a topical antifungal cream once or twice a day. Use an antifungal powder once the infection has cleared. Avoid tight-fitting clothing and activities that promote excess friction and sweating. Boxer shorts can help prevent excess sweating.

For infections of the soles of the feet and palms of the hands, try applying a topical antifungal cream twice daily. If that doesn't work you may need to take oral antifungal drugs. For nail infections, you may need to see your doctor for a prescription medication. Nails tend to be resistant to topical treatments. You may need to have material from your nails cultured.

Bacterial Infections

Bacteria can infect the outer layer of your skin, the epidermis, or the second, deeper layer of skin, called the dermis. Superficial bacterial infections can usually be treated easily. However, when bacteria infect the deeper layer of the skin and make their way to underlying tissue, the outcome can be more serious.

Impetigo

Impetigo is an infection of the outer layer of skin, the epidermis, caused by the *Staphylococcus aureus* bacteria.

■ SYMPTOMS

An impetigo infection appears as a yellow-crusted spot on a red base. It often affects the face and hands. Sometimes it may also blister.

■ WHAT TO DO

A localized impetigo infection can be treated with an antibacterial ointment, such as mupirocin or bacitracin. Once the skin infection has cleared up, your doctor may want to take samples from your nostrils, groin, or other parts of your body to make sure the bacteria are not lurking there, ready to infect again.

Erythrasma

Erythrasma is caused by the bacteria *Corynebacterium minutissimum* that tends to infect folds of the skin, especially under the arm and in the genital regions.

■ SYMPTOMS

Erythrasma manifests itself as a brownish itchy patch of skin. It tends to look like some fungal infections. Under ultraviolet light, these patches emit a red fluorescent glow. The rash usually does not produce any discomfort or pain. It can sometimes itch and sometimes causes a breakdown of skin tissue.

■ WHAT TO DO

If symptoms do occur, talk to your doctor. Erythrasma can be treated successfully with the antibiotic erythromycin.

Erysipelas

Erysipelas is an infection that affects the deeper dermal layer of skin tissue. The grave danger with this infection, especially for someone with diabetes, is its tendency to spread quickly.

■ SYMPTOMS

Erysipelas initially appears as hot, red, hive-like spots on one side of the face, but it can spread to other parts of your body. You may also develop fever and may feel run-down.

■ WHAT TO DO

Notify your doctor right away if you notice any of the symptoms of erysipelas. If you cannot reach your doctor, get to the nearest hospital right away. You will most likely require intravenous therapy with antibiotics.

Carbuncles and Furuncles

Carbuncles and furuncles are caused by the *Staphylococcus aureus* bacteria. The bacteria often colonize in the nose and then spread to the skin, usually infecting hair follicles.

■ SYMPTOMS

Infected hair follicles can develop into larger and deeper infections called furuncles. These can then progress to carbuncles, larger lesions that often occur on the back of the neck. Carbuncles appear as warm, tender, boil-like swellings that sometimes drain pus.

■ WHAT TO DO

If your infection is mild, it may be easily cured with antibiotic therapy. If the infection is more severe, you may need surgical drainage in addition to antibiotics.

Cellulitis

Cellulitis is an infection caused by *Streptococcus aureus.* It tends to occur more frequently in people with diabetes and the symptoms are usually more severe.

■ SYMPTOMS

Cellulitis occurs as a red, tender swelling of the feet or legs. It occasionally affects other parts of the body and tends to spread superficially.

■ WHAT TO DO

If you experience symptoms of cellulitis, contact your doctor, who will prescribe an antibiotic. Cellulitis responds well to antibiotic therapy. Your condition may appear to get worse in the first 24 hours, but after 36 to 48 hours symptoms should begin to improve. If there is no improvement from antibiotics, contact your doctor right away. Your doctor may need to reevaluate your situation and look for possible microorganisms that may be resistant to the antibiotic you are taking. Your doctor will also be on the lookout for a more serious infection, such as necrotizing fascitis and cellulitis (see below). If these infections are not caught in the very early stages, you will need an intravenous course of antibiotics.

Necrotizing Fascitis and Cellulitis

Necrotizing fascitis and cellulitis are life-threatening infections that occur in the soft tissues below the skin. They are caused by a mixture of pathogenic bacteria. Something that is necrotizing can cause the death of cells. Necrotizing fascitis infects soft tissues down to the fascia, the connective tissue that covers your muscle. Necrotizing cellulitis usually affects the muscles. Necrotizing infections are very serious and spread quickly, destroying healthy tissue along the way. They often result in gangrene. Fortunately, these infections are fairly rare. They are more likely to appear in patients with impaired circulation following some sort of trauma. They can also result from deep infections, especially in the legs and genital or rectal areas. Fournier's gangrene is a necrotizing infection that affects male genitals.

■ SYMPTOMS

Symptoms include severe pain, the appearance of blisters, and bleeding into the skin.

■ WHAT TO DO

Contact your doctor immediately or seek emergency help if you experience any of these symptoms. You will need to be treated at once. Your doctor will need to remove any dead tissue by surgical debridement. This will be followed with an aggressive course of intravenous antibiotics.

Abscesses

An abscess is a localized, confined area of infection. It tends to occur at the insulin injection site and is apparently caused by using contaminated needles.

■ SYMPTOMS

Symptoms include an area of skin, often red and swollen, that contains pus.

■ WHAT TO DO

Depending on the size of your abscess, your doctor may need to drain it and then treat it with an antibiotic solution. To prevent abscesses, always use clean sterile needles and syringes. Also clean your injection site and the tops of any vials that you use over again with alcohol or antiseptic.

Reactions to Diabetes Medications

Insulin

Local allergic reactions to insulin used to be more common when beef and pork insulins were in common use. However, the purer human recombinant forms of insulin are making this problem a thing of the past. Historically, repeated injections of insulin can cause indentations at the injection site. This condition, known as lipoatrophy, occurs less often with newer, purified insulins. Over the years, fat may accumulate at the injection site in a condition known as hypertrophy. (For more on injection site problems, see page 123.)

■ SYMPTOMS

Symptoms of a local reaction to insulin include burning at the injection site, followed by a local outbreak of hives. This reaction, which usually fades in hours to days, can be immediate or delayed. Generalized skin reactions and anaphylactic shock are extremely rare.

Lipoatrophy is characterized by indentations at the injection site due to the loss of fat under the skin. Hypertrophy appears as lumps in the skin near the injection site.

■ WHAT TO DO

Most injection site problems can be overcome by switching to human insulin and rotating the injection site.

Sulfonylureas

Sulfonylurea drugs are oral agents commonly used to treat type 2 diabetes. Older sulfonylurea drugs may create more problems than newer, second generation drugs. Common effects are skin rashes, which usually appear in the first few months of therapy in 1 to 5 percent of patients.

■ SYMPTOMS

Symptoms of an allergic reaction to a sulfonylurea drug include a rash that looks like measles. Hives are more likely to occur after exposure of the skin to the sun and are more frequently found with tolbutamide and chlorpropamide use. If you drink alcohol with one of the older sulfonylureas, you may experience a flushing of your skin, especially your face. This is less common with newer sulfonylurea drugs.

■ WHAT TO DO

The measles-like rash when taking sulfonylureas usually disappears after a few months of therapy. Report any skin rash to your doctor. If you are experiencing any other kind of rash or skin irritation, your doctor can reevaluate your medication and decide if another drug would suit you better.

Chapter 14
Solving Men's Problems

All men experience changes as they grow older. Some changes are emotional and others physical. But perhaps the most troubling changes for many men are those that affect sexual function. Most men experience some degree of sexual dysfunction at one time or another. But if you have diabetes, the problems can be more difficult to handle. This is due to a combination of both biological and psychological factors.

A sexual encounter involves four important events: desire, arousal, orgasm, and satisfaction. Both emotional and physical factors affect each of these stages. For men with diabetes, the emotional and physical burdens of the disease can take their greatest toll on desire and arousal. Diabetes can be both physically and emotionally overwhelming. There are so many things to worry about, so much to do to manage the disease, that you may feel too emotionally drained to even want to think about having sex.

Often, complications of diabetes can interfere with the physical aspects of sexual performance. For example, men with diabetes often have problems with circulation and neuropathy. This can directly interfere with the mechanics of achieving an erection. As a man with diabetes, you are also more likely to be on medications that can trigger penile failure.

But there is good news. Doctors and scientists are beginning to get a better understanding of the biology of sexual function and have developed breakthroughs in using drugs to treat erectile dysfunction. They are also beginning to understand more about how changing male hormone levels affect not only your libido, but also your insulin sensitivity and blood glucose levels. As a result, you may be better able to take steps to keep your blood glucose levels under control and enjoy a healthy sex life.

Problems with Desire

Desire can be defined as the wish or the motivation to have a sexual encounter. Society tends to stereotype all men as being ready for sex at the drop of a hat. But that is not an accurate description of any man, whether he has diabetes or not. However, as a man with diabetes, you are more likely to have more health problems in general. This can leave you feeling unmotivated for sex in the first place. Or you could find that you can't even think about sex because you are overwhelmed with the emotional burden of dealing with diabetes. You may find that this happens occasionally, frequently, or all the time. As if that's not bad enough, diabetes can reduce the amount of testosterone your body produces. This can make you feel less energetic and less interested in sex.

Testosterone may also affect the way insulin does its job. As testosterone levels decline, you may experience more insulin resistance and have a harder time keeping your blood glucose levels under control. This, in turn, can make you feel worse physically and further decrease your sexual desire.

■ SYMPTOMS

If you are feeling low sexual desire, you may experience it in different ways. You may feel no motivation for sex with anyone at any time. This might indicate you have a medical problem, such as low testosterone, or it could be a reflection of your general state of health. Maybe you are taking medication that interferes with your libido.

If, however, you feel desire for someone other than your partner, or feel the urge to masturbate, there could be a problem with your current relationship. Maybe your partner no longer excites you. Maybe your arguments leave you too drained for sex.

Your low libido could also reflect feelings you have about yourself. Maybe you are feeling depressed or anxious about something. Maybe you are feeling stressed out by work. Maybe the emotional toll of dealing with diabetes leaves you zapped of all energy for sex.

■ WHAT TO DO

First, ask yourself if your low libido is really a problem. If your partner doesn't want sex, then maybe you can coexist peacefully without it and find joy in some of life's other pleasures.

If, however, you desire sex with someone other than your partner, you may need to address problems with your relationship. Perhaps psychological or marital counseling would help the problem. If you are suffering from depression or anxiety, psychological counseling may also help.

If you do not want to give up sex, and the relationship is not the problem, then talk to your doctor. She will need to conduct a thorough examination to determine whether other medical problems might be contributing. Your doctor will also want to review all the medications you may be taking to see if any might be inhibiting your desire.

Your doctor will also determine whether or not your body has adequate amounts of testosterone. If your body doesn't make enough testosterone, you could be a candidate for hormone therapy.

■ TREATMENT

Before considering any sort of hormone therapy, your doctor may first try to eliminate any medications that may be inhibiting your sexual desire. Do not discontinue any medication on your own without first consulting your doctor. This could threaten your life. Your doctor will probably try switching you to another medication that does not have the same side effects.

If you have a reduction in the amount of testosterone your body produces, your doctor may suggest hormone therapy. Testosterone can affect libido and lack of it may contribute, at least in part, to any sexual difficulties you might be having. Your doctor can measure your testosterone levels and determine whether you would benefit from replacement therapy. Testosterone can be given by injection or through a transdermal patch. Testosterone injections are less desirable because they produce high levels at injection and then drop to very low levels before the next injection. Patches are applied over muscles, such as those on the arm or shoulder, or on the scrotum, although more success is reported with the muscle patches. The patch seems to produce testosterone levels that most closely approximate those found in the body.

Patients taking testosterone supplements report having more energy, a better mood, and increased strength, libido, and sexual function. Disadvantages are skin irritation and itching, but these usually go away.

If you do take supplemental testosterone, make sure to monitor your blood glucose levels frequently and ask your doctor whether any adjustments in your insulin doses or oral medications are necessary. Low testosterone is associated with insulin resistance. Therefore, as you increase your testosterone levels, you may find an improvement in your insulin sensitivity and may find that you need less insulin. Check with your doctor before making any changes, however, and don't change any doses without first checking your blood glucose levels.

Erectile Dysfunction

Erectile dysfunction or the fear of erectile dysfunction can be a major problem for most men. You have erectile dysfunction, or impotence, if you cannot consistently maintain an erection long enough to have sexual intercourse. All men are bound to have problems maintaining a hard penis from time to time. And as you age, the problem may occur more frequently. But if you have diabetes, you may be especially concerned over the problem of erectile dysfunction, and with good reason.

The tough facts are that the incidence of erectile dysfunction increases as you age. The older you are, the more likely you are to experience occasional or complete penile failure. And if you have diabetes, you are likely to develop erectile dysfunction 10 to 15 years earlier than men without diabetes. A full 50 to 60 percent of all men with diabetes over the age of 50 have some sort of problem with erectile dysfunction.

It is not easy to figure out what causes erectile dysfunction. Certainly several biological components have to be functioning properly. A host of factors, including external stimuli, emotions, hormones, circulation, and nerves, all play a role in achieving and maintaining a penile erection. A normal erection occurs when the brain receives a signal that makes you become sexually aroused. This could be provoked by the sight of an attractive person, catching a glimpse of your spouse in the shower, having your penis stroked, or even something you are thinking about. In the normal flaccid state, the muscles of the penis are contracted, allowing only a small amount of blood to enter the penis. When you are aroused, the nerves of your autonomic nervous system release chemicals known as neurotransmitters. These chemicals cause the penis muscles to relax, which allows blood to flow in and makes the penis hard.

If you have poor circulation, blood flow to the penis can be impaired and that can prevent an erection. Or if your nerves are damaged, they may not be able to deliver the signal to your penis that you are feeling aroused, and you may fail to get hard. And certain medications can impair your ability to have an erection. Psychological factors also play an important role. If you have had a failure because of physical reasons, you may become anxious and that could make it more difficult to become erect. The stress of managing your diabetes could be overwhelming and that can also affect your ability to feel aroused. It is often difficult to tell which of these is the greater problem.

Fortunately, there are now a wide variety of medications available that can help you achieve sexual satisfaction. In addition, there are several steps you can take to reduce the likelihood that you will experience sexual problems.

■ SYMPTOMS

If you have a problem achieving and sustaining a penile erection long enough to allow you to have intercourse, you may have some degree of erectile dysfunction. If you are able to have erections most of the time that allow you to have sexual intercourse, you probably don't have erectile dysfunction. There are a variety of factors that can get in the way of an erection on occasion. But if penile failure consistently keeps you from enjoying sexual relations, then you have erectile dysfunction. The bottom line is that if you perceive it to be a problem, then it is a problem and needs to be addressed.

Erectile dysfunction may have nothing to do with feelings of desire. Your general state of health, mental outlook, level of hormones such as testosterone, and blood glucose levels can all affect how you feel and whether or not you feel sexual desire. If you are unable to feel sexual desire, you do not necessarily have erectile dysfunction. Usually, men with erectile dysfunction have a healthy libido.

■ RISKS

Many factors can put you at risk for erectile dysfunction. It could be due to purely physical or medical factors such as heart disease, circulatory problems, high blood pressure, high cholesterol, or neuropathy. If you have suffered any injury to the penis or genital region, this could also interfere with erection. Having poor blood glucose control over time can also increase your risk of erectile dysfunction.

Psychological factors can also make erectile dysfunction more likely. These include depression, anxiety, and low self-esteem. Emotional factors can also come into play. Perhaps you are having problems with your partner, are bored, or harbor some resentment or anger about issues outside of the bedroom. These problems can feed on each other and make the problem worse. Maybe one day you started out feeling overtired and stressed from work and were unable to perform. This can make you anxious and even increase your stress level, making it even more difficult the next time you attempt intercourse.

Medications you may be taking for other conditions can also interfere with your ability to have an erection. Common culprits are blood pressure medicines, such as beta-blockers and diuretics, some antidepressants, some antianxiety drugs, and some stomach ulcer medications. Even drugs such as alcohol or marijuana can interfere with erectile function. Cigarette smoking can also increase your risk of penile failure, because it contributes to poor circulation. The table on page 319 shows some common medications that may be contributing to the problem.

■ WHAT TO DO

If you are having problems maintaining erections, contact your health care provider. These issues can be difficult to discuss, but be aware you are not alone and should not feel embarrassed. This is a medical issue, and just as you would talk to your doctor about having difficulty breathing, you can talk to your doctor about the function of your penis.

Your doctor will first want to figure out whether your problem has a physical basis and will most likely conduct a thorough physical exam. Your doctor might want to know when your last successful erection occurred, how often you experience erectile failures, whether you are able to have an erection with masturbation, or whether you experience any nocturnal erections. If there are no physical barriers to erection, your penis will normally become hard several times during the night, during REM or dream sleep. You can conduct a little self-test to see whether you experience these nocturnal erections. Before you go to

MEDICATIONS ASSOCIATED WITH MALE ERECTILE DYSFUNCTION

Antihypertensives (High blood pressure)	1. Diuretics 2. Vasodilators 3. Central sympatholytics 4. Ganglion blockers 5. Beta-blockers 6. ACE inhibitors 7. Calcium channel blockers
Antiandrogens (Testosterone)	1. Estrogens 2. Luteinizing hormone–releasing hormone agonists
Anticholinergics	1. Atropine 2. Propantheline 3. Diphydramine
Antidepressants	1. Tricyclines 2. Monoamine oxidase inhibitors 3. Serotonin re-uptake inhibitors
Antianxiety Drugs	1. Benzodiazepines 2. Phenothiazines 3. Butyrophenones
Miscellaneous	1. Alcohol 2. Marijuana 3. Cocaine 4. Barbiturates 5. Nicotine 6. Cimetidine 7. Clofibrate 8. Digoxin 9. Indomethacin

bed, you can wrap a strip of paper around your penis and secure it with a small piece of tape. (Do not wrap a whole strip of tape all around your penis, however.) If you have a nocturnal erection, then the piece of paper will be broken in the morning.

Your doctor will want to know whether you are taking any medications that could be contributing. Make sure to bring a complete list of all your medications, even over-the-counter drugs or herbal remedies, to your doctor's appointment. Your doctor will also want to know about any emotional or psychological issues that could be bothering you. Are you having marital difficulties? Are you under an unusual amount of stress at work? Have you lost interest in your partner? If psychological factors are contributing, it is more likely that your difficulties came on suddenly. If there is a psychological cause, for example, you may be able to maintain an erection while masturbating or you may experience nocturnal erections, but you may be unable to sustain an erection when you are trying to make love to your wife. If impotence is due to physical factors, it is more likely that you have been experiencing a gradual decline in performance over the past several months or years. If your problem is purely physical, you may be unable to sustain an erection under any circumstances.

■ TREATMENT

Before your doctor prescribes a treatment, she will want to determine what is causing the problem. It will be important to distinguish between a physical source or a psychological source of the penile failure. There are certain tests your doctor can conduct to get at the source of the problem. In addition to standard lab tests, including a urinalysis and blood glucose test, your doctor will also measure the level of hormones, including testosterone, in your blood.

Your doctor can also test your erectile response to the injection of a drug that will induce an erection if you have a normally functioning penis. If you are injected with one of these drugs, often a prostaglandin, and you fail to have an erection, your doctor can conclude that your erectile problem is due to poor circulation. If you have an erection, then your problem could be due to nerve damage or to psychological factors. If your problem is psychological or neurological, you may find relief in one of several oral or injected drugs now on the market that affect the signaling system in nerves that lead to erection. If your problem is due to poor circulation, these drugs will probably not be as effective.

Other treatment options included abstinence and surgery. If your problem is due to poor circulation, you and your doctor need to discuss whether your heart and circulation system are strong enough to withstand the levels of exertion and excitement that may be brought on by the prolonged sexual intercourse that may result from successful therapy.

Before reviewing the treatment options, your doctor will first try to eliminate any medications that may be causing your erectile dysfunction. You should not stop any suspect medication without your doctor's supervision. Discontinuing a needed heart or high blood pressure medication without medical supervision could be life-threatening. Instead, your doctor may want to try switching you to another medication that will not cause erectile dysfunction. In fact, some medications for heart disease or high blood pressure may actually enhance erectile function.

If you have eliminated suspicious medications and your doctor believes that sexual activity will not harm your health, then there are several treatments you can consider: abstinence with or without psychological counseling, injectable or oral medications, mechanical devices, or surgical implants.

Abstinence

This may hardly seem like a treatment. But before resorting to medication or surgery, you may want to consider whether you can make adaptations in your life to get along without erections. This could mean finding new ways to experience sexual pleasure for you and your partner. You may also want to combine this with psychological counseling to explore whether there is a nonphysical cause of your erectile dysfunction. You may also choose this course if you and your doctor decide that you may have other medical problems that would make sexual activity unwise.

Medical Therapy

There are several drug therapies available that can induce a penile erection. Yohimbine is an old remedy, heralded for more than a century as an aphrodisiac. It comes from the bark of the yohimbe tree. This drug seems to be most successful in men who still have erections, but have problems with rigidity. It has not been extensively tested in men with diabetes, because they typically do not seek treatment until they have lost complete ability to sustain erections.

The recently released drug sildenafil (Viagra) has created the greatest media interest. It was originally tested in volunteers as a blood pressure medication with lackluster results. Researchers were alerted to its erectile potential when the research volunteers refused to give up the drug. A little detective work revealed that it could induce erections.

Viagra can be taken in pill form and stimulates and maintains an erection 30 to 60 minutes after being swallowed. The erection persists for about an hour and appears to work in up to 80 percent of patients. Side effects include headache, diarrhea, flushing, low blood pressure, and disturbed color vision.

Other drug therapies include apomorphine, which works on the centers in the brain that trigger erection. It seems to work in 70 percent of people with mild erectile dysfunction. Phentolamine (Vasomax) is a drug that had been used in an injectable form, but it is now being introduced in pill form. It can improve erections in about 40 percent of mild cases.

Injectable forms of the erectile drug alprostadil are in popular use throughout the country. This drug can be injected 20 minutes before sex and lasts for more than an hour. The big drawback to this approach is the pain of having to stick a needle directly into your penis. One novel way around this is the suppository form of alprostadil known as Muse. This is inserted into the tip of the penis in the urethra 5 to 10 minutes before sex and provides an erection that lasts an hour. It can be used twice a day, but it is not safe if used with a pregnant partner. Drawbacks include pain reported by some patients and low blood pressure.

Mechanical Devices

Another, perhaps less palatable, treatment for erectile dysfunction is a mechanical vacuum device. The device consists of a long, clear plastic tube, a vacuum pump, and a constriction band. The plastic tube is slipped over the penis and the vacuum pump is turned on. This pulls blood into the penis to achieve an erection. Once the erection is complete, a rubber band is placed at the base of the penis to maintain the erection. These devices are especially useful in patients with vascular disease. Side effects include a feeling of coldness or numbness during erection and difficulty ejaculating because of the ring.

Surgical Implants

Surgical implants have been in use for more than 30 years, but with the advent of newer drug therapies they seem to be on the decline. Many different implant models are available. They are usually inflatable or a semirigid rod. All can make the penis hard on demand, but they differ on how soft they allow the penis to become after intercourse. The drawback is that they have to be surgically implanted and there is a risk of infection. Patients with diabetes are especially susceptible to infection. Also, the components of the devices can be broken or the fluid in the prosthesis can leak. Patients also report reduced sensation, reduced penile length, and frequent pain.

■ PREVENTION

The best way to prevent erectile dysfunction is to take steps to prevent impairment of the circulatory system and damage to the nerves. This can be done by keeping your blood glucose levels as close to normal as possible over the long term. You can further preserve erectile function by keeping your blood pressure and cholesterol levels under control. If you smoke, stop smoking. Eat a healthy, balanced diet, try to reduce the stress in your life, and get plenty of exercise. If you do have to take medications for other conditions, ask your doctor whether they can affect erectile function.

Sexual Activity and Blood Glucose Control

The act of sexual intercourse is much like any physical activity or exercise. Depending on the level of physical exertion, it can burn up to 600 calories. Make sure when you engage in sexual activity you are adequately prepared to avoid the risk of hypoglycemia. If your blood glucose level is normal or low before engaging in sexual activity and you burn up a significant number of calories during sex, you may develop hypoglycemia. Be aware that you may need an extra snack after sex, just like after any other exercise. In addition, many people with diabetes have circulatory problems. You may want to check with your doctor to make sure that your body can withstand the level of exertion required for sex.

■ SYMPTOMS

Symptoms of hypoglycemia include shakiness, nervousness, sweating, irritability, impatience, chills, clamminess, rapid heartbeat, anxiety, light-headedness, hunger, sleepiness, anger, stubbornness, sadness, lack of coordination, blurred vision, tingling or numbness in the lips or tongue, nightmares, crying out during sleep, strange behavior, confusion, delirium, and unconsciousness.

■ WHAT TO DO

If you have any of the symptoms of hypoglycemia, especially if you have engaged in sexual activity, test your blood glucose level right away. If your blood glucose level is below 60 mg/dl, you need to treat the hypoglycemia. Eat about 10 to 15 grams of a fast-acting carbohydrate snack. You may find it handy to keep a snack on your nightstand to eat after engaging in intercourse. Better yet, share a snack with your partner.

If you use an insulin pump, you may want to unhook it during periods of sexual activity, to avoid having your blood glucose levels fall too low. How long you can safely keep it off depends on how active you are. If in doubt, test your blood glucose level.

Ask your doctor about what blood glucose levels are safe for you following sexual activity, especially if you go to sleep right away. If you engage in sex before bedtime, you may also want to cut your nighttime insulin dose. Talk to your doctor about the best way to handle this.

If you show any signs of a severe hypoglycemic reaction, your partner may need to give you a glucagon injection or seek emergency help for you. Make sure your partner knows the signs of severe hypoglycemia and is knowledgeable about how to administer glucagon.

■ PREVENTION

The best way of preventing hypoglycemia is to keep close tabs on your blood glucose levels. Before initiating any sexual activity, as with any exercise, check your blood glucose level. Ask your doctor about the level at which you should take an extra snack. A general guideline is to eat a carbohydrate snack if your blood glucose level is less than 100 mg/dl. Remember that any physical activity, including sex, can trigger hypoglycemia several hours after you engage in it.

Chapter 15
Solving Women's Problems

Diabetes can pose unique challenges to women. Some of these challenges are purely medical. For example, women with diabetes are more prone than women without diabetes to urinary tract and vaginal infections that can create risks to overall health. Women with diabetes may experience a host of medical problems when faced with the prospect of becoming pregnant. If you are a woman, you may also notice that diabetes affects your menstrual cycle, which in turn can affect your diabetes and blood glucose control. And older women with diabetes may face special problems as they proceed through menopause.

Diabetes presents many emotional challenges of particular concern to women, particularly as it relates to sexuality. A woman's sexuality is a complex mix of emotional and physical factors. Diabetes can affect a woman's emotional and physical state of well-being and thus may have a significant impact on her sexual well-being. However, medical literature presents a confusing picture of what impact diabetes has, if any at all, on a woman's sexual relations.

You may already be aware that women with diabetes face special challenges when it comes to sex. If you have diabetes, you are at greater risk of developing medical problems. When you are not feeling well physically, you are more likely to feel emotionally drained or overwhelmed, depressed, or anxious. And when you are not feeling emotionally healthy, your are even less likely to feel sexually comfortable. Sexual function depends on both physical and emotional factors and diabetes can impact both.

Sexual Relations

For both women and men, problems with sex can have many causes. A sexual encounter involves four important events: desire, arousal, orgasm, and satisfaction. Each stage of sex can be affected by both emotional and physical factors. You may have problems with one aspect of the sexual response, but not others. Your physical state of well-being can affect your emotional state and vice versa. For example, you may be feeling ill because of physical factors and have no desire for sex. This can create conflict with your sexual partner. If you have difficulties in the relationship and are unable to talk about your feelings, this can create stress, make you feel less healthy in a physical sense, and have even less desire for sex. This can, in turn, trigger more difficulties in the relationship. It is often difficult to determine the original source of the problem or whether physical or emotional factors are to blame. Usually they are intricately intertwined.

Women with diabetes are especially at risk for sexual problems. Some women with type 1 diabetes have difficulty becoming aroused. Sexual arousal and vaginal lubrication both depend on an increased flow of blood to the vagina, a process that requires healthy nervous and circulatory systems. Inadequate blood flow to the vagina can cause irritation and pain during sexual activity.

Many women with type 2 diabetes tend to have low sexual desire, poor vaginal lubrication, difficulty reaching orgasm, and less satisfaction. Overall, women with type 2 diabetes tend to be less satisfied with almost every aspect of their sexual relationships compared to women without diabetes. These problems are likely due to a combination of psychological and physiological factors.

Problems with Sexual Desire

Women in general, and women with diabetes in particular, often report problems with sexual desire. Desire can mean different things to different people. For the most part, desire means having the motivation or the wish for a sexual encounter. It can be triggered by something external, such as viewing an erotic movie or feeling the embrace of a special person. Desire depends on having sufficient levels of certain hormones in your blood, but it can also be influenced by other physical and emotional factors.

■ SYMPTOMS

Problems with desire can manifest themselves in different ways and it is important to figure out where they are coming from. You may feel no motivation for sexual relations at all with anyone. This might indicate a physical problem. Or you could have no desire for sex with your current partner. This might indicate a problem with the relationship. Maybe you have been fighting or are unable to communicate your feelings on any of a variety of subjects. Maybe you are unable to agree on money and cannot put those feelings aside in the bedroom.

Your lack of desire may also stem from feelings about yourself. Maybe you are feeling depressed and find it difficult to get motivated about anything. Maybe you are overwhelmed from dealing with diabetes and have no emotional energy left for anything else. If you are obese, you may have a negative image of your body and feel little desire to initiate sex. If you have low self-esteem, you may also be unmotivated to initiate a sexual encounter. Other feelings, such as anxiety, can also inhibit desire. Maybe you are worried about becoming pregnant or being infected by a sexually transmitted disease.

A lack of desire for sex can also have physical roots. Maybe you suffer from some of the complications of diabetes and do not have the physical energy to feel desire. Maybe you have mobility problems and sex is the last thing on your mind. Maybe your blood glucose levels are not well controlled, leaving you feeling overtired, irritable, or just not quite right. Maybe menopause has left you with little desire and you just don't understand why.

Other emotional factors can also affect your desire for sex. Some may be obvious and others more subtle. The bottom line is that if the thought of a sexual encounter does nothing for you, then you may have a problem with sexual desire.

■ WHAT TO DO

First, ask yourself whether it is even a problem. If you have a partner or spouse who very much wants regular sexual encounters, then it could cause stress in the relationship and create problems. If you yourself wish that you had more desire and feel that you are missing something you once enjoyed, then it could be a problem. But if you don't have a partner or your partner has no desire for sex, then you should ask yourself whether your low libido is a problem. You may want to seek the advice of a professional therapist to assess this situation and to make sure that you and your partner are not denying your true feelings. Many people can live quite happily without sex, but for others, the lack of sex can create problems when you would least expect it.

If you decide that living without sexual desire is not an option for you, then talk to your doctor or health care professional about what may be causing your low libido. Your doctor may want to first conduct a thorough examination to rule out any obvious physical factors. Any physical condition, such as circulatory problems, difficulty breathing, neuropathy, a bladder or yeast infection, or poor blood glucose control, that makes you feel unwell or generally ill may affect your physical desire. Certain medications may also affect your libido. Together with your doctor, try to determine what physical factors could be affecting your sexual desire. Try to figure out what factors you can do something about and which problems you may have to learn how to accept.

Also talk to your doctor about any emotional problems that could be affecting your desire for sex. If you have any symptoms of depression or anxiety, for example, you may benefit from individual psychological counseling and/or medication. If you and your partner are experiencing any relationship difficulties, marital or couples counseling may help. It is important that your partner understands what you are going through. It is also important that your partner understands what makes you feel aroused.

You can also help stir up your feelings of desire and achieve a positive state of mind by maintaining a healthy, active lifestyle. Try to eat a balanced diet and keep your blood glucose levels as close to normal as possible. Get some sort of exercise. Pursue those activities and interests that bring you joy and add balance to your life.

Problems with Arousal

Sexual arousal is closely related to sexual desire. It is difficult to feel physically aroused if you have no desire. However, it is possible to feel desire but be unable to become physically aroused. Arousal often follows naturally from a stimulus such as a visual image or physical touch in combination with feelings of desire. Arousal depends on both emotional and physical factors, such as the emotionally charged excitement of anticipation as well as the physical process of increased blood flow to the genital tissues. The physical outcome of arousal in women is vaginal lubrication.

■ SYMPTOMS

For women, the most obvious sign of a problem with sexual arousal is poor vaginal lubrication. This is analogous to erectile dysfunction in men and occurs commonly among women with both type 1 and type 2 diabetes. Vaginal lubrication can also be affected by the phase of the menstrual cycle. During the ovulatory phase, many women secrete vaginal fluids with little sexual stimulation. Between periods of ovulation and menstruation, the vagina may be much dryer. In evaluating your ability to secrete vaginal fluids, also pay attention to your menstrual cycle and/or hormonal status.

■ WHAT TO DO

Talk to your doctor if you are experiencing any problems with sexual arousal. Vaginal dryness itself can have other causes and can, in turn, inhibit physical arousal. For example, certain medications may cause vaginal dryness, which can make physical intercourse uncomfortable. Vaginal infections can also interfere with feelings of sexual arousal. Your doctor will want to make sure that no medical conditions are interfering. Neuropathy and poor circulation, for example, could also inhibit sexual arousal.

Women who are postmenopausal may experience a general tendency toward vaginal dryness. If you have vaginal dryness, you may want to consider using a vaginal lubricant that can increase your feelings of sexual arousal. Postmenopausal women find that taking estrogen supplements also increases vaginal secretions.

Also, talk to your partner about what provokes feelings of arousal. If you are able to become aroused during masturbation, but not with your partner, there may be something you are doing to yourself that you could teach your partner to do. Many women are also helped by having their partners perform oral stimulation before vaginal intercourse.

Maybe you need more foreplay, but your partner is into quick sex. A candid talk with your partner about what brings you pleasure can go a long way in enhancing sexual arousal.

Problems with Achieving Orgasm and Satisfaction

Orgasm is a primarily physical culmination of sexual stimulation, but it is affected by both physical and emotional factors. Orgasms are controlled by the nervous system and consist of a series of rhythmic contractions of the muscles and tissues of the vagina and genital region.

■ SYMPTOMS

Some women experience pain during or after intercourse, especially when there is not enough lubrication. This condition is known as dyspareunia. Other women may experience vaginismus, an involuntary contraction of the vaginal muscles during intercourse. This is literally a tightening up of the muscles of the vagina in response to penetration by the penis. Still other women may be unable to reach climax because of medical problems that inhibit physical activity. Other women may fail to achieve orgasm for unknown reasons.

■ WHAT TO DO

If you become physically aroused, but have problems achieving orgasm, talk to your doctor to rule out any physical reasons. If you are obese or have problems with your heart or respiratory system, for example, you may not have the physical stamina required to achieve orgasm. If this is the case, you may benefit from a medication or exercise program designed to improve heart and lung function. Obesity puts an extra burden on your heart and lungs and can make orgasm difficult, even without underlying heart or lung disease. Talk to your doctor about weight-loss reduction programs. If your ability to achieve orgasm is inhibited by vaginal dryness, a vaginal lubricant may help. Talk to your doctor about these and other possibilities.

Also talk to your partner about your feelings toward orgasm. If your partner typically climaxes before you, ask him to take steps to first ensure your satisfaction. Sometimes women need more foreplay and stimulation than men. Some women find it easier to orgasm in certain positions than in others. If you are always on the bottom, try lying, sitting, or kneeling on top, for example, because this position gives you more control. You might also find greater satisfaction lying on your side facing your partner during sex.

You may also need more clitoral stimulation than you are currently receiving. Many women find it difficult to achieve orgasm through penile-vaginal thrusting alone. Talk to your partner and try experimenting with different types of stimulation to see what works for you. If you have desire for sex but difficulty reaching orgasm, a candid talk with your partner may be in order.

If pain during intercourse is interfering with orgasm, there are some exercises you can do on your own. A group of muscles called the pubococcygeal muscles often tense up during intercourse and can cause pain. You can feel them when you try to stop the flow of urine while urinating. You can also locate them by inserting a finger into your vagina. Now if you squeeze the same muscles, you can feel a slight vaginal contraction. Once you know how to contract them, you can practice squeezing them for a count of three and then releasing them. Repeat this 10 times in a session, several times each day. If you are feeling pain during intercourse, try squeezing and releasing before and during intercourse to relax the muscles.

If you have talked to your partner and your general care practitioner and are still feeling pain during intercourse, you may need to visit your gynecologist. Your gynecologist will check whether there is any tenderness around your vagina or pain deep in your vagina, as well as the general health of the mucous membranes around the vagina. If you have any tenderness, burning, or pain with sexual stimulation, you may have a condition known as vulvar vestibulitis. If you have this condition, the glands around the vaginal opening may be inflamed. If you feel pain only on deep thrusting, you may have endometriosis, pelvic adhesions, abnormalities of the uterine ligaments, or ovarian cysts. None of these conditions is specifically associated with diabetes, but one or more could be contributing to your problem.

Also, don't forget to pay attention to your blood glucose levels. High blood glucose levels can lead to neuropathy. Often, symptoms of neuropathy are improved with better blood glucose control. This could affect your ability to orgasm, since it is under control of the nervous system. If you don't already do so, try to incorporate regular exercise into your daily routine. Sex is a physical activity and the better your physical condition, the better you will be able to enjoy its pleasures.

Sexual Activity and Blood Glucose Control

The act of sexual intercourse is much like any physical activity or exercise. Depending on the level of physical exertion, it can burn up to 600 calories. Make sure when you engage in sexual activity you are adequately prepared to avoid the risk of hypoglycemia. If your blood glucose level is normal or low before engaging in sexual activity and you burn up a significant number of calories during sex, you may develop hypoglycemia. Be aware that you may need an extra snack after sex, just like after any other exercise. In addition, many people with diabetes have circulatory problems. You may want to check with your doctor to make sure that your body can withstand the level of activity required for sex.

■ SYMPTOMS

Symptoms of low blood glucose include shakiness, nervousness, sweating, irritability, impatience, chills, clamminess, rapid heartbeat, anxiety, light-headedness, hunger, sleepiness, anger, stubbornness, sadness, lack of coordination, blurred vision, tingling or numbness in the lips or tongue, nightmares, crying out during sleep, strange behavior, confusion, delirium, and unconsciousness.

■ WHAT TO DO

If you have any of the symptoms of hypoglycemia, especially if you have engaged in sexual activity, test your blood glucose level right away. If your blood glucose level is below 60 mg/dl, you need to treat the hypoglycemia right away. Eat about 10 to 15 grams of a fast-acting carbohydrate snack. You may find it handy to keep a snack on your nightstand and eat after engaging in intercourse. Better yet, share a snack with your partner.

If you use an insulin pump, you may want to take it off during periods of sexual activity to avoid having your blood glucose levels fall too low. How long you can safely keep it off depends on how active you are while it is off. Test your blood glucose level to be sure.

Ask your doctor about what blood glucose levels are safe for you following sexual activity, especially if you go to sleep right away. If you engage in sex before bedtime, you may also want to cut your nighttime insulin dose. Talk to your doctor about the best way to handle this.

If you show any signs of a severe hypoglycemic reaction, your partner may need to give you a glucagon injection or seek emergency help for you. Make sure your partner knows the signs of severe hypoglycemia and how to administer glucagon.

■ PREVENTION

The best way of preventing hypoglycemia is to keep close tabs on your blood glucose levels. Before initiating any sexual activity, as with any exercise, check your blood glucose level. Ask your doctor about the level at which you should take an extra snack. A general guideline is to eat a carbohydrate snack if your blood glucose level is less than 100 mg/dl. Remember that any physical activity, including sex, can trigger hypoglycemia several hours after you do it.

Menstrual Cycles

If you are a woman between the ages of 12 and 50 or so, chances are that you are keenly aware of the all-important task your body performs every month—preparing an egg that is ripe for fertilization. And if you have diabetes, you may also feel its effects in more ways than one. Not only are you subject to the changes in mood brought about by fluctuating hormones, but you may find that ovulation wreaks havoc with your efforts at blood glucose control.

Ovulation is precisely executed, thanks to the carefully timed release of estrogen, progesterone, and other hormones. The follicular phase of your monthly cycle starts the day your period begins. This lasts for 12 to 14 days until ovulation, when you release an egg. During the early part of this phase of the cycle, the female sex hormones estrogen and progesterone are at their lowest levels. Then the follicle-stimulating hormone (FSH) is released and this turns on the production of estrogen. This causes your ovaries to release an egg midway through your cycle. Once the egg is released, you enter the luteal phase of your cycle. A second hormone, luteinizing hormone (LH), causes the secretion of estrogen and progesterone. These hormones thicken the lining of the uterus in anticipation of egg fertilization. If the egg is fertilized and implants, pregnancy proceeds. But if the egg is not fertilized, the ovary stops making estrogen and progesterone. This causes the uterus to shed its lining, and you have your period.

If you are like many women with diabetes, this high level of estrogen and progesterone about a week before your period can make it difficult to control your blood glucose levels. That may be because too much estrogen can make your cells more resistant to your own insulin or the insulin that you inject. Some doctors think that this change in blood glucose control before your period is just because you tend to eat more during this part of the cycle. But others think that there is a real change in how your body responds to insulin at this time.

But what does this mean for you? It means that if you notice that it is more difficult to control your blood glucose levels before your period, it's probably not your imagination. Many women have high early morning blood glucose levels only to have a low mid-morning value. Other women have consistently high blood glucose readings. Some women may not even notice a change. The trick is to recognize how your body's menstrual cycle affects your blood glucose control.

■ SYMPTOMS

You may notice erratic patterns of blood glucose control during your menstrual cycle. Most commonly, you may notice that your blood glucose levels are higher during the luteal phase, or the week before your period. It is not unusual for your blood glucose levels to be higher than normal for 3 to 5 days and then return to normal when menses begins. This may occur even if you are following the same eating and exercising routines. You may also notice a dip in blood glucose levels in the late morning.

■ WHAT TO DO

If you are not sure whether your blood glucose levels are affected by your menstrual cycle, you can do a little detective work to find out for sure. If you are already keeping track of your blood glucose levels on a daily basis, take a look at your log book. Mark down the dates at which your menstrual period began each month for the past 6 months, if you can remember. If you don't know for sure or have not kept good records of your blood glucose levels and dates of menstruation, now is a good time to start.

Start with a calendar or a logbook specifically designed for keeping track of blood glucose levels. Write down all your blood glucose readings on a daily basis. Also make note of the day your period starts each month. If possible, jot down any notes about how you feel. If you get any symptoms of premenstrual syndrome (PMS), jot them down. If you notice any sort of moodiness, bloating, fatigue, cramps, food cravings, or weight gain, make a note of it. Also make notes of how you are feeling on other days in the month. Be honest about how you are feeling, whether you are close to having your period or not.

After you do this for a few months, review your records. Do you notice a pattern? Do your blood glucose readings remain more or less stable from day to day throughout the month? Or do you notice a different pattern before your period begins? If you notice any abnormal blood glucose levels—either too high or too low—around the time you get your period, first think about controlling the symptoms of PMS. Maybe you don't feel moody or irritable before your period and don't think you have PMS. However, it could be affecting you in more subtle ways, and this could affect your blood glucose levels.

You can take the following steps at first to try to control the symptoms of PMS during the week before your period begins. Try to change one thing at a time. This will help you figure out which of the following steps is most effective at helping you control the symptoms of PMS and whether any of these measures improves your blood glucose control.

- Follow your meal plan as closely as possible. Too much salt can cause you to retain water and make you feel bloated, so limit your salt intake. If your food is too bland, try using pepper, garlic, cayenne, chopped herbs, onions, or scallions to spice up your meals.

- Eat at regular intervals. Don't skip meals or put off eating. If you eat erratically, your blood glucose levels could swing too much. These swings in blood glucose levels could worsen some of the emotional and physical symptoms of PMS, which could in turn worsen your blood glucose control.

- Limit your intake of alcohol, chocolate, and caffeine. They can affect both your blood glucose levels and your emotional state.

- Try to exercise regularly. You may feel lethargic before your period and this may be the last thing you want to do. But regular exercise can diminish mood swings, prevent weight gain, and make it easier to control blood glucose levels.

Controlling the symptoms of PMS may not be enough to avoid swings in blood glucose levels before your period. If your morning blood glucose levels are still higher than normal, take the following steps.

- Add some extra exercise to your daily routine. This may help clear some of the extra glucose from your blood. However, be careful you don't overdo it and trigger an episode of hypoglycemia. Make sure to monitor your blood glucose level after any period of exercise and then again a few hours later.

- Avoid eating any extra carbohydrates. If you feel the urge to snack, keep a supply of fresh veggies handy. Celery, radishes, and cucumbers can be tasty if you dip them in a fat-free dip such as salsa.

- If you use insulin, ask about gradually increasing your dose during your premenstrual week. This should be done in small increments so that insulin levels are higher the last few days of your cycle, at the same time that your blood glucose levels tend to rise. It may only take 1 or 2 additional units of insulin. As soon as menstruation begins, return to your usual dose of insulin to avoid hypoglycemia.

While some women may experience high blood glucose levels before menstruation, others may find that blood glucose levels tend to dip. If this is the case for you, try these tips.

- If you exercise regularly, try to reduce—but do not eliminate—the amount you exercise.

- Try to increase your carbohydrate intake modestly. Don't make the mistake of adding a lot of junk food to your diet. Add healthy, low-fat foods to your diet.

- If you use insulin, ask your doctor about decreasing the amount of insulin you take a few days before your period begins. This should be done in small increments. A decrease of only 1 or 2 units may do the trick.

Some women report that their blood glucose levels swing before their periods. Some report a high morning blood glucose level and then a low midmorning blood glucose level. This mid-morning dip may be a response to the morning hyperglycemia. See if this is a reproducible pattern for you. If so, talk to your doctor about the best way to handle it. You may want to try incrementally increasing your evening dose of insulin or decreasing your bedtime snack to prevent morning hyperglycemia. This may take care of both your morning hyperglycemia and your midmorning hypoglycemia. You may also have to make some adjustments in your morning routine to prevent the midmorning hypoglycemia. This could mean decreasing your insulin slightly or increasing your food intake slightly. Talk to your doctor about the best way to approach this problem.

If your periods are irregular, you may find it difficult to predict when your period will start. Some women can predict it from the first signs of PMS. Maybe your breasts become a little sore a week before your period starts. For other women, these signs are not so obvious and it may work better to chart your ovulation. Even when your periods are irregular, if you are ovulating, ovulation invariably occurs 14 days before your period. So if you can pinpoint the date of ovulation, you can be on the lookout for symptoms of PMS a week later. Many women can tell when ovulation occurs by paying attention to vaginal secretions. Your vaginal discharge tends to be thicker and stickier when you ovulate, often taking on the consistency of egg whites. However, for many women with diabetes, this may be more difficult to notice, due to problems with vaginal dryness.

Another way to predict ovulation is to measure your temperature the first thing in the morning before you get out of bed. After your period, your temperature should remain the same until just before you ovulate. It will dip about 0.5 degrees then rise a degree or two. It will remain elevated until just before your period, when it returns to normal. Your ovulation occurs on the same day you see the rise in temperature, just after a small dip. With training, you can begin to recognize your body's signals and know when you are ovulating and when you will begin to menstruate. This can provide you with another tool in dealing with changes in your blood glucose control on a daily basis.

You can also invest in an ovulation prediction kit, available at most pharmacies. These kits measure the hormones in your morning urine to predict when you are ovulating. However, they are quite costly.

Contraception

Contraception, or birth control, is really not much different for a woman with diabetes than for a woman without diabetes. However, if you do have diabetes, it may be even more important for you to choose a method with high effectiveness and minimal risk. You should only become pregnant if your blood glucose levels are under tight control and if you are prepared to handle the physical and emotional burden of carrying a baby. Blood glucose levels can affect a baby's development as well as your own health, so unless you are prepared for pregnancy, do a little research to find the birth control method that works for you.

Oral contraceptives, intrauterine devices (IUDs), and barrier methods such as the diaphragm and condom are all effective ways to prevent pregnancy when used correctly. The rhythm method relies on predicting ovulation and avoiding intercourse during fertile periods. This is not a desirable method of birth control for someone with diabetes. If you are 100 percent sure you do not want children or if you have already completed your family, you may want to consider sterilization. But be aware that this procedure is almost impossible to reverse.

As a woman with diabetes, you will want to be especially careful with birth control methods that alter hormone levels. These include oral contraceptives, injectable contraceptives, and contraceptive implants. Some of these methods can affect blood glucose control. And some oral contraceptives can be affected by diabetes medications.

Birth Control Pills

Birth control pills, or oral contraceptives, are the most popular and effective contraceptives on the market today. The content of birth control pills has changed substantially since they were first introduced decades ago. Today's birth control pills are safer and more effective than ever because they contain lower doses of hormones. But in deciding whether or not they are right for you, make sure that the risks do not outweigh the benefits.

Three types of pills are available today. Monophasic birth control pills contain fixed amounts of estrogen and progesterone that are taken through your entire menstrual cycle. Triphasic pills contain doses of estrogen and progesterone that vary every 7 days. Progesterone-only pills contain only progesterone and are taken daily. This type of contraceptive is also available in an injectable form as Depo-Provera and in implantable capsules as Norplant. These forms of progesterone-only contraceptives last for several months. Before committing to one of these longer-lasting forms, consider trying a pill form of progesterone-only contraceptive first. That way, if you do develop some difficulties you can discontinue the medication right away.

Maybe you have heard that birth control pills are not a good idea for someone with diabetes. This may or may not be true for you. Short-term studies have shown that today's newer low-dose birth control pills are safe and effective for people with diabetes, but no long-term studies have been done. If you are healthy and have type 1 or type 2 diabetes and you are controlling your diabetes with insulin, monophasic or triphasic pills may work perfectly fine for you. The progesterone-only pills can affect your blood glucose levels if you are on insulin, so you have to monitor them carefully and perhaps switch to a monophasic or triphasic pill. If you have type 2 diabetes and are controlling it through diet alone, you probably should avoid progesterone-only forms of birth control because they may cause you to need insulin treatment.

If you find that your blood glucose levels vary throughout your menstrual cycle as a result of changes in insulin sensitivity, then the monophasic pill may be your best bet. This pill contains the same amount of estrogen and progesterone every day of the month. This can level out the ebb and flow of hormones in your blood throughout the month and minimize swings in blood glucose levels. On the other hand, triphasic pills contain varying amounts of hormones and may cause greater swings in blood glucose levels throughout the month.

■ RISKS

Oral contraceptives can be risky for some women with diabetes. Oral contraceptives can increase the risk of blood clot formation in some people. If you smoke, are over the age of 35, have high blood pressure, or have a history of heart disease, stroke, or peripheral vascular disease, oral contraceptives are not a good choice for you. Smoking clogs up your arteries, which greatly increases the risk of blood clot formation. Do not start with an oral contraceptive unless you first quit smoking. If you develop high blood pressure while on the pill, your risk of retinopathy and kidney disease will increase. Also, if you show signs of poor blood glucose control, such as a high HbA_{1c} level, or if you often have symptoms of dehydration, oral contraceptives may be a poor choice, because they increase your chance of forming blood clots.

Oral contraceptives may not be a good choice if you have type 2 diabetes and are controlling your blood glucose levels with troglitazone (Rezulin). Troglitazone can decrease the effectiveness of estrogen-containing pills by 30 percent. If you are on a low-dose pill and taking troglitazone, you may experience bleeding between periods or may even become pregnant. Talk to your physician about changing your birth control method if this is the case.

■ WHAT TO DO

If you do decide to use an oral contraceptive, test your blood glucose levels frequently, especially during the first few months. You may find that the pill changes your insulin sensitivity and you may need to adjust your insulin dose. Keep good records so that you and the members of your health care team can decide whether any changes in food, activities, or insulin dose are needed.

Also, ask your doctor about having your glycated hemoglobin, blood pressure, cholesterol, and triglyceride levels checked 3 months after you begin oral contraceptive therapy. You should continue to be checked out on a regular basis.

Intrauterine Device (IUD)

An intrauterine device (IUD) is a small T-shaped object that is inserted by your doctor into your uterus. Currently two types of IUDs are in use in this country: a plastic T-shaped device that releases progesterone that must be replaced each year and a copper-containing T-shaped device that can remain in your uterus for up to 9 years. You ovulate as normal, but if any egg is fertilized, the device prevents the embryo from implanting in your uterus. An IUD must be surgically implanted and can remain in place for more than a year at a time. When properly inserted, they are 97 percent effective at preventing unwanted pregnancy.

■ RISKS

The IUDs, particularly those containing progesterone, have been under scrutiny for increasing the risk of vaginal infections. However, that claim remains debatable. They have been blamed for a higher incidence of pelvic infections and should not be used by anyone who plans on having children in the future. They are not recommended for any women who have multiple sex partners. You may experience more menstrual pain and menstrual irregularities with an IUD.

■ WHAT TO DO

If you would like to consider an IUD, talk it over with your diabetes care provider and gynecologist. You must have it inserted and removed by a trained professional. If you experience any pelvic pain, contact your doctor at once. Also, check periodically that it is still inserted properly. This can be done by inserting a finger into your vagina and feeling for the string up against the cervix. If you can't feel anything, the string may have slipped up into the uterus. Use backup contraception until you have your doctor check it. If you feel a hard object, it may have slipped out and you should have it removed by your doctor. Contact your doctor also if you have any signs of vaginal or pelvic infection, foul-smelling discharge, fever, or if you believe you may be pregnant.

Barrier Methods

Barrier methods physically prevent the sperm from traveling to the uterus and Fallopian tubes. Barrier methods are more effective when used with spermicidal foams or jellies. The best barrier methods are the diaphragm used with spermicide jelly and the condom used with a spermicide foam. The diaphragm is a shallow rubber cup that is coated with a spermicide jelly and can be inserted by you or your partner. It must be left in place for 6 hours following intercourse.

Male condoms are thin penis-shaped tubes of latex rubber that are rolled onto an erect penis. When the male ejaculates, the sperm remain in the condom and are unable to enter the woman's vagina. Condoms are more effective when used in combination with spermicidal foam. Typically a woman inserts an application of foam into the vagina before intercourse. Condoms alone have a 15 percent failure rate but are 97 percent effective when used with foam.

A female condom is another type of barrier method. It is larger than the male condom and is inserted into the vagina before intercourse. When removed after intercourse, it takes the sperm with it.

■ RISKS

The greatest risk of barrier methods is user failure. Usually, when these methods fail, it is because the user has failed to insert or use it properly. Some women complain about a higher number of vaginal infections while using the diaphragm, but this has not been scientifically documented. Some people also experience an allergic reaction to the latex used in most condoms. Condoms can reduce sensitivity for the male and must be put on the penis in the middle of lovemaking, which many see as a drawback. Also, the condom must be handled carefully to avoid tearing.

■ WHAT TO DO

Barrier methods can be very effective if used properly. The best combination is to use a barrier method along with a spermicide. An added advantage is that barrier methods, particularly the condom, protect against sexually transmitted diseases, including AIDS. This is especially important for someone with diabetes.

Before you use a barrier method of birth control for the first time, have your health care professional show you how to properly use it. Diaphragms must be fitted by your doctor and are only available by prescription. It is important to have your diaphragm refitted regularly, especially if you have had a baby or have had a big gain or loss of weight.

Sterilization

Sterilization is available for both males and females. Sterilization should not be performed unless you are absolutely sure you do not want to have children or already have all the children you want. For women, the operation is performed by a surgeon, who ties off the Fallopian tubes (called tubal ligation). This prevents eggs from reaching the uterus and thus prevents pregnancy. For men, a vasectomy can be performed, which prevents the release of sperm into the seminal fluid. Some men opt to store their sperm prior to surgery.

■ RISKS

Vasectomy and tubal ligation pose no great risks, other than those of any kind of surgery. Sterilization has no hormonal, metabolic, or vascular side effects. The greatest risk for permanent sterilization is its permanence. Do not opt for this approach unless you are absolutely sure.

Pregnancy

It's not impossible to have a healthy pregnancy and a healthy baby if you have diabetes. But careful planning and establishing healthy habits and good blood glucose control are essential before you become pregnant. All your baby's major organs are formed during the first 8 weeks of pregnancy. That's before many women even know they are pregnant. If your blood glucose levels are out of control during this period, your baby could be seriously affected. That is why it is so important to have a full physical and an evaluation of your blood glucose control before you even begin trying to conceive.

■ RISKS

If you have diabetes, both you and your baby face additional risks compared to a woman who does not have diabetes and her baby. But those risks are not insurmountable.

In rare cases, serious diabetes-related problems can pose a significant risk to you or your baby. If you have severe cardiovascular disease, kidney failure, or crippling gastrointestinal neuropathy, think through your decision very carefully. Pregnancy can make these conditions worse, or it can lead to life-threatening conditions such as a stroke or heart attack.

Certain medications can risk the health of your baby. If you take sulfonylurea drugs, for example, you will have to discontinue them because of the potential for causing birth defects. Your doctor may suggest switching to insulin. Also, certain medications, such as ACE inhibitors, that you may be taking for other conditions will have to be switched to safer medications because of the potential danger for your baby.

The greatest risk to your baby is unstable blood glucose levels. This is especially critical during the first 3 months when all the baby's organs are developing.

■ WHAT TO DO

Before You Conceive

First, schedule a pre-pregnancy visit with your primary care doctor, obstetrician, diabetes educator, and other members of your health care team. You will want to discuss any specific risks you need to be aware of, any concerns you may have about the risks to your baby, and how to achieve and sustain good blood glucose control both before and during your pregnancy.

Your doctor should complete a thorough physical examination before you become pregnant. You will be evaluated for evidence of high blood pressure, heart disease, kidney disease, nerve disease, and eye disease. If you have any of these problems, they should be treated before you consider pregnancy. Your doctor will probably take a blood sample and measure your glycated hemoglobin. This will tell how good your blood glucose control has been over time. If you have type 1 diabetes, your thyroid function should also be evaluated. If you have had diabetes for more than 10 years or have any signs of heart disease, such as chest pain on exertion, your doctor may suggest an electrocardiogram.

Your doctor will also look for signs of neuropathy. Neuropathy can affect how your heart and blood pressure will respond to the physical demands of pregnancy. It can also affect how well your body nourishes both you and your baby, so make sure your doctor knows if you have any signs of neuropathy. Your doctor will also examine your kidney function. If you have a history of kidney problems or poor blood glucose control, your kidney function can worsen during pregnancy. Problems with your kidneys can put you at risk for a difficult pregnancy, including edema and high blood pressure. Also visit your ophthalmologist for a thorough eye examination. Untreated diabetic retinopathy can also worsen during pregnancy.

You and your doctor will want to discuss the possibility of practicing tight blood glucose control before you get pregnant. Before you commit to the awesome burden of pregnancy, you want to make sure you can achieve blood glucose levels that are as close to normal as possible. If you plan on waiting until after you are pregnant, it may be too late. Your baby's organs will begin to develop before you even know you are pregnant.

Talk to your doctor about whether tight control will work for you. In one study, women who practiced tight control reduced the risk of birth defects to only 1 percent, compared to 10 percent for those who began intensive therapy after the pregnancy had begun. You should begin your intensive management well before becoming pregnant. If you have type 1 diabetes, this means adhering to a program of several insulin injections per day and testing your blood glucose level six to eight times per day. If you have type 2 diabetes, you may need to begin insulin therapy and may need to test your blood glucose level two to three times each day. If you have never used insulin before, the best time to develop your program is before you become pregnant. Your doctor will evaluate how well you are controlling your blood glucose levels by measuring your glycated hemoglobin. When your day-to-day blood glucose measurements and your long-term glycated hemoglobin measurements indicate that your blood glucose levels are under control, your doctor will probably advise you and your partner to stop using birth control and try to get pregnant.

Once You Are Pregnant

One of the most important aspects of your pregnancy care is to maintain good blood glucose control. You and your doctor should set reasonable blood glucose goals that you can follow. During the first 3 months, maintaining good blood glucose control will ensure the proper development of your baby's organs. During the last 6 months, your good blood glucose control will prevent your baby from growing too large, a condition known as macrosomia. Having a big baby may seem like a good thing, but it can cause complications during birth. Women with diabetes often have larger-than-normal babies because of all the extra glucose in their blood. However, this is not as big a problem as it was in the past, because today more women practice tighter blood glucose control. If your baby is too large, there is a greater risk of having a Caesarian section to avoid the danger of trying to push a large baby through a small birth canal. This could result in shoulder damage to the baby or respiratory distress. To avoid this risk to your baby and the possibility of a

Caesarian section (C-section), keep your blood glucose levels close to normal throughout the entire pregnancy.

If you are not using insulin, you may have to do so for the first time to maintain good blood glucose control. If you are already using insulin, be prepared to make adjustments in the timing, dose, and type of insulin you may be used to using.

Good nutritional habits are essential during pregnancy for anyone, but even more so for a woman with diabetes. This can be especially challenging during the first trimester if you are experiencing any kind of nausea or vomiting. You should schedule a visit to your dietitian even before you become pregnant, and then continue visits on a regular basis. Your dietitian will devise a plan for you based on your weight, your weight gain during pregnancy, and your blood glucose goals. Your dietitian may suggest eating five or six small meals a day to keep your blood glucose levels stable and to prevent nausea.

If you do develop nausea, eat dry crackers or toast before rising and eat small meals every 2 1/2 to 3 hours. Avoid caffeine, fatty foods, and salty foods. Drink fluids between meals, not with meals. Take prenatal vitamins after dinner or at bedtime, and always carry a fast-acting carbohydrate snack with you.

It is important to remain physically active during your pregnancy. This will not only help you better control your blood glucose levels, but also help you handle the physical demands of labor and speed your recovery once your baby is born. Talk to your doctor about what types of exercise are safe and appropriate. Of course, the best time to begin an exercise program is before you become pregnant.

Your doctor will probably encourage you to monitor your blood glucose levels several times a day. If you take insulin, you may start out testing only before meals during the first trimester and add after-meal testing during the second and third trimesters. Suggested times for testing may be once before each meal, 1 hour after each meal, at bedtime, during the middle of the night (around 2 a.m.), and before any exercise or physical activity, including sex.

If you have type 2 or gestational diabetes and are controlling your blood glucose levels through diet alone, you may not have to monitor quite as often. Instead, your doctor may suggest that you monitor before each meal, 1 hour after each meal, and before you go to bed. Always test before you exercise.

In addition to your regular doctor's visits, you will need to visit your obstetrician more often than most women, perhaps on a weekly basis. Your obstetrician may suggest amniocentesis, screening for neural tube defects, regular ultrasounds, and fetal heart rate monitoring.

Giving Birth

If you have practiced good blood glucose control throughout your pregnancy, are in good general health, and your baby is not too large, there is no reason you can't have a normal vaginal delivery. However, even with good blood glucose control, your baby may still be too big for your birth canal. Many women without diabetes face this dilemma. You and your doctor will have to evaluate whether a vaginal delivery or C-section is safer. Much will depend on the size of your baby at birth, the size of your birth canal, the state of your placenta, and your overall general health. If you have any complications that could endanger your life or that of your baby, your doctor may recommend a C-section.

Your doctor will also be on the lookout for other complications that may arise during pregnancy. Your blood pressure will be checked at every visit. Sometimes during pregnancy, a serious condition known as preeclampsia occurs. This condition is marked by high blood pressure and tends to occur more often in women with diabetes than in those without diabetes. Preeclampsia can threaten the life of both mother and baby. If you show any signs of preeclampsia, your doctor may recommend an early delivery, probably by C-section.

Labor is hard work, but it can be especially tricky for someone with diabetes. You will not be allowed to eat during labor because of the possibility of eventual C-section. This can be difficult if your labor is prolonged, because you need the energy to get you through labor and delivery. Some hospitals allow women to drink juice during labor, but others allow only water. Your blood glucose levels need to stay close to normal throughout the whole process, preferably below 120 mg/dl. Your blood glucose levels will be monitored frequently throughout labor to ensure this. You will most likely have an intravenous catheter inserted so that fluids or calories can be given as needed. You can be given insulin as injections or through an IV, but most women don't need insulin during active labor.

Being hooked up to monitors and IV lines can tie you down during labor. Most obstetricians and midwives believe that walking around during labor is good for you and the baby. Lying flat on a bed may be the last thing you want to do. If you are having a vaginal delivery, you want to let gravity help in the process of moving the baby down the birth canal. Also, the more active you are in labor, the better chance that you can use active muscles to contract and push the baby out. Many women find that moving around helps to deal with the pain of labor. Talk to your doctor in advance about what to expect in labor. Will you be strapped to a bed the whole time or will you be allowed some mobility? Make sure your doctor understands what is important to you. However, if your doctor feels that you will need more monitoring and restriction during labor, it is best to discuss this in advance. Make sure you have a clear understanding of what to expect during labor before you go to the hospital. Also discuss the possibility of C-section even if you are attempting a vaginal delivery and know what to be prepared for.

Once your baby is born, he will be watched closely for certain conditions. Your baby is at high risk for hypoglycemia and will be monitored for blood glucose in the first 4 to 6 hours after delivery. Jaundice is also common in newborn babies, and your baby may be treated with light therapy to overcome this condition. If your baby was delivered too early or is much larger than is normal for his or her age, your pediatrician will be on the lookout for any respiratory problems.

After Delivery

If you have type 1 or type 2 diabetes, your blood glucose levels will be monitored regularly in the hospital. Your insulin requirements will depend on whether you begin eating regular meals right away or are limited to liquids and IV feedings. If your blood glucose levels are low, you may be given a snack right away or will be given glucose intravenously. If you are not yet eating solid food, you will need less insulin. You may very well need less insulin during the first 3 to 4 weeks. After 1 to 2 months, you will probably be able to go back to the same diabetes management plan that you followed before becoming pregnant.

In the meantime, your insulin and dietary needs will depend on whether or not you are breastfeeding, how quickly you get back to eating regular meals, and how quickly you resume your normal activities. You have just been through a very stressful, physically challenging ordeal. During this period your blood glucose levels may swing wildly. The hormones in your body and your whole body metabolism are undergoing a great change. While you are in the hospital, you will be given food and insulin as required and will be monitored carefully. But going home may be a scary prospect.

Make sure that before you go home, you meet with your doctor and go over a diabetes management plan to follow in the immediate postpartum period. Ask your doctor the best way to make adjustments for swings in blood glucose levels. This plan should take into account whether or not you will be breastfeeding. Also, meet with your dietitian, who should devise a meal plan for you that will take into account your caloric needs, especially if you are breastfeeding. With a new baby, you will have to be especially careful about hypoglycemia. During this period it is especially important to test your blood glucose levels frequently. This is true even if you have type 2 diabetes and are not taking insulin. If you feel hypoglycemia coming on, test right away and treat it if necessary. If you can't test, you may want to eat a carbohydrate snack anyhow. Keep plenty of fast-acting carbohydrate snacks close at hand.

You should schedule a follow-up visit with your diabetes care doctor soon after leaving the hospital to assess how well you are adjusting to your new schedule. This is an emotionally joyous, yet stressful, period and you will need all the help you can get. You may also consider arranging for visits from a home health care nurse in the first few weeks, while you make the adjustments to your new life.

Breastfeeding

Breastfeeding may seem like a bother, especially if you are trying to deal with your own changing needs. But in many ways, breastfeeding is more convenient than bottle-feeding. You can feed on the spot with no preparation. And breast milk is the ideal food for your baby. Babies who are fed breast milk for at least 3 months are less likely to develop diabetes themselves. Your body uses up a lot of energy and this can cause your blood glucose levels to fluctuate. However, some women find that breastfeeding makes blood glucose control a little easier. You may be able to eat a little more and require less insulin without having your blood glucose levels rise too high. Make sure to pay attention to the possibility of low blood glucose. Test your blood glucose level frequently, even if you are not taking insulin, and keep fast-acting carbohydrate snacks close at hand. When you nurse your baby during the day or in the middle of the night, have a snack and glass of water or milk handy. You can have your snack as the baby feeds.

Make sure to schedule a follow-up visit with your dietitian soon after you come home from the hospital. Your dietary needs will change if you are breastfeeding, and your dietitian can help you make the necessary adjustments. You will want a plan that provides you and your baby with adequate nutrition, but at the same time helps you lose any weight you put on during pregnancy. All this, while you maintain normal blood glucose levels.

Breastfeeding may seem challenging for any woman, but it can be especially so if you have diabetes. But as many women with and without diabetes can attest, the convenience, personal satisfaction, and benefits to your baby far outweigh these minor challenges.

Gestational Diabetes

Even if you don't have diabetes at the beginning of your pregnancy, there is a slight chance that you will develop insulin resistance about halfway through your pregnancy. Usually, sometime between the 24th and 28th week of pregnancy, your doctor will give you an oral glucose tolerance test. You will be asked to drink a glass of a high-glucose fluid, and your blood glucose levels will be monitored at 1-hour intervals for 1 hour or 3 hours. If your blood glucose levels do not come down as quickly as someone without diabetes, your doctor may determine you have gestational diabetes.

Approximately 2 to 3 percent of all pregnant women develop gestational diabetes. You may have it for one pregnancy, but not for another pregnancy. For some reason, your body develops a resistance to insulin. It may be due to the high levels of hormones circulating in your body, or the additional stress placed on your body during pregnancy, or a combination of factors. Whatever the reason, you have developed a temporary resistance to insulin that will most likely go away once the baby is born.

■ RISKS

If you have gestational diabetes, the greatest risk is to the growth and development of your baby. Fortunately, by the time gestational diabetes develops, all your baby's organs and systems have formed. But if you do not control your blood glucose levels, your baby may grow too large, and a condition known as macrosomia occurs. If your baby is larger than normal and/or your birth canal is too narrow, your baby could be at risk for damage to the shoulder or respiratory distress during delivery.

If you develop gestational diabetes, you are at increased risk of developing diabetes later. You have an almost 70 percent chance of developing gestational diabetes during another pregnancy. You also have a 40 to 60 percent chance of developing type 2 diabetes in 5 to 15 years, compared with a 15 percent risk for someone who has not had gestational diabetes. If you are obese and have had gestational diabetes, your chances of developing type 2 diabetes can be as high as 75 percent. You can reduce your risk of diabetes to 25 percent by keeping your body weight within healthy limits and getting plenty of exercise.

■ WHAT TO DO

If your doctor determines that you have gestational diabetes, you should see a dietitian or nutritional counselor right away. Your doctor can recommend someone for you. Gestational diabetes can usually be controlled by adhering to a meal plan aimed at keeping blood glucose levels close to normal while providing for the nutritional needs of you and your baby. Your meal plan will probably recommend that you avoid refined sugar, maintain a suitable calorie intake, and eat a higher amount of protein. You should continue your regular prenatal vitamins.

You and your doctor will discuss a blood glucose monitoring plan that works for you. Some doctors may advise monitoring your blood glucose level 4 to 6 times per day, much like a person with type 1 or type 2 diabetes would do. Other doctors find that measuring your fasting and 2-hour postmeal blood glucose level on a weekly basis works just fine. If your fasting blood glucose level is consistently under 105 mg/dl and your 2-hour postmeal level is less than 120 mg/dl, then following your diet plan and keeping close tabs on your baby's development is probably sufficient.

If your fasting and 2-hour postmeal blood glucose levels are too high, then your doctor may advise that you begin insulin treatment. If your fasting blood glucose levels are greater than 105 mg/dl, you will probably be asked to take a bedtime dose of intermediate-acting insulin, usually no more than 10 units initially. If your postmeal blood glucose levels are above 120 mg/dl, you will probably be advised to take a mixture of intermediate and short-acting insulins in a 2:1 ratio. Typically, you might take 30 units of such a mixture before breakfast. Although it is rare for gestational diabetes, you should be aware of the signs of hypoglycemia. If you believe you are going through a low blood glucose reaction, test your blood glucose and eat 10 to 15 mg of a carbohydrate snack. If you are unable to test, have the snack anyhow and call your doctor.

As your pregnancy proceeds, your obstetrician will see you on a weekly basis. You will probably be asked to monitor fetal movement yourself. Your doctor will also monitor the baby's growth by periodic ultrasounds and will also conduct fetal heart-rate monitoring from time to time.

If you stick to your diet, exercise moderately, and keep good blood glucose control throughout the rest of your pregnancy, there is no reason that you should not have a normal delivery. Talk to your doctor about any special concerns you might have as your delivery date approaches.

After delivery, your blood glucose levels should return to normal. You should be tested for diabetes on a regular basis. The best way to prevent type 2 diabetes from developing is to keep your weight down, exercise frequently, and eat a well-balanced, low-fat diet.

Menopause

Menopause is a process, not an event. It is the natural way your body responds to a changing physiology. It can be a trying period for most women both emotionally and physically, but if you have diabetes, it can be even more challenging.

Menopause proceeds slowly, often spanning a period of 5 to 10 years. It begins as your body slowly decreases the production of estrogen and progesterone, the hormones that regulate your menstrual cycle and set the stage for pregnancy. When this happens, ovulation and menstruation become irregular. You may find that you ovulate one month and have a period, but then may go several months without any period or signs of ovulation. Some women begin menopause before 40, but others continue to ovulate and menstruate well into their 50s or even 60s. The average age for most women to have their last period is 51.

This may be a difficult time if you have diabetes. Maybe you have finally figured out how to adjust your eating schedule, insulin plan, and exercise routines around your hormonal fluctuations. You have learned how estrogen and progesterone can affect your blood glucose levels. Progesterone tends to decrease insulin sensitivity and estrogen tends to increase it. With these hormone levels now changing, your blood glucose control can be thrown way off balance.

■ RISKS

As you go through menopause, you may face new risks, and some of the risks of diabetes may become more serious. Diabetes itself, for example, increases your risk for heart attack and stroke two to four times above that for people without diabetes. Estrogen protects against heart disease. As your estrogen supply diminishes, your risk of cardiovascular disease increases. After menopause, women without diabetes have the same risk of heart attack as men. If you are a postmenopausal woman with diabetes, you have twice the risk of heart disease and stroke as a man without diabetes.

When you lose estrogen, levels of total cholesterol tend to rise, and good cholesterol tends to drop. If you do not practice good blood glucose control, your cholesterol levels can become even worse. You also face a greater risk of osteoporosis after menopause.

Women with diabetes face a greater risk of yeast and vaginal infections than women without diabetes, and as you pass through menopause, your risk can increase even further. Without a good supply of estrogen to keep the vaginal lining healthy, yeast and bacteria have an easier time growing there uncontrolled.

■ SYMPTOMS

Symptoms of menopause include hot flashes, moodiness, short-term memory loss, and wide swings in blood glucose levels. You may have more episodes of low blood glucose that are stronger and more frequent, especially during the middle of the night. Sleep is often disturbed. You may also notice more vaginal dryness and pain during intercourse.

■ WHAT TO DO

If you begin to experience some of the symptoms of menopause, there are several steps you can take to minimize the discomfort, keep your diabetes on an even keel, and prevent the worsening of the complications of diabetes. First and foremost, monitor your blood glucose levels regularly and keep your blood glucose under control. Make sure your doctor and dietitian know what you are experiencing. You may need adjustments in your insulin plan, your meal plan, or perhaps your oral medication.

If you are prone to vaginal and bladder infections, bathe regularly and try to keep fecal bacteria from coming into contact with your urethra or vagina. Try including a low-fat yogurt in your diet. Some doctors believe the bacteria in yogurt can keep the yeast in your digestive tract at bay and prevent vaginitis. The extra calcium in yogurt is an added bonus in preventing osteoporosis.

Consider hormone replacement therapy. This can be a difficult decision that requires careful consideration of the risks and benefits. Estrogen can decrease the risk of heart disease, stroke, osteoporosis, and vaginitis, but it can also increase the risk of breast and uterine cancers. Progesterone given along with estrogen can diminish the risk of uterine cancer. Your risk of dying from heart disease may be greater than your increased risk of cancer induced by hormone therapy. To make this decision, you may need to discuss your options with your doctor. If you have a family history of heart disease, you may very well benefit from hormone replacement therapy. However, if there is a strong risk of breast cancer or blood clotting in your family, you may not want to increase that risk by taking hormone supplements.

If you do opt for hormone replacement therapy, be aware that you may have to readjust your blood glucose management plan to accommodate the additional hormones. Estrogen increases insulin sensitivity, but progesterone decreases it. You and your doctor should discuss an approach that works best for you.

After menopause, make sure to keep up with your regular diabetes care plan of good blood glucose control, regular exercise, and a healthy eating plan. You may also want to consider adding some tests or taking some tests more frequently.

- Have your glycated hemoglobin tested four times a year. This will tell you and your doctor how well you are controlling your blood glucose over time.

- Have your lipid and cholesterol levels checked four times a year. The progesterone in hormone replacement therapy can sometimes cause your cholesterol levels to rise.

- Have yearly eye exams and kidney function tests.

- Have a yearly mammogram to detect breast cancer. This is especially important if you are receiving hormone replacement therapy.

- Have a yearly Pap smear and gynecological exam to detect cancer of the cervix, uterus, endometrium, and ovaries.

Osteoporosis

As you go through menopause, you lose estrogen. Estrogen can protect against osteoporosis, or porous bones. This condition is more common in women as they age, and if you have diabetes, you may face an additional risk of osteoporosis.

■ RISKS

Your risk of osteoporosis as you age increases if you are a smoker, thin, fair-skinned, have experienced early menopause, have been on steroid therapy, or have had prolonged bouts of high blood glucose levels. Your risk is further increased if you do not take in enough calcium, have a history of anorexia or bulimia, or have a diet high in alcohol and caffeine or very low in fat.

■ SYMPTOMS

Osteoporosis does not really have symptoms, unless it affects the bones of the back. If this happens you may experience backache or notice that you are becoming shorter or more round-shouldered. In rare cases you may experience a sudden onset of severe back pain.

■ WHAT TO DO

The best way to prevent osteoporosis from occurring or getting worse is to engage in regular weight-bearing exercise. This can help build up your body mass and bone density. Talk to your doctor or exercise physiologist about what might work for you. Even lifting 1-or 2-pound weights can help improve your bone strength. This needn't require any overexertion. For many exercises, you can sit in a chair and lift a 1-pound weight repeatedly. Consult with an exercise specialist to learn how to lift weights correctly, or read Miriam Nelson's *Strong Women Stay Young* (Bantam Books, 1997).

If you smoke, stop smoking. Smoking can prevent calcium absorption by your bones and leave your bones fragile and thin.

Eat a balanced meal plan that has enough calcium, phosphorus, and vitamin D. Talk to your dietitian about what foods will provide these nutrients. Of course, the time to begin eating better is even before osteoporosis sets in. If you do not do so already, keep your blood glucose levels under control.

Consider hormone replacement therapy. Estrogen prevents the loss of calcium and bone deterioration. Talk to your doctor about whether the benefits outweigh the risks for you.

Chapter 16
Solving Kids' Problems

For Kids

Some kids are tall, some short, some stocky, some skinny. Some kids have brown eyes and some kids have blue eyes. Some kids get sunburns and some kids get suntans. Some kids get cavities and some kids don't. Some kids wear glasses and other kids wear braces. And some kids have diabetes. Maybe you are one of those kids.

The truth is you are just like any other kid on the planet. No one is exactly the same, not even identical twins. We all have differences and that's what makes each one of us special. And one of the things that makes you special is having diabetes. That doesn't mean there is anything wrong with you as a person. It just means that there is something a little different about the way some of the cells in your body work. The cells of your pancreas have been damaged and don't work as they should. They don't produce the insulin your body needs. Your body needs insulin to let glucose, or sugar, into your cells. Your body breaks down, or digests, most of the food you eat into glucose. The cells in your body need glucose to give them the energy to work right. You're not that much different than the kid next door who can't see right. He needs glasses to help his eyes do their job. You need insulin to help your cells do their job.

Diabetes is not easy. You already know that it takes extra effort to keep everything in balance. You have to pay attention to what you eat, figure out how much insulin you need, and measure your blood glucose levels. But the good news is that when you do these things, you are learning to live a healthy lifestyle. And that's just what everyone else is trying to do, whether they have diabetes or not. Maybe you're even a little luckier than most kids, because you are forced to eat good foods and take care of yourself. That may make you even healthier than kids who don't always eat what they should.

Managing Your Daily Routine

Diabetes can change the way you go through your daily routine: eating, drinking, playing, going to school, along with testing your blood glucose and taking insulin. Doing all the right things can take a little getting used to. But once you figure it out, you can get through each day just like any other kid.

Whatever you do during the day and night, you want to keep your blood glucose from getting too high or too low. If it gets too high or too low, you will feel sick. Eating food makes the glucose level in your blood go up. Insulin and exercise makes it go down. If you have diabetes, your body doesn't make the insulin your body needs, so you have to give yourself insulin. Your body needs food and glucose to be able to do all the things it is supposed to. So as you go through your day you have to eat enough food to give your body the glucose and nutrients it needs, but not so much that your blood glucose level goes too high. You also have to take enough insulin so your body can use the glucose, but not enough to make your blood glucose level go too low.

Eating

This might be the hardest part about having diabetes for you. You go to lunch and the kid next to you gets a big fat brownie for dessert and you're stuck with an apple. You wish you could have a brownie or cookies for dessert. And often you might get tired of always having to eat healthy foods. It just doesn't seem fair.

■ WHAT TO DO

If you have a hard time eating what you should, or don't like that you never get to have a treat you like, talk to your parents. Try not to complain in a whiny voice. Instead ask nicely, "Mom (or Dad), do you think we could do something about my meal plan?" The time to ask is not when it's an hour before dinner and you are begging to have a chocolate bar. Talk about it when you are both happy and calm. Ask your mom or dad if you could meet with your dietitian and figure out a meal plan that lets you have a treat you like every now and then.

Your dietitian is the person who figures out the best way to plan your meals. Sometimes people with diabetes are told to follow the same meal plan that everyone else follows. But not everyone likes the same things. It is hard to stick to a meal plan that doesn't include any of your favorite things and makes you eat a lot of foods you don't like. Your dietitian should ask you what kinds of foods you like, what kinds of foods you don't like, whether you like to eat just a few big meals, or whether you like to eat a lot of small meals. Your dietitian might be able to work out a plan that lets you have a lot of snacks instead of eating a lot at each big meal. Your snacks should be healthy, but they should also be things that you like.

And your meal plan ought to let you have a special treat every now and then. That doesn't mean you will be able to eat a lot of junk food all the time. But maybe it will be easier to stick to your plan if you know you will get a little treat sometimes. Your dietitian may also be able to give your parents some special recipes. Maybe you can't eat a certain candy or cake because of all the sugar or fat in it. But maybe your parents can make you some snacks that taste good, and don't hurt your blood glucose control. If you are able to eat meals and snacks that include the foods you like, it might not be so hard sticking with your meal plan.

Just remember that the foods you eat are not any different than what people without diabetes eat. You don't have to eat special diabetic foods. You just need to eat healthy foods. And that's just what everyone else on the planet should be doing. You are getting a head start at healthy eating because you know how important it is to eat the right foods.

Testing

This might be another thing you don't like that much about having diabetes. You have to poke your finger several times a day to get a drop of blood to test it for glucose. It may not be much fun, but it's the way you and your parents can tell if you're doing okay. It's sort of like having your temperature taken when you're sick. If your glucose goes up too high or down too low, you will feel sick. As long as you and your parents have a way to keep track of your glucose, you will feel okay and can do all the things you like to do, just like any other kid.

■ WHAT TO DO

The worst part about testing is the way it feels when you have to poke yourself. Most kids get used to it. But if it still hurts when you get poked, ask your parents to find you a lancet that doesn't hurt that much. You are probably already using an automatic lancing device. If you are not using an automatic lancing device, make sure you get one. Tell your parents to look for one with shallow penetration. These work better for kids. Try different ones until you find one that doesn't hurt. Also poke a different finger each time so your fingers don't get too sore. Some kids poke and test themselves and some kids have their parents do it. Try both ways and see which you like best.

It may seem like you are testing all the time. You might not like that, especially if you are in the middle of doing something fun. But remember, the more you test, the better you are able to keep your blood glucose levels normal. Good times to test are before breakfast, lunch, and dinner, before you go to bed, and 2 hours after each meal. Sometimes you might even have to test in the middle of the night. You should do extra tests when you are sick or have your parents do it for you. Also, test before doing any sport or physical activity.

Insulin

Insulin works like a little teeny key. It finds the "locks" on the cells in your body that need glucose and unlocks the door to let the glucose into the cell. Without the energy they need, cells like your muscle cells and brain cells don't have the energy to help you move, grow, and think. Your doctor has worked out a plan to give you enough insulin during the day to let you use the glucose in the foods you eat. Your plan gets you more insulin before your meals. If there is too much or too little glucose in your blood, you will feel sick. So your insulin plan has to make sure to take care of just the right amount of glucose. That's why it is important to stick to your plan. Don't ever skip doses, even if you don't feel like taking a shot. Don't skip planned meals and snacks, even if you think you're not hungry. You have to keep the food and insulin balanced with each other.

What you might not like about insulin is having to give yourself shots. It will take a little getting used to. You might feel more comfortable if your parents do it for you, especially if you are new to diabetes. But eventually you will need to learn to do it yourself, because your parents can't always be with you.

Where do you inject insulin? Your skin is a layer of cells that covers and protects your body. If you inject your syringe into your skin, insulin won't get to where it needs to be. Just underneath the skin is a layer of cells called the subcutaneous (or sub-Q) layer that contains a lot of fat. This is where you want to inject insulin. When you inject insulin here, it goes into your body at a steady rate. This will help keep too much or too little glucose from staying in your blood.

There is sub-Q tissue all over your body. The places for injecting insulin are:

- Your arm—the upper outside part

- Your thighs—the front and sides

- Your buttocks

- Your back—just above your waist (this might be a hard place to reach, though, and you may need a little help)

- Your stomach—except for the area around your belly button (be sure to inject here if your glucose level is high)

If you inject in the same place every time, after a while it might start to hurt, or you could get bumps forming there. To make sure this does not happen, change the place where you inject each time. This is called site rotation. Your doctor can help you figure out a plan for rotating sites. You might want to do your morning shots in your arm and your evening shots in your leg, or the other way around. If you do this, try to always do your morning shots in one place and your evening shots in the other place. That's because insulin can get into your body faster from some places than others and you want to make sure you do the same thing every time, so your glucose levels don't go too far up or too far down. But if you are doing your morning injections in your arm, change the exact spot each time.

If you have a hard time giving yourself your own shots, talk to your parents. Ask them to let you try something like the Inject-Ease injector or other kind of injection aid. This is a special kind of syringe. The needle stays inside the unit so you don't even see it. When you press the button, the needle goes in very quickly so it doesn't hurt. It's easy to use and many kids—even little kids—can use it themselves.

Some kids find it easier to use a pump. A pump is something you keep strapped to you all the time. It holds a supply of insulin and pumps it into your body at a steady rate. The insulin goes through a piece of tubing to an insertion site. This is sort of like a needle that you leave there for a few days. Every few days you move your insertion site somewhere else. With a pump you don't have to worry about shots all the time. You just press a button before your meal to give yourself a little extra insulin. You can take your pump off when you are doing sports. If you think you might be interested in trying a pump, talk to your parents. It might make things a lot easier for you.

Special Events

Once you get used to eating right and giving yourself insulin, you might think having diabetes is not all that bad. You and your parents have probably worked out ways to make blood testing, eating, and insulin injections fairly easy. But then something comes up. You want to stay overnight at your friend's house or you are invited to a birthday party or want to go on an overnight camping trip with your scout troop. You might be afraid you can't do these things. But if you plan things in advance, you should be able to do anything any other kid can do.

■ WHAT TO DO

Any time you want to do something out of the ordinary, make sure to come up with a plan. Exactly what goes into your plan depends on what you are expecting to do and how you handle things every day. When you make your plan, try to keep things as normal as possible.

If you are just going to a party for a few hours, talk to your parents about whether you need to test and when to do it. If there are going to be special treats served, talk about what you can eat and how you can fit it into your meal plan. If snacks will be served, count what you eat as one of your snacks. Test before you eat to make sure your glucose is not too high. You should be able to eat what others are eating, as long as you account for it and don't overdo it. If you work out that you can have a cupcake, don't have three. You may need to change some of your other meals or your insulin dose. If you drink soda, make sure to drink diet soda. Or better yet, drink water. If you are eating hamburgers or pizza, make sure to count it as one of your regular meals. Your parents will probably want to talk to whoever is in charge of the party to make sure the food and activities will fit in with your plan.

If you are going to stay overnight somewhere, you also need a plan. If you are staying at a friend's house, make sure your friend's parents know what you need to eat and when, when you need to test, and when you need to take your insulin. Sometimes if you are having too much fun it is easy to forget and it helps to have someone who can remind you. Make sure your friend's parents know how to tell if your blood glucose is too high or too low. As long as you stick to your plan and count any snacks you have as you do for anything else you eat, you should be able to have a fun time.

If you are staying overnight in the woods or having some sort of adventure, you want to plan for it the same way. Make sure to pack plenty of snacks. Pack all the supplies that you normally need for testing blood and taking insulin in a special bag and keep it close to you. A fanny pack works well, especially if it is insulated. If you are going with a big group, you might want to pack extra supplies and give it to your leader or whoever is in charge. Make sure that whoever is in charge knows how to test your blood and knows when you should test, eat, and inject your insulin. Plan your meals in advance just like you would plan your meals at home. If you need any foods that won't be served to the whole group, make sure to bring along your own supply. Wear a watch so you know when you should test, eat, and take insulin. Also, if you are doing anything physical, like hiking a mountain or paddling a canoe, you may need extra snacks. Make sure to test your blood before and during any physical activity and eat extra snacks if your blood glucose falls too low. Always carry a pocket carbohydrate snack. Ask your mom or dad to talk to your doctor about whether you should also bring a glucagon kit.

Sports and Activities

If you like sports, dance, or anything physical, there is no reason you shouldn't be able to do it. In fact, exercise is good for people with diabetes. It helps keep your blood glucose from going too high. Exercise uses up glucose for energy and makes your blood glucose go down. You just want to be careful you don't let it go down too low.

■ WHAT TO DO

You can do just about any sport you want to if you just plan ahead. Depending on your activity, your parents may want to ask your doctor whether you need to adjust your insulin dose. They will also want to make sure your coach or whoever is in charge knows about your diabetes.

Before you start any game or activity, test your blood glucose. If it is too low, have a quick snack and drink lots of water. Pay attention to how you are feeling. If you start to feel shaky or dizzy, tell whoever is in charge and sit down for a few minutes. Test your blood glucose if you feel funny at any time. Also test after you have been doing the game or activity for 30 minutes, especially if it is a nonstop activity, like soccer. Even if you are just running around on the playground, you may have to stop, test, and have a snack. If you are using an insulin pump, you will probably be able to take it off while you are playing. All athletes (even Michael Jordan) should stop and have a break every now and then to drink some water and have a snack. You are no different. Play smart and you should be able to have fun just like everyone else.

Handling Emergencies

Every now and then, even if you take special care to test often and watch what you eat, sometimes your blood glucose may go too high or too low. Usually when that happens you won't feel right. If you pretend you are feeling okay when you aren't, you could start to feel much worse. This could be dangerous. The best way to keep things from getting worse is to take action right away.

■ WHAT TO DO

If you don't have enough glucose in your blood, you can get something called hypoglycemia, or low blood glucose. This can happen when you have too much insulin, too little food or carbohydrate, too much exercise, or if you eat your meal too late. You may start to feel shaky or nervous. You might start sweating or feel chills and a little clammy. You may feel very hungry and light-headed. You may also feel sad, angry, or confused. You can also get a stomachache or your tongue or lips may feel funny. When you are sleeping, you might have nightmares.

If you feel any of those things, make sure to tell an adult at once. You should test your blood right away. If your blood glucose is below 60, eat a snack without delay. If you don't have time to test, eat a snack anyhow. You could have a few glucose tablets, a half a can of regular soda or a small glass of orange juice. Or have 5 to 10 jelly beans, Lifesavers, or gumdrops. This should bring your blood glucose back up. After you eat, test 10 to 15 minutes later. If your reading is still low, have another snack. If you are playing or running around, stop and test.

If you take these steps and rest a while, you should feel better in no time. If you don't feel better, make sure to tell someone. If your glucose drops too low, someone else will have to take over. Make sure your friends or people you are with know what to do if you have low blood glucose.

You can also start to feel bad if you have too much glucose in your blood. When this happens you have hyperglycemia, or high blood glucose. This can happen if you eat too much, don't take enough insulin, or skip an insulin dose. When your blood glucose is too high, you may feel extremely thirsty. Your mouth may feel very dry. Your skin can feel warm and dry even though you aren't sweating. You can even feel sleepy or confused. You might just feel funny or not quite right. Any time you don't feel like you usually do, tell an adult, and test your blood glucose. If it is over 250, tell an adult right away. You may also have to do something called a ketone test. If your glucose is too high you may have to take some extra insulin. But don't take any extra insulin without talking to an adult first.

Dealing with Your Friends

At first you may feel funny about your diabetes around your friends. You may feel kind of left out, maybe even a little weird. Or, maybe you'll feel kind of special. Your friends will want to know about your diabetes. Tell them what you know about diabetes and make sure they understand that they can't "catch" it. It's not like a cold or the flu.

Tell them how you test your blood and inject insulin. You can even show them if you want to. Most kids will find that interesting and even kind of cool. They will think it's neat that you do these tests and take these shots every day. If you have a pump, show them how that works. Once your friends understand something about diabetes, they won't treat you any differently than anyone else.

If someone does treat you unfairly, talk about it with your teacher or parents. Usually people act strangely only when they don't understand something. If you sit down and talk with that person and explain your diabetes to them, that will probably make them understand. Insulin gives you that extra help you need. You're no different in that way than someone who has to wear glasses or braces. But sometimes people are just mean. If you run across people like that, just ignore them. There are plenty of other people around who want to be friends.

Dealing with Your Family

Sometimes having diabetes can change things in the family. Maybe your parents treat you differently. Maybe it seems like they boss you around too much or don't let you do the things you used to. Maybe it seems like they nag you. Maybe your parents seem nervous and you start to feel nervous too. It can be hard when you are treated differently and you may start to feel bad, too. But this is normal. Even when you are sick in bed with the flu or a cold, your parents worry and maybe even fuss a little too much. When you have diabetes, your parents worry about you. It's because they love you and want you to feel good. If you don't like they way they are treating you, talk to your parents. Tell them how you are feeling. This can help everyone feel a little better.

If you have brothers and sisters, things can change for them too. When you found out about your diabetes, you probably got a lot of attention. This probably made your brothers and sisters feel left out. They may have even felt that your parents loved you more. That can make them feel bad and start treating you badly too. Even though they love you and care about you, they are not used to being left out. If you see your brothers and sisters treating you differently, try to be understanding. After a while everything will probably go back to normal. If things really get out of hand, talk to your parents about it. Sometimes your siblings act just the opposite. They care about you too and worry about you. They may follow you around all the time. It might even start to bug you. If this happens, don't worry about it. Tell them you are okay and want to be treated like you always were. Just understand that they act that way because they care.

Dealing with Your Feelings

When you found out you had diabetes, you probably felt a lot of different feelings. Maybe you were feeling sick before you knew, and finding out it was diabetes was a relief. No wonder you were feeling so crummy! Maybe you were a little scared. You knew that diabetes was serious and your life would never be the same. Maybe you felt odd, like you had something no one else did and you really didn't like feeling different. Or maybe you even felt special. You may have received extra attention and maybe even now you get special treats that no one else gets.

Once you began to work with your diabetes, maybe things settled down a little. You got used to testing your blood, giving yourself shots, and eating a little differently. Maybe you realized it wasn't all that bad. Still, every now and then, maybe you get sick of always having to worry about what you are supposed to eat and get tired of having to test your blood all the time. Sometimes you might even feel downright angry. It's okay to feel that way sometimes. You will have good days and bad days, like any other kid or any other grown-up. Sometimes you feel bad and it has nothing to do with your diabetes. Just make sure that if something really starts to bug you, you talk to your parents. A lot of times, there are things about your diabetes you don't like, such as never being able to have the snacks you want. But often you can work out ways around this so you can make your diabetes easier to live with. Your parents can be your best friends when it comes to sorting out your feelings. Talk with them, and you can probably figure out a way to work things out.

For Teenagers

If you are a teenager, you have to deal with all the problems that anyone else with diabetes deals with. But as a teenager, you may also have special concerns. Whether you have had your diabetes since childhood, or are newly diagnosed, you may start to resent all the attention your diabetes gets. You just want to live like any other teenager. You want your parents to recognize that you are getting older and you can take of yourself. That's normal for any teen, whether you have diabetes or not. And as you go through the teen years, life is full of its ups and downs. Sometimes you want your parents near and sometimes you don't want to be seen with them. But if you have diabetes, life can be even more challenging. Your parents may dote on you more than other parents. And your diabetes may produce even more emotional ups and downs than for most kids.

Becoming independent is hard for any teen, but even more so if you have diabetes. Your parents are probably even less willing to let go, when they are so concerned. The best way for you to get them to stop bugging you, if that is a problem, is to show them that you can take care of yourself. Keep good records of your blood glucose and show them those records. Show them how you take care of any special situations and discuss any problems you may run into. Sometimes enlisting their aid is the best way to show them you can take care of yourself. If you feel they are being overbearing, don't confront them when everyone is upset. Instead, approach them at a calm moment and have an honest talk about your concerns. If you show that you can handle your diabetes in a mature manner, they will probably treat you like the mature person that you are.

Teens face other problems, too. Maybe you want to fit in and don't like appearing different from the other kids. You don't want your friends to think you are some kind of freak. You may react to this pressure by skipping your blood tests, skipping insulin doses, or eating things you shouldn't be eating. But if you ignore your diabetes care plan, you could put yourself in a dangerous situation. If you are trying to fit in like everyone else, the worst thing you want to do is throw your blood glucose out of control. If you take care of your blood glucose, you can live just like any other teen and do all the things that everyone else does. But if you trigger an emergency episode of hypoglycemia or hyperglycemia, you could set yourself apart more than any simple blood test would.

The best way to deal with diabetes is to talk to your friends about it. Tell them what you do to take care of it. If you have to test or take insulin and don't feel comfortable around others, excuse yourself and do it in a bathroom or a private room. If you get tired of having to eat all the right things, then talk to your parents or your dietitian about ways to accommodate your particular tastes in your meal plan. You can have a treat every now and then if you make the right allowances or take a little extra insulin. But talk to your health care team about the best way to do this. If you need flexibility, think about trying an insulin pump to free you up.

Making the transition from childhood to adulthood can be tumultuous. You may feel down and out on occasion. This is normal. Sometimes life just stinks and you are going to feel bad. Allow yourself to have those feelings from time to time. Whether you are 14 or 40, you are likely to feel depressed sometimes. But if you have feelings of sadness, hopelessness, or despair that just won't go away, you may have a more serious problem. Here are some danger signs to look for:

- significant weight loss or gain (without trying to lose or gain)

- increase or decrease in appetite

- sleeping more than usual

- moving slower than normal or being in constant motion

- feeling extremely tired all the time

- feeling worthless, hopeless, or guilty, for no specific reason

- having a hard time concentrating or studying

- having thoughts about death or suicide

Any time you experience any of these feelings and it goes on for more than a few weeks, you may have depression. Don't ignore these feelings or hope that they will go away. When this happens, you might be likely to neglect your diabetes care and this could jeopardize not only your health but your life as well. Even if you think those around you don't care, it is not true. Be assured that your parents, family, and friends love you very much. There are some things you can do to help yourself when you are feeling depressed:

- Keep a journal. Write down your thoughts and feelings.

- Participate in some sort of sport or physical activity. Try yoga or another form of meditation.

- Call a friend or talk to your parents or other understanding adult.

- Have fun. Sometimes life with diabetes can seem so serious. Try to relax and do some things you really enjoy.

- Try doing some volunteer work. Talk to kids younger than you about having diabetes. Build a house with a community group. Work in a soup kitchen. Sometimes it helps to see that others are struggling just like you. Doing your bit to help out can help your outlook, too.

If you try some self-help measures and nothing seems to work, you may need to talk to someone who is experienced with helping people work through their problems. If you can, talk to your parents about your feelings. If you can't do that or feel like they don't understand, find another adult you feel comfortable with: a guidance counselor, your diabetes educator, your clergyman, or one of your friend's parents. Sometimes things may be just too much for you to handle alone. It can help to talk to someone who understands. You may want to talk to a professional counselor who can help you sort through your feelings. In some cases, antidepressant medication may help you through a rough spot. (For more on depression and coping, see Chapter 19.)

For Parents

The best way to deal with your child's diabetes is to learn all you can. Read some of the other chapters in this book and talk to your child's doctor and diabetes educator. Read the rest of this chapter to get an idea what your child may be going through. Check out all the resources you can (including the section in the back of this book). In general, you will want to learn about how to test your child's blood glucose, how to give insulin, and how to figure out an insulin injection plan. The most important thing to remember is that every child is different. What works for one may not work for another. Your job is to find out how *your* child experiences diabetes and what are the best ways to help.

You should meet with a diabetes educator for help in coordinating your child's diabetes care. You will also want to meet with a dietitian and figure out a healthy eating plan. Make sure to take into account your child's particular likes and dislikes. You and your child should not feel that having diabetes means having to eat differently than anyone else. All kids should be eating healthy food, whether they have diabetes or not. In fact, you will help your child and your family if you eat the same foods. You will be able to work out with your child's dietitian ways to include special treats in the meal plan. You will just have to take time to make sure your child with diabetes is balancing meals with his insulin schedule and physical activities.

Talk to your child's teachers about any special needs your child will have in school. Once you and your child figure out the daily routine and work out ways to deal with special events and circumstances, you'll both feel better knowing you can cope with diabetes.

Your Attitude and Feelings

Finding out your child has diabetes can come as a great shock. You may feel disbelief, sadness, or even guilt. You may feel that it's just not fair, or you may feel overwhelmed, wondering if you can give your child the care he needs. Life is stressful anyhow and being a parent today is demanding enough. It may seem at some point that you just won't be able to handle it all.

Once you learn enough about diabetes, you will soon realize that your child should be able to live just like any other kid. It is just a matter of balancing your child's meals with insulin injections and physical activities. Perhaps the most difficult part for a parent is learning how to adjust and come to terms with your feelings.

Be aware that your child is watching you for guidance. If you accept your child's diabetes in stride, so will your child. But if you react with anxiety, apprehension, and fear, so will he. Try to maintain a sense of calm as much as possible, and deal with diabetes matter-of-factly. At the same time, be sensitive to your child's fears or concerns. The more you and your child know about diabetes, the more relaxed you will both be.

If you are overanxious and nervous about your child's diabetes, your child will sense your fear. Don't try to do everything for your child. Let your child have some say in his diabetes care plan. At the same time, don't overindulge your child. If you let your child skip a blood test or insulin because you don't want him to feel so tied down by diabetes, you'll do your child a great disservice. You have to treat certain things as a given, with no questions asked. As soon as your child realizes that certain procedures are not negotiable, he won't try to get you to let him off the hook. If you don't provide enough discipline, your child will learn that he doesn't have to pay attention to diabetes care. The best way is to establish good diabetes care habits early and matter-of-factly, so that they become a way of life.

Of course, you also want to make sure that you don't become too much of a perfectionist when it comes to your child's diabetes care. Don't make your child feel guilty if blood glucose readings are out of range, but take steps to remedy the situation and try to prevent it from happening again. Don't use words like "cheating" or refer to glucose readings as "good" or "bad." Instead, discuss your child's blood glucose level as "low," "normal," or "high." Try to work out ways to adjust diet and exercise that give your child flexibility and allow him some special treats every now and then. As long as things remain in balance and precautions are taken, your child should be able to have a cupcake at a birthday party or go to the movies with a friend. You just need to develop a plan for handling these situations. If you are too inflexible, your child is bound to rebel at some point. Set the attitude that you can work with your child to develop a plan that works for his lifestyle.

Your child's level of involvement and responsibilities will change as he matures. During your child's infancy and toddlerhood, you will have complete responsibility for all aspects of care. That doesn't mean you shouldn't involve your child, however. You have to be in charge of the timing of insulin shots or blood tests, but you can let your child pick the injection spot or choose which finger to poke. This is a good way to get your child used to having a say in his care, and it will ultimately help your child to take greater responsibility as he gets older.

When your child begins preschool, you are still responsible for making sure he is eating according to plan, testing when needed, and taking the right amount of insulin at the right time. However, during this period, your child can begin to take over some of these tasks. Many 3-year-olds can learn to conduct a blood test and do their own finger pokes. By age 12, most children can take their own insulin. Your child can manage this even sooner with an insulin injection aid, such as Inject-Ease. You may also consider getting your child an insulin pump to give him greater flexibility and independence. It is important through this period that your child learn responsibility, because he will often be with friends or at school and out of your watchful field of vision.

Adolescence is probably the most challenging period for both teens and parents. Even if you are the world's most perfect parent, there will be times when your child resents you. This is a normal part of establishing independence. Once you and your child are educated about diabetes, you should both participate in treatment decisions. Adolescents may try to deny their diabetes in an effort to fit in and appear just like everyone else. They may have a tendency to skip insulin doses, ignore their meal plans, and even falsify blood glucose readings.

It is not uncommon for an adolescent to feel depressed. Eating disorders, especially among girls, are not uncommon. One particularly dangerous type of eating disorder is to skip insulin, which enables your child to eat and not gain weight. If you start to suspect that your child is developing any sort of coping problems, don't hesitate to seek the help of a professional counselor. You may suggest that your child go to visits to a diabetes educator on his own. This may help him develop a sense of responsibility about diabetes care. When your child is treated more like an adult, he may act more like an adult. It is important that your child understands the importance of good diabetes care and recognizes that it is his responsibility to take charge of that care.

Handling Emergencies

Once you and your child work out a diabetes care plan, your child should be able to live just like any other kid. However, it is important that you and your child be aware of signs that could signal an emergency situation. Severe hypoglycemia or hyperglycemia are both dangerous situations. It is important that both you and your child recognize the warning signs. Hypoglycemia can affect the brain and lead to unconsciousness and coma. Hyperglycemia can lead to a life-threatening situation known as diabetic ketoacidosis. The key to preventing either situation is to recognize the warning signs, test blood glucose right away, and treat promptly. Talk to your doctor in advance about what you should do if your child's blood glucose levels fall too low or rise too high.

Hypoglycemia

Any time your child's blood glucose level falls below 60 mg/dl or whatever value your child's doctor suggests is too low, your child may have hypoglycemia. Signs of hypoglycemia include nervousness, shakiness, sweating, irritability, impatience, chills and clamminess, rapid heartbeat, anxiety, light-headedness, and hunger. When hypoglycemia begins to affect the brain, your child may also appear sleepy, angry, uncoordinated, or sad. He may also experience nausea, blurred vision, tingling or numbness in the lips or tongue, nightmares, crying out during sleep, headaches, or strange behavior. In severe stages, confusion, delirium, personality changes, and unconsciousness can occur.

If your child is experiencing any of the symptoms of hypoglycemia, have him test his blood glucose right away. If you don't have time to test, treat anyhow. Usually anything below 60 mg/dl requires treatment, but check with your child's doctor to see what value requires treatment for your child. To treat, give your child a fast-acting carbohydrate snack: 2 to 5 glucose tablets, 2 tablespoons of raisins, half a can of regular soda, 4 ounces of juice, or 5 to 10 jelly beans, Lifesavers, or gumdrops. In general, you want to give your child 10 to 15 grams of a fast-acting carbohydrate. Wait 10 to 15 minutes and test again. If his blood glucose is still low, give another dose of carbohydrate. If your child shows any signs of severe hypoglycemia (confusion, delirium, or unconsciousness), he needs emergency help right away. Call your doctor and/or call for emergency help. The quickest way to get blood glucose levels up is to give an injection of glucagon. Ask your child's doctor to show you how to give a glucagon injection and under what circumstances you should give it. This will require a doctor's prescription. Make sure your child wears jewelry identifying him as a person with diabetes at all times. (For more information about hypoglycemia, see Chapter 2.)

Hyperglycemia and Diabetic Ketoacidosis

If your child's blood glucose level rises too high, he could develop hyperglycemia and diabetic ketoacidosis. This is a life-threatening condition that requires immediate attention. Symptoms of hyperglycemia include extreme thirst, dry parched mouth, and sleepiness or confusion. Your child may also have warm dry skin with no sweating. If you notice any of these symptoms, have him test his blood glucose right away. If it is over 250 mg/dl, also have him test his urine for ketones. If your child has moderate to high levels of ketones, call your doctor right away. Also call your child's doctor if your child has a lack of appetite, stomach pain, vomiting or feelings of nausea, blurry vision, fever, difficulty breathing, or a fruity odor on his breath. Call your child's doctor if your child has a blood glucose reading over 350 mg/dl whether or not there is evidence of ketones. If your child has a blood glucose reading over 500 mg/dl, take him to an emergency room right away. (For more information about hyperglycemia and diabetic ketoacidosis, see Chapter 3.)

Chapter 17
Solving Eating, Exercise, and Weight Problems

It's easier said than done: eat healthy foods . . . control your blood glucose levels . . . get plenty of exercise. If it were that easy, we wouldn't have a nation in which so many adults are considered obese. You know the reality: food that's bad for you tastes good. And exercise, which is good for you, is hard work. But the truth is, if you have diabetes, you have to take the best care of yourself you can. So how do you eat the right foods, get enough exercise, and keep your blood glucose levels in balance all at the same time? There is no simple answer that will work for everyone.

If you have type 1 diabetes, you probably don't have to lose weight. But you do have to develop a meal plan and follow that plan to balance your food intake with your insulin schedule and physical activities. If you have type 2 diabetes, you have probably been told two things: losing weight will help you achieve better glucose control by reducing insulin resistance, and it will also help prevent many of the complications of diabetes. That's true. So not only do you have to balance your food intake to match your physical activity and perhaps insulin or oral medication, but you also have to try to lose weight. And on top of all that, you're supposed to exercise, too. It may seem like too much to handle. Maybe you've tried before and found it overwhelming, so you just gave up. Or maybe you have already gotten on track with healthy eating habits, but you just need to learn how to fine-tune your plan.

Whatever your reasons for wanting to eat better, it is important to keep one thing in mind. Healthy living for someone with diabetes is not any different from that for someone without diabetes. You need to first set your goals and decide what you ultimately want to achieve. Do you want tight control? Or do you want something that gives you more leeway? Do you want to lose weight, or are you happy with your current weight? How much exercise do you want to incorporate into your daily routine?

The next step is to meet with a dietitian and perhaps an exercise specialist to figure out the best way to put your plan into action. In developing a plan to reach your goals, make sure your goals are realistic and that you take a path toward reaching those goals that suits you. Maybe you're the type of person who likes to go cold turkey and start right away with your bigger goal. Or maybe you really would do better if you broke down your bigger goal into smaller, more manageable steps. Whatever your style, the key is to work with the members of your health care team to develop a healthy living plan that works for you.

Setting Goals

Whatever your goal, there is good news. You don't have to go on a crash diet and you don't have to make a whole bunch of changes at once. Your goal is to develop new lifestyle habits that you can follow for the rest of your life. It may not happen overnight. The key is to set realistic goals that you can reach. Don't set goals you know you can't achieve, because you will set yourself up for failure. And work toward those goals over time. Take small steps at first, and eventually you may find that you can change the way you live.

You may want to set new goals for healthy living if one or more of the following statements is true:

- You are recently diagnosed with diabetes.

- You are not happy with your blood glucose control.

- You are experiencing frequent bouts of hypoglycemia or hyperglycemia.

- You have noticed any worsening of your complications or blood glucose control.

- Your glycated hemoglobin measurement is higher than desirable.

- You are becoming more insulin resistant.

- You experience any other changes in your feelings of well-being.

First, assess where you are. Start with those aspects of your general health that are important to you. You might start with your weight, your blood glucose levels, your cholesterol level, or your exercise level, for example. Think about where you are now and where you want to be. Do you want to improve your blood glucose control? What blood glucose levels are reasonable for you? Do you want to practice tight control? Or would it be more reasonable for you to just shoot for blood glucose levels between 90 and 180? Do you want to start exercising more? Would you like to run a marathon, or would you just be happy if you could walk around the block? Would you like to lose weight? How much? All your excess weight, or just enough, say 10 percent, to improve your insulin resistance?

In setting goals, it is important to be realistic. Are you the type of person who likes to exercise? Will it be easy for you to cut back on the fat or the number of calories in your meal plan? Do you rise to the challenge of hard-to-reach, long-term goals? Or would you have more success with smaller, more attainable goals? If you spend some time now thinking about what would work best for you, you'll probably have more success achieving your goals.

Weight Goals

If you are overweight, why is losing weight so important? Other than genetics, the biggest risk factor for developing type 2 diabetes is obesity. A full 80 percent of people with type 2 diabetes are obese. By medical standards, being obese means weighing more than 30 percent of your ideal body weight. In contrast, most people with type 1 diabetes are of normal weight. If you have type 2 diabetes and you are overweight, the best thing you can do is try to shed some weight. Many people with type 2 diabetes find that losing weight helps to restore insulin sensitivity and makes blood glucose levels easier to control. You don't even have to lose all your extra weight. Many people find that losing just 5 to 10 percent of their total weight is enough to see improvements in managing their diabetes. That means that if you weigh 200 pounds, losing 10 to

20 pounds could improve your blood glucose control, blood pressure, and cholesterol levels and reduce the risk of heart disease.

Just why being overweight triggers diabetes is not known for sure. But scientists do know that when you eat more than your body needs, you store the extra energy in your fat cells as triglycerides, a form of fat. As you store more body fat, the size and number of fat cells increases. For some reason, having too much fat, especially if your fat reserves are distributed more on your upper body, diminishes your body's ability to use insulin. When your body can't use insulin as it should, you have insulin resistance. At the same time, carrying too much extra fat places a burden on your pancreas and it can't make enough insulin. If you get rid of some of your extra body fat, then you can increase your insulin sensitivity. That means your body can use insulin better, and your pancreas may be able to make more.

Your doctor can help you decide what a healthy weight for you should be. You and your doctor will probably consult certain tables and formulas devised by the government, health insurance companies, and health experts. These tables are based on scientific studies that suggest that carrying too much weight increases the risk of certain diseases, such as heart attack, stroke, diabetes, and early death. Not all studies agree on what weight is ideal for reducing the risk of disease. But there is a general consensus that if you keep your weight within a certain range, your chances of remaining healthy are improved. Remember these weights are not absolutes, but rather guidelines as to what a healthy weight could be.

Blood Glucose Goals

The goal for many people with diabetes is to maintain blood glucose levels as close to normal as possible. Your goals will be individualized for you, but if you have diabetes, the American Diabetes Association (ADA) recommends target blood glucose levels of 80–120 mg/dl before meals and 100–140 mg/dl at bedtime.

Does this mean you should strive for the same levels? Maybe. Or maybe these goals are not realistic for you. For example, these goals may not be appropriate for someone at risk for hypoglycemia. If you are elderly or live alone, keeping your blood glucose too low may put you at risk for hypoglycemia. Small children should probably not strive for these goals either, because they do not always recognize the symptoms of hypoglycemia. A more appropriate goal for children may be in the target range of 100–200 mg/dl. It's important to meet with your health care team to set your own personal goals.

A good place to begin is to see where you are now. Monitor your blood glucose level before each meal and 2 hours after and record your results. Do this for a week to make sure they are consistently within the same range. This tells you where you are now. How close are you to the goals recommended by the ADA?

Now write down an acceptable range of goals that you would like to strive for. Your own personal goals should take into account your age, activity level, lifestyle, overall health, and motivation level. Do you want to practice intensive control, for example, to achieve near-to-normal blood glucose levels? This requires a significant effort, but the rewards are substantial. Do you have the time to devote to this? Or is your lifestyle too demanding to allow monitoring 7 times a day? Are you willing to risk a greater chance of diabetes complications to follow a more moderate blood glucose control program?

If your blood glucose levels are not well controlled now, it may simply be too much to expect to get them consistently below 120 or 140 mg/dl. Maybe, for now at least, it would be more realistic to try to keep them within the range of 70 to 200 mg/dl. This may be an achievable goal for you. Then, as time goes on you and you learn to manage your diabetes, you may find that you could shoot for blood glucose levels between 70 and 175 mg/dl. Whatever you and your doctor decide, it is better to have a goal that is achievable than no goals at all or goals that are impossible to attain.

Fitness Goals

Whether you are a fitness fanatic or a couch potato, you are probably well aware that exercise is good for you. You probably know that exercise can help you lose weight and that it is good for your heart. But did you also know that if you exercise regularly, you may lower your blood glucose levels and improve your insulin sensitivity? Over time, regular exercise will also bring down your glycated hemoglobin levels. This is especially true if you have type 2 diabetes. Not only does exercise burn up calories, it can also lower triglyceride levels, increase HDL (the "good cholesterol") levels, and improve circulation, an important consideration for someone with diabetes. This is because the most devastating complications of diabetes develop from poor circulation.

Some people are miserable without a 5-mile run every day. But for others, a 5-yard walk to the refrigerator is a major effort. Most likely, you fall somewhere in between. Unfortunately, many sedentary people know that exercise is good for them, and maybe have even tried it, but it is just too much work and not much fun. If this sounds like you, maybe it is time to revisit the issue.

Exercise can be more fun than work! Think of something you really love to do. Lie on your back and float in the pool? Add some laps and you've got a swimming program. Talk to your neighbor? Walk a few blocks with him while you talk and you won't even notice you're exercising. In setting up an exercise program and setting your goals, make sure to find something you like to do and proceed slowly. A good workout should be invigorating and slightly challenging, but not miserable. If you find that you are in pain the whole time, stop for a few minutes and take a rest. Or find a new activity, one that actually makes you want to get out of bed in the morning, not roll over and go back to sleep. Anything that makes you feel terrible the whole time is not going to make you want to go back and do it again.

The trick in setting goals and finding the right activity is to choose something you like well enough to incorporate into your new lifestyle. After all, any activity you do is better than doing nothing at all. Start at an easy level, and remember that the more you do something, the easier it gets. Once a given activity or activity level feels so easy that you no longer feel challenged, then step up the level of intensity or distance. However, if you push yourself too far or too fast or set unrealistic goals, you will set yourself up for disappointment.

Before starting any exercise program, see your doctor for a thorough exam. Make sure the activity or program you have in mind will not endanger your health. Think about what you want to accomplish through exercise or any physical activity and bring your list of goals into your doctor's appointment. Maybe you just want to lose weight or keep your weight at the same level. Or you might want to improve your blood glucose control or cholesterol level. Maybe you would like to increase your energy level and just want to feel better. Perhaps you would like to improve your blood pressure or bring down your resting heart rate. Whatever your aim, write it down.

Now make a list of all the things you like to do that involve movement of some sort. Imagine that someone gave you a free hour each day. What would you do with it? You don't have to choose a traditional exercise like running, biking, or swimming. Maybe you like bowling, gardening, walking, bird-watching, drawing, riding horses, or playing music.

Now look at your list. Start with your favorite activity and commit to doing it three times a week. Or make a commitment to do something different every day. If your list of favorite activities isn't very long, think about what you really like to do. Is it watch TV? Read? Listen to music? If so, think about incorporating some sort of activity into them. If all you really want to do is watch TV, think about setting up a chair or bench and lifting weights while you watch. You can buy a treadmill and walk while you listen to music.

Now, bring your list of goals and your favorite activities to your next doctor's appointment. Tell your doctor what you have in mind in terms of exercising. If you have never exercised much or are trying to develop a new program, you might benefit from a few visits with an exercise physiologist or personal trainer who has experience with people with diabetes. But before you begin, your doctor and your trainer should know what you like to do and what you hope to accomplish. And make sure you are physically up to the challenge. You will also want to coordinate your exercise program with your meal plan and insulin or oral medication treatment schedule.

Making a Plan

On your next visit to your doctor or diabetes educator, bring in the list of all your goals. This should include any weight loss or weight maintenance plans, blood glucose control goals, and exercise goals. Discuss with your team member whether these are realistic goals and talk about developing a plan of action. You may want to schedule visits with other members of your team to help you achieve those goals. Your dietitian can help you develop a meal plan, understand food labels, control your weight, and deal with obesity. Your exercise physiologist can help you develop an exercise program, and your diabetes educator and doctor can help you balance your insulin, oral medication, meals, and physical activities.

Your Meal Plan

It is time to develop a meal plan that you can follow. If you have diabetes, you probably have one or two things you hope to accomplish. You probably want to have a meal plan that will keep your blood glucose levels under control. If you are overweight, you may want to control your calorie and fat intake to allow you to lose some weight. Whether you have 5 pounds to lose or 200 pounds, the trick is to take it off slowly and keep it off. You don't want to diet, because as soon as you go "on" a diet, there is a danger that you'll go "off" your diet. Instead, gradually change the way you eat so that you develop healthy habits that will be with you for the rest of your life. A successful meal plan starts with foods that are healthy and nutritious, includes foods that taste good, keeps your blood glucose levels under control, allows for special treats, leaves you feeling satisfied and fulfilled, and helps you to lose weight, if desired.

■ WHAT TO DO

To start, schedule a visit with your dietitian. Before your visit, have a goal in mind, whether it is to lose a certain amount of weight, keep your blood glucose levels within a certain range, or lower the fat and cholesterol levels in your blood. When you come to your first visit, bring your list of goals with you.

During the week before your visit, eat as you normally would, but write down everything you eat, how much you ate, and when you ate it. Also record your blood glucose levels before each meal and 2 hours after your meals. This will give your dietitian an understanding of you, your meal patterns, the foods you like, and how these foods affect your blood glucose levels. Also, if you are trying to lose weight, this will help determine your total caloric intake. The idea is to burn off more calories than you take in. If you are eating a certain amount and staying the same weight, your dietitian can calculate how many calories you need to lose weight. A reasonable weight loss rate is 1 or 2 pounds per week. Since each pound equals 3,500 calories, you will have to reduce your total food intake by at least 500 calories a day. So if you are used to eating 3,000 calories a day, you should eat 2,500 each day to lose 1 pound a week, or 2,000 calories per day to lose 2 pounds each week. Whatever your eating pattern is, recording the exact foods you eat will give your dietitian an idea of where to start.

Once your dietitian has an idea where you are coming from, she will probably recommend a meal plan. This plan will be individualized for you. Some dietitians use plans in the form of an exchange menu. You will be given an outline of how many food exchanges you can have at each meal or snack time. You will also be given a list of different foods and how much of each food counts as each exchange. Or your dietitian may teach you how to count the carbohydrates in the foods you eat, and tell you how many carbohydrates you should eat at each meal or snack.

Make sure that the foods you like are on your meal plan. Most diets fail because they are only temporary, and because they forbid so many foods. The more you think about the foods you can't have, the more you want them. Finally, when you get frustrated, depressed, or just plain hungry, you eat whatever you want without looking back. You can avoid this pattern if you build some of the foods you love into your meal plan. For example, if you know you always have a dish of ice cream after dinner, ask your dietitian how to account for this. The best way is to plan in advance. Make an allowance in your meal plan for your special treat and count up its fat and carbohydrate exchanges. This way you can still have some of your favorite foods without feeling that you have failed. With time, you may even find that you crave junk foods less and begin to find more pleasure in the foods that are more nutritious.

In addition to giving you a sample meal plan, your dietitian can also help you figure out:

- how to count food exchanges or servings and make allowances for different foods

- how many calories you should eat each day

- how much carbohydrate you can eat each day and still keep your blood glucose levels within your target range

- how many grams of fat you should eat each day

- new ideas for breakfast, lunch, dinner, and snacks

- how to adjust your meals or medications for exercise

- what foods to have on hand for hypoglycemia and how much of each food you should eat

- how to manage your diabetes when you travel

- how to handle changes in your meal plan when you're sick

- how to handle eating out

- how to change your eating pattern if you want to practice tight glucose control

Despite your best efforts, problems are bound to arise from time to time. Maybe you're traveling out of town and can't stick to your meal plan. Your schedule gets delayed, you're invited to a big holiday bash, or you're afraid to refuse the boss' homemade cheesecake. Maybe you're meeting your client for dinner at 7, even though you usually eat at 5:30. Your dietitian can help you plan for these situations. For example, if you can't change the timing of your insulin dose, eat a piece of fruit or another carbohydrate snack at your usual mealtime. Then account for the snack in your daily tally. Always carry snacks with you. You never know when you will get stuck in traffic or in a meeting that runs over-time.

Sometimes you need to readjust your meals in advance. For exam-ple, if you are invited out to a 10:30 brunch when you usually eat break-fast at 7, eat an early-morning snack at your normal breakfast time. At brunch, eat what is left of your breakfast allotment along with part of your normal lunchtime allotment. Save the rest of your lunchtime allot-ment for a snack in 2 hours or so. If you're having a late dinner, eat your bedtime snack at your normal mealtime, then eat your meal a little later. If you take insulin, you may have to adjust your short-acting doses to account for these changes.

Exactly how you do this depends on your particular meal plan. In general, you will want to take your short-acting dose of insulin before your big meal. Talk to your doctor or diabetes educator in advance about the best way to do this for your particular meal plan. Often it will mean delaying your dose of short-acting insulin to coincide with your delayed meal.

Eating more often than usual is common around holiday times. You're around food all day long and it may be too difficult to wait until dinnertime to have just a little something to eat, especially when every-one around you is eating. When this happens, try dividing your total food for the day into snack-sized meals. Then you can spread the food out a little more, even nibbling here and there without guilt, as long as you account for it. You can join in the fun without going over your allotted amounts.

You may find that you want to eat more than you usually do on certain special occasions. Sometimes just going out to a new restaurant, having friends over, or eating Thanksgiving dinner may tempt you to overeat. Ask your doctor if you can make adjustments in your insulin or exercise program to allow for the occasional larger-than-usual meal. If you know in advance that you will be eating a big dinner, for example, find out whether it would be advisable to skip a snack or reduce your lunchtime meal beforehand. Depending on your meal plan and insulin schedule, you might be able to eat less at lunch and take a lower dose of short-acting insulin at that time, and eat a little more at dinner along with a little more insulin. Or it might be enough to add an extra workout after dinner. Ask your doctor what is advisable for you, on occasion, and exactly how to make these adjustments.

Understanding Food Labels

A food labeled "50 percent fat-free" sounds great until you realize that means it is still 50 percent fat. It's not always easy sorting out all the food claims as you are trudging through the grocery store aisles, trying to make healthy food choices. You may think you are doing a good job only to discover that you have been had. A box of cookies may have a banner proclaiming it to be low in fat, but if you read the food label carefully, you discover that it is loaded with lots of extras, such as added sugars that will throw your carbohydrate count out of whack. Reading food labels may seem impossible at first, but once you and your dietitian come up with a food plan that balances the amount of calories, fat, saturated fat, cholesterol, carbohydrate, fiber, and sodium in your diet, you may find food labels to be very helpful. Each packaged food item you buy will list all these nutrients on its label, and will take some of the guesswork out of meal planning for you. You just need to know what to look for.

■ WHAT TO DO

When you shop, ignore the fancy claims on the front of a container. Instead, flip it over until you find the panel labeled "Nutrition Facts." There you will find the serving size, the number of calories per serving, and the calories from fat. Make sure to pay careful attention to the serving size. A bag of potato chips may seem like a low-fat, low-calorie dietary bargain until you realize that what you thought was one serving is actually 4 servings!

Reading Labels

If you look at the sample label shown below, you will also notice additional information. Below the information on calories, you will also find information about the grams of fat, cholesterol, sodium, and carbohydrate in one serving. To the right of these values, you will find the % Daily Value. This tells you how much of the total recommended daily intake you will use up when you eat one serving of this food. These numbers assume you are eating 2,000 calories each day. The actual percentages may be higher or lower, depending on your total calorie intake. The label also tells you that 1 cup of chili counts as 1 starch exchange, 3 lean-meat exchanges, and 1 vegetable exchange. This will help you in deciding whether the chili will fit into your meal plan.

However, in planning your meals, you might also take a closer look at the fat content in deciding whether this would be a good choice for your meal. The chili label, for example, tells you that if you are eating

NUTRITION FACTS

Serving Size 1 cup (235 g)   Servings Per Container 2

Amount Per Serving			Vitamin A	35%	Vitamin C	2%
Calories 260 Calories from Fat 72			Calcium	6%	Iron	30%

	% Daily Values
Total Fat 8g	13%
Saturated Fat 3g	17%
Cholesterol 130mg	44%
Sodium 1,010mg	42%
Total Carbohydrate 22g	7%
Dietary Fiber 9g	36%
Sugars 4g	7%
Protein 25g	

*Percent Daily Values are based on a 2,000-calorie diet. Your Daily Values may be higher or lower depending on your calorie needs.

Ingredients: water, beef, tomatoes, modified food starch, chili powder, salt, sugar, flavoring

1 Starch Exchange, 3 Lean-Meat Exchanges, 1 Vegetable Exchange

2,000 calories each day, 1 serving, or 1 cup of chili will provide you with 8 grams of total fat, 3 grams of saturated fat, 72 calories from fat, and 13 percent of your recommended fat allowance for the day.

If you eat the whole can (2 servings), you would be eating 144 calories from fat. This amounts to 26 percent of your daily fat limit. This is not necessarily out of line, if you pay attention to what else you eat with the chili and what you eat during the rest of the day. If you eat your chili with a salad with reduced-fat or fat-free dressing, a whole-grain roll or slice of bread, and fruit or fat-free frozen yogurt for dessert, this could be a healthy meal choice. Make sure you don't garnish the chili with high-fat foods, such as cheddar cheese or sour cream, or eat it with tortilla chips and corn bread. Whatever you add must be accounted for. However, it is very easy to keep the chili meal to under 30 percent of your total fat intake for the day. Of course that means that your other meals and snacks combined should not exceed 70 percent of your total daily fat allowance.

In addition to watching your fat intake, you should also pay attention to the carbohydrate content of the food you eat. If you look at the chili label again, you'll notice that one serving of chili provides 22 grams of carbohydrate or 7 percent of the total number of carbohydrates you are trying to eat each day (if you eat 2,000 calories a day, that is). If you look under the heading "Total Carbohydrate" on the left side of the panel, you can see that it is broken down into the different kinds of carbohydrate. For the can of chili beans, the total carbohydrate includes 4 grams of sugars. All sugars are listed in the Nutrition Facts, whether they are added to the food or occur naturally in a food. This means that the lactose that occurs naturally in yogurt and the fructose found naturally in fruit juice will show up as sugars on the food label.

As far as the chili is concerned, it does not supply much of your daily requirement for carbohydrate. Even 2 cups of chili will only give you 14 percent of your total daily requirement. However, if you add the low-fat choices mentioned above—salad, bread, and fruit or frozen yogurt—your total carbohydrate will be closer to 26 percent of the recommended daily intake. This can make your meal a healthy choice.

In addition to information on the nutritional content of food, you may also find a variety of health claims, usually in bold letters on the front of the label. Food manufacturers can only make health claims that are supported by scientific research. For example, you may see labels that suggest the following:

- Calcium can prevent osteoporosis.

- Fiber-containing foods such as grains, fruits, and vegetables can help prevent cancer.

- Fiber-containing foods such as fruits, vegetables, and grain products can protect against heart disease.

- Saturated fats can increase the risk of cancer.

- Lack of folic acid in pregnant women can increase the risk of birth defects.

Sometimes food manufacturers make claims about the nutritional value of their foods that can be more than a little confusing. For example, it is not always obvious what "all-natural" or "lite" means exactly. Here's what some of these claims really mean.

- *Calorie-free* means that the product has less than 5 calories per serving. Make sure to pay attention to what constitutes a serving.

- *Low calorie* means the food has less than 40 calories per serving.

- *Light* or *lite* means that the food has one-third less calories or 50 percent less fat than the food with which it is being compared, usually the same product with the full amount of calories.

- *Less* and *reduced* usually refer to a decreased amount of calories, fat, sugar, salt, or other ingredient. To use this label, the food must be at least 25 percent lower in calories or other ingredients compared to the full-calorie or nonreduced version. When these words are used on a label, the actual percentages must also be included, as in "50 percent less salt" or "fat reduced by 25 percent."

- *Cholesterol-free* means that the food must contain less than 2 milligrams of cholesterol and 2 grams or less of saturated fat per serving. Vegetable oils have no cholesterol, but are 100 percent fat.

- *Low cholesterol* means that a food contains 20 milligrams or less of cholesterol and 2 grams or less of saturated fat per serving.

- *Low-fat* means that a food must have 3 grams or less of fat per serving.

- *Fat-free* means that a food has less than 0.5 grams of fat per serving.

- *Low saturated fat* means that a food has 1 gram or less of saturated fat per serving and not more than 15 percent of its calories from saturated fat.

- *Low sodium* foods contain 140 milligrams or less of sodium per 100 grams of food. Sodium can be found in other forms besides ordinary table salt, or sodium chloride. For example, monosodium glutamate (MSG), sodium bicarbonate (baking soda), sodium nitrate, and sodium citrate all contain sodium. Sodium also occurs naturally in some foods.

- *Very low sodium* foods contain 35 milligrams or less of sodium per 100 grams of food.

- *Sodium-free* or *salt-free* means that a food has less than 5 milligrams of sodium per 100 grams of food.

- *Light in salt* means that an item has 50 percent less salt than the regular version.

- *Sugar-free* means that the item has less than 0.5 grams of sugar per serving. It can contain artificial sweeteners, however.

- *No Added Sugar, Without Added Sugar, Dietetic, No Added Fat,* and similar phrases really have no meaning. A phrase like this simply means that something has been changed or replaced. It could contain less sugar, less fat, less salt, or less cholesterol than the regular version of the same product. This label can be misleading. The only way to tell for sure what it means is to read the Nutrition Facts label. You may think a package of dietetic cookies has no calories, but it may very well be that the only thing missing is salt. It could have just as much sugar or fat as the regular version.

- *Natural* can also be misleading. When used on meat and poultry labels, it means that no chemical preservatives, hormones, or similar substances have been added. But on other food labels, it has no particular meaning.

- *Fresh* can only be used to describe a raw food that has not been frozen, heat processed, or preserved in some way.

What to Look for When Shopping

When shopping for the foods you will eat, it pays to read the food labels. But how do you know what you should buy? It can all seem very confusing. Here are some tips to single out those food items that will fit in well with your healthy living plan.

- *Bread.* Look for low-fat varieties that list whole grains as the first ingredient on the label.

- *Cereal.* Choose brands that list whole grains first on the label and contain 3 or more grams of dietary fiber per serving, 1 gram or less of fat per serving, and 5 grams or less of sugar per serving.

- *Crackers and snack foods.* Look for whole grains as the first ingredient listed on the label and 2 grams or less of fat per serving. Usually 5 to 10 crackers constitute a serving. Good examples of low-fat snacks are pretzels or plain popcorn that has been air-popped with no added cheese or butter and that contains 2 grams of fat or less per serving. Try to keep sodium content under 400 milligrams per serving.

- *Rice, pasta, and whole grains.* Use converted, brown, or wild rice of any type (watch out for high-fat flavored rice mixes). Look for fresh or dried pasta with no added filling, preferably those made with whole-grain flours. Try to avoid pastas or noodles that contain eggs and fat.

- *Frozen desserts.* Look for those that contain 3 grams or less of fat per 4-ounce serving (1/2 cup). Low-fat frozen yogurt, low- or fat-free ice cream, and frozen fruit juice bars with less than 70 calories per bar are all good choices. Avoid food made with cream of coconut, coconut milk, or coconut oil, which are all high in saturated fat. Count the carbohydrates as part of the meal's allotment.

- *Milk and yogurt.* Choose fat-free or 1 percent milk, buttermilk made from fat-free milk, and low-fat and non-fat yogurt that is artificially sweetened.

- *Cheese.* Look for fat-free milk and reduced-fat cheeses that contain less than 6 grams of fat per ounce. Good choices include fat-free mozzarella and low-fat Farmer's cheeses, fat-free or low-fat ricotta cheese, and fat-free or 1 percent fat cottage cheese.

- *Red meat.* Beef, veal, and pork are all labeled by the animal, body part, and type of cut. For example, "pork loin chops" are chops from the loin of the pig. The grade of meat is based on its fat content. Prime cut is the highest in fat, and Choice or Select is lower in fat. Pick lower fat grades of meat, such as Choice and Select, and choose lean body parts, such as round or sirloin beef, tenderloin pork, or leg of lamb.

- *Luncheon meat.* When shopping for luncheon meats, choose lean or 95 percent fat-free meats. Look for those that contain 30 to 55 calories per ounce and contain less than 3 grams of fat per ounce.

- *Poultry.* Breast meat is the best choice, because it contains the least amount of fat. Removing the skin before cooking will cut the fat content by 50 to 75 percent and the cholesterol content by 12 percent. Salami, bologna, hot dogs, and bacon made from chicken and turkey aren't necessarily low in fat. In fact, the fat content can be quite high. Check the label and choose those that are less than 30 percent fat.

- *Seafood.* Choose fresh fish and shellfish. Look for clear eyes, red gills, and shiny skin and avoid those with a "fishy" smell. Shrimp is usually shipped frozen to preserve freshness. When choosing canned fish, look for fish packed in water or rinse the oil off thoroughly. Look for low amounts of sodium.

- *Vegetables.* Your best bets are fresh and frozen vegetables without any sauces or flavorings. When using canned vegetables, drain and rinse them thoroughly to remove excess sodium.

- *Fruit and fruit juice.* Choose fresh, frozen, or dried fruit, preferably without any added sugar. When buying juice, look for those that are 100 percent pure fruit juice. Fruit juices made from concentrate can come fresh, canned, bottled, or frozen. Labels that say "made with 100 percent juice" or "juice drink" are not 100 percent juice themselves and may contain other ingredients. Check the label.

- *Margarine and oil.* Choose olive, canola, soybean, safflower, sesame, sunflower, or corn oils. Look for those brands that list these or "vegetable oil" first on the label and that contain 1 gram or less of saturated fat per serving (usually 1 tablespoon.) Use any fat sparingly.

- *Salad dressings.* Choose reduced-calorie and fat-free types of dressings.

- *Sour cream and cream cheese.* Look for fat-free or light types of sour cream or cream cheese. Instead of regular sour cream, try using fat-free or low-fat yogurt, either plain or flavored with chives, herbs, and spices.

- *Soup.* Try low-sodium, reduced-fat varieties. In preparing cream soups, use fat-free or low-fat milk or water.

- *Cookies and cakes.* Look for brands that contain 3 grams or less of fat per 100 calories. Angel food cake is made without fat and has no cholesterol. When making cakes, you can cut out cholesterol by using egg substitutes. You can substitute applesauce or fat-free yogurt for oil in some recipes. Many cake mixes now include directions for low-fat and low-cholesterol variations. Again, count the carbohydrates as part of the meal's allotment.

Losing Weight

Many people with diabetes, especially type 2 diabetes, would like to lose weight. But how much? You may decide that you want to lose just enough weight to improve your insulin sensitivity. Many people with type 2 diabetes find that losing just 10 to 20 pounds can improve blood glucose control, blood pressure, and cholesterol levels. Some people with type 2 diabetes even find that by losing all of their excess weight, they are able to stop taking their medications.

■ WHAT TO DO

The key to losing weight is burning up more calories than you take in. Follow your meal plan and exercise schedule. Once you have set your goals, the biggest problem is getting started. Make sure your goals are realistic. It may seem like too much to think you have to lose 100 pounds and start a marathon training program. And it probably is. Instead, take small steps. For example, for the first week, try to eliminate 250 calories from your total intake each day and increase your physical activity to burn up an extra 100 calories each day. That could be as simple as giving up that slice of apple pie at lunch and taking a 1-mile stroll every evening. Once you get used to it, you can add more exercise or further decrease your calorie intake to lose more weight. Or you can just keep on at the rate you're going. Even with this modest change, you could lose a pound every 10 days. Most doctors recommend losing 1 or 2 pounds a week. It may not seem like much, but over the long haul, those pounds can add up.

If you find you're not making much progress with your meal and exercise plan, try some of the following suggestions:

- For a solid week, write down everything you eat. Don't leave out anything. You want to get an honest assessment of what you're actually eating. Make sure you describe each food and the serving size. Use a calorie chart to figure out how many calories and grams of fat you are currently eating each day.

- During the same week, write down all the physical activities you do. Even walking up and down the stairs or working in your garden or cleaning your house is exercise.

- Now look over your weekly log and see if there are any obvious things you can change. Did you really need to eat those cookies on the way home from the grocery store? Make it a rule never to eat anything without sitting down at the table, and see if that eliminates some unnecessary snacking. If you are used to a dessert every night, see if you can find a low-calorie version. Try to eliminate just one high-calorie food each day, if the idea of a severe calorie restriction unnerves you. This will help you get going. Once you get motivated and start to feel the rewards, talk to your dietitian about other ways you can cut calories.

- Think about ways to increase your physical activity. If you are already walking a mile each day, think of increasing it bit by bit. A general rule of thumb is to start with a comfortable level of activity and increase it by 10 percent each week. Try to get to the point where you are exercising for 30 minutes each day, or walking 2 miles each day. Talk to your doctor before increasing the intensity or frequency of your exercise program.

- Think about adding weight training to your routine. When you lift weights, you increase your muscle mass and your muscles burn more fat all day long during everything you do. You don't need to lift much—a 1- or 2-pound weight used for several repetitions can do wonders.

- Look around your home to see how you can change your habits to promote a healthier lifestyle. If chocolate chip cookies call out to you in the middle of the night, don't keep them in the house. If you have a hard time resisting a bag of chips while watching TV at night, munch on celery sticks instead. Every time you feel the urge to go get a snack, walk up and down the stairs, or do another round of weight lifting.

- Make it easy to exercise. If you have a treadmill or a stationary bike, keep in the living room where you watch TV, not stuck in the hall closet. Instead of munching those chips on the couch during the late show, sit on your bike and pedal for a few minutes. If you like to work out in the morning, have your exercise clothes laid out the night before, so you don't make an excuse and roll back over in bed. Make healthy habits easy.

- Set smaller goals. Don't think of losing 200 pounds. Think of losing 10 or 20 pounds and then reassess once you have reached that goal. Once you lose 5 pounds, tell yourself, "If I can lose 5 pounds, I can lose 10 pounds," and "If I can lose 10 pounds, I can lose 20 pounds." Once you get going, it is easier to continue. Make those first steps easy.

- Think about changing portion sizes. If you can't stand the idea of giving up some of your favorite foods, have little servings of them instead, and ask your dietitian to account for them in your meal plan. Always ask yourself before you eat those last three bites or reach for another helping, "Am I eating this because I am truly hungry, or am I eating this out of habit, because it's there?"

If, despite your best efforts, you are having a hard time losing weight, ask your doctor about appetite suppressants. Appetite suppressants are only recommended for people who are significantly overweight and who have health problems that result from being obese. Make sure to discuss the side effects of any medication you take with your doctor. Many medications are available for weight loss, some of which work and are safe. Few weight-loss medications are safe for the long term, but carrying around a load of extra weight is not safe either. To get the most out of your weight-loss medication, it should be used along with your approved meal plan and exercise schedule. Usually, weight loss with medication begins to plateau at about 6 months.

However you plan to lose weight, you are bound to have setbacks on occasion. Don't beat yourself up about them. Instead of looking back and chastising yourself as you seek comfort in a bowl of ice cream, think ahead. Visualize the person you want to become and try to use that image to get you back on track. Once you start losing weight and exercising more, you may find that you like being able to walk up the stairs without huffing and puffing. Pat yourself on the back for how far you have come and keeping moving toward your goal.

Exercise

If a drug company hawked a pill that made you lose weight, improved your circulation, protected you against heart disease and stroke, improved your blood glucose control, and made you feel great, people would be lining up in the streets to buy it. How much would you pay for such a miracle drug? A dollar a day? Five dollars? Well, the truth is, exercise is as good as any pill, and depending on what activities you choose, it can even be a lot of fun. This is one miracle cure that really lives up to its advertising. And the best part is that it's free.

Active movement, the kind that gets your heart pumping and makes you breathe deeper, improves blood flow to your blood vessels, improves your cholesterol profile, and protects against heart disease. For people with diabetes, this is good news in itself. But there is an added benefit. Exercise also helps clear glucose from your blood, both while you are exercising and several hours after. If you use insulin, this could mean that you need less insulin on the days you work out. If you have type 2 diabetes, regular exercise along with a healthy diet could mean that you can control your diabetes without insulin or oral agents, or that you can get by with less medication.

■ WHAT TO DO

Take your goals for exercise to your doctor or diabetes care team. After your meeting, you should be able to answer the following questions:

- How often should I exercise?

- What times of the day or week are best for me?

- How long should my exercise sessions be?

- How hard should I exercise?

- Should I stick to the same routine each day, or should I vary the length and intensity of my workouts?

- How should I gauge how hard I exercise? Should I count my heart rate? What heart rate should I aim for?

- Are there any activities I should avoid?

- Are there symptoms (of hypoglycemia, heart disease, or muscle strain, for example) that I should look out for?

- What special precautions should I take?

- Do I take less insulin or change my injection site before I exercise?

- How do I modify my meal plan?

- Will oral agents affect me differently if I exercise?

Choosing an Exercise

In choosing any exercise, pick one that you like to do. The simplest is walking. It is cheap, nonstrenuous, and something you can do with a friend. Even if you would like to do something more vigorous eventually, walking is a good way to get started. Start walking 5 to 10 minutes at first and gradually increase your time. Try to get to the point where you walk for at least 30 minutes or 2 miles. Walk at a pace that is both enjoyable and invigorating for you. And if you want something more aerobic, just walk faster, incorporate hills, or throw in a little jogging.

You might prefer jogging because you only have to work a short time to get an invigorating workout. To start jogging, make sure you can comfortably walk for 30 minutes or 2 miles. Then eventually jog for a little portion of your normal walk until you are out of breath. Walk until you feel more rested, then jog a little more. Every day you will find that you can comfortably jog more and more. You may want to switch to all jogging, or you may want to stick with a jogging-walking combination.

Before you start jogging, make sure to check it out with your doctor. Invest in a good pair of supportive, well-padded running shoes. Your shoes should feel comfortable the first time you put them on. Consider having your podiatrist check their fit before you use them. Avoid running on concrete—try the track at a local school or a nature trail. If you feel any pain in your feet or legs, stop running and walk. Rest or take a few days off before starting again.

A good workout session should include 5 to 10 minutes of warm-up exercises and gentle stretching. During the warm-up phase, move slowly at first, using low-intensity, easy movements. You can stretch gently, but don't bounce. You are more likely to hurt yourself by doing this with cold muscles. You can follow this with at least 20 to 30 minutes of aerobic activity. When you are first starting, however, don't overdo it. If you are not used to an aerobic workout, try getting your heart rate up for just 5 to 10 minutes. Then increase a little each day or each week.

The aerobic session is the fun part. It should rev you up and get your heart pumping, but it should not be so intense as to cause shortness of breath, weakness, or intense pain. One easy guideline to follow is that during your workout, you should still be able to carry on a conversation with your workout partner. After the aerobic portion, end with a cool-down activity and gentle stretching. To see improvement, you will want to work out at least 3 to 4 times per week. If you are engaged in intense physical activity, you might want to alternate days of intense workouts with days of rest or light activity.

You might want to alternate days of aerobic activity with days of strength training and muscle toning. Weight training has come a long way. It's not just for Arnold Schwarzenegger-wanna-be's anymore. Anyone—young, old, male, or female—can benefit from weight training. It is a good idea to alternate weight training with aerobic activity. There are several approaches to weight training. It can be as simple as a few light hand-held weights in your living room or as complex as membership at an expensive, well-equipped gym. Most weight-training programs involve sets of weight-lifting exercises. Each set consists of a series of repetitions. When you first start, do just one set each session. Eventually, work your way up to 3 to 6 sets each session.

As you become stronger, you will also find that you can lift more weight. Add more weight a little at a time. A general rule is to use a weight that you can repeat 8 to 12 times. At the end of your reps, you should feel like you can't do anymore. If you are straining at 8 reps, you are using too much weight. If you are still raring to go after 12 reps, you need to add more weight.

Just make sure that whatever you do suits your style. If you are social and more motivated by others joining in, think about joining a health club, taking an aerobics class, or exercising with a friend. If you like to do things on your own, think about investing in some exercise tapes or home gym equipment and working out in your own home. However, be careful about exercising alone. You will have to be extra careful that you avoid hypoglycemia, both during and after exercise.

Avoiding Hypoglycemia

If you have type 1 diabetes, you have to plan carefully when you exercise. You need to guard against having your blood glucose levels fall too low, as well as having them rise too high. During moderate exercise that doesn't last too long, your blood glucose levels may fall during and after exercise. This is because the glucose in your blood is being used up faster than your liver can release it. This is one of the benefits of exercise. But if you don't have much glucose to begin with or you exercise too long, you could have an episode of hypoglycemia. To avoid this, make sure you test your blood glucose level before you exercise. If you work out for a long time, you may even want to test in the middle of your workout. If your blood glucose level is below 100 mg/dl before you work out, eat at least 15 grams of a fast-acting carbohydrate. Then test 15 to 30 minutes later. Don't start exercising until your blood glucose is at least 100 mg/dl. Check with your doctor to find out a safe blood glucose range for you to exercise in.

Avoiding Hyperglycemia

If you exercise too vigorously or if you have not given yourself enough insulin, you could develop hyperglycemia. Sometime during vigorous exercise, your nerves signal your liver to release stored glucose. This can cause your blood glucose levels to rise. If your blood glucose is a little on the high side to begin with, overly vigorous exercise can trigger hyperglycemia. If your insulin levels are low, this can happen with even moderate activity.

If you are exercising vigorously, think about testing in the middle of your workout. You may also want to consider eating a snack during the workout. Try a snack that is low in fat and has 20 to 25 grams of carbohydrate. You may need to repeat your snack every 30 minutes for extended workouts.

If your blood glucose goes over 250 mg/dl, stop exercising and test your urine for ketones. If you have moderate to large ketone levels, this means you do not have enough insulin. You will need another injection of insulin. Do not resume exercise until ketone levels return to trace amounts.

In general, you don't want to exercise within an hour of your last regular insulin injection. Try to avoid exercising when your insulin is working hardest. You also want to avoid exercising when your insulin levels are at their lowest. An intermediate time point is usually the best. Talk to your doctor about the best time to work out with your insulin and eating schedule.

If you have type 2 diabetes, regular exercise can improve your blood glucose control. If you use insulin, you may have to follow the same precautions as someone with type 1 diabetes. Check your blood glucose levels before exercising. You will want to avoid treating low blood glucose with extra snacks if you are trying to lose weight. Instead, try to time your workouts at your normal snack time or an hour or so after your meals.

Staying Motivated

Probably the hardest part of any exercise program is staying motivated. Here are a few tips to help you get started and stick with it.

- Schedule your workout and stick to your schedule. Think of your workout as an important part of your day, as important as a meeting with your boss or doctor. Make it a regular part of your daily life. If you decide to forego your workout, write out a written excuse and post it on your bulletin board. Sometimes the act of writing down an excuse makes you throw it away and exercise anyway.

- Work out with a partner. Some days you might have a hard time rolling out of bed. But knowing your exercise buddy is sitting there waiting for you makes it easier to stick to your schedule.

- Cross-train. This means doing a different type of exercise each day instead of the same old thing day in and day out. Combine walking and swimming, for example, or lifting weights and jogging. This is more fun and it will help you avoid injury.

- Set realistic, specific goals. Don't expect to lose a lot of weight or run a mile or two without stopping right away. Set goals you can build toward. Set both long-term ("I plan to lose 20 pounds this year") and short-term ("I plan to exercise 4 times this week") goals.

- Reward yourself. No, don't go eat a hot-fudge sundae for walking a mile. But do let yourself do an easier workout every now and then. Treat yourself to a massage for each week you stick to your schedule or exceed your goals. Buy yourself a new pair of walking shoes or a new exercise outfit if you keep at it for a month.

- Track your progress. Keep a log of all your activities. Make note of how you feel. Also find a way to measure any weight loss, change in appetite, or how much medication you need. Noting positive changes may help you keep going.

A Word of Warning

If you have any kind of proliferative retinopathy, see your eye doctor before starting any physical activity. Get your retinopathy treated and your doctor's okay before any exercise. If you have peripheral neuropathy, you should avoid exercises that jar your feet, such as running, jogging, or high-impact aerobics. You may injure your tissues and joints without knowing it. Instead, think of biking or swimming, or light walking. If you have autonomic neuropathy, don't exercise without your doctor's okay. Your body may have a hard time compensating for the exertion of exercise. You may risk dehydration, hypoglycemia, and low blood pressure. You might be able to do light walking, but check with your doctor first. If you are pregnant, ask your doctor if you should modify your exercise routine.

Chapter 18
Solving Lifestyle Problems

Diabetes is unlike most other diseases or serious conditions. Many diseases are curable or treatable. You seek treatment, put the condition behind you, and get on with your life. Other diseases are chronic, with no sunny outlook, simple cure, or available treatment. But diabetes falls somewhere in between. It is treatable, and if properly managed, you can live a long and healthy life. But managing diabetes takes a lot of work.

You may find that your biggest problem with diabetes is adjusting to it. Whether you have type 1 or type 2 diabetes, you have probably found that you need to change your lifestyle, perhaps drastically, and let healthy living become a way of life for you. This requires a delicate balancing act as you try to integrate healthy habits into your day-to-day routine, without letting diabetes consume you. But it can be done. It's a matter of accepting your new lifestyle as part of who you are as you go through the daily tasks of living, balancing your needs with those of your family, friends, and career, and gathering the support you need from those around you.

Managing Your Daily Routine

Your biggest challenge in managing diabetes may not be dealing with life-threatening emergencies. Rather, it may simply be managing your daily routine, day in and day out—learning to plan your activities around your meals and insulin or medication schedule, whether you a dealing with a demanding boss or a screaming toddler. The key to successfully managing your diabetes is to fully accept your condition, realize that you are in charge of controlling your diabetes, arm yourself with information so that you understand how diabetes affects your body, develop a plan for managing your diabetes, and learn how to adapt your diabetes care plan to changing needs.

■ WHAT TO DO

The first step toward managing diabetes is to fully accept your condition. Many people enter a stage of denial (see Chapter 19) and are reluctant to come to terms with all the demands of the disease until they are confronted with a medical emergency. If you ignore or deny that you have diabetes, you may ultimately put yourself in a position in which diabetes may restrict your life and make day-to-day living more difficult. For example, if you ignore your blood glucose levels and develop diabetes complications, you may find you have leg problems that affect your mobility. But if you come to terms with diabetes and find a way of dealing with it, day-to-day living can be as smooth as or even smoother than that of someone without diabetes.

The next step in managing diabetes is to realize you are ultimately in charge of your own life, including your diabetes. You cannot rely on a doctor to give you a magic pill to make it go away or hope that someone else will tell you what to do. It is up to you to develop a plan of action that works for you. By taking charge of your daily management plan, your meal plan, and your medication schedule, you can find a plan that works for you.

The next step in figuring out a way to manage your daily routine is to arm yourself with information. Ask your doctors lots of questions and don't worry that you are taking up their time. Talk to your diabetes educator who can explain all the ins and outs of diabetes. Read all you can. Talk to other people with diabetes. Make sure you understand how diabetes affects your blood glucose level, and how insulin, your food, and physical activities all connect to affect your blood glucose levels. Once you understand how this works, you can begin to make the necessary adjustments so you can manage your daily routine.

Managing day-to-day living is tough for anyone these days. Sometimes, it seems as though nothing ever goes smoothly. And if you have diabetes, life is even more of a challenge. The key is to accept and understand your diabetes. Then work with your health care team to develop a management plan that accommodates your lifestyle. Is your life structured, or do you prefer to go with the flow? If you are comfortable with a predictable routine for eating, testing, injecting, and exercising, then you may find it easy to manage your daily routine. But if your job is anything but predictable and you never know from minute to minute when you'll get a chance to eat lunch or get home, then you will need a plan that allows some flexibility. For many people with diabetes, using an insulin pump can allow for the needed flexibility.

One of the most important things in managing diabetes is to incorporate ways of making adjustments. If you're running late for dinner or are shuttling your kids to soccer and ballet, what do you do? If you're out late visiting friends and oversleep the next day, how can you handle that? What if you have those days when you just don't feel like doing anything? A key ingredient in making adjustments in your daily routine is to test your blood glucose level frequently. And always keep a carbohydrate snack at hand for those times your blood glucose level falls too low.

When you talk to your doctor or diabetes educator, make sure to bring up those real-life situations that tend to occur during your days and ask about how you can make the necessary adjustments. Once you realize that you can live a real life and learn how to make the changes to accommodate different situations, the idea of maintaining your diabetes management plan day in and day out may seem less daunting.

Diabetes and Your Family

When you develop diabetes, you are not the only one dealing with the disease. Your whole family is affected by your new lifestyle and what they do influences how you manage your condition. How you schedule your meals, time together, and family activities will all depend, to some extent, on your diabetes care schedule. Your family members will also have to become familiar with how to recognize and handle emergency situations.

■ WHAT TO DO

The first step in integrating diabetes into your family life is to make sure your family members understand diabetes, what causes it, how it's treated, and how important it is to keep blood glucose levels under control. It may seem like an inconvenience for your kids to have to eat at a certain time if they would rather stay out and play for another hour. But if they realize the importance of eating according to a schedule, they may be more cooperative. It may be tempting to put off a meal "just this one time," but if your family members understand that doing so can have serious consequences in both the short and long term, they will be more willing to accommodate your schedule and more supportive of your efforts to keep your blood glucose levels under control.

Of course, balancing diabetes with family life may require some give and take on your part, too. If you can't miss your daughter's performance as the rainbow in the class play, even though it comes at lunchtime, you can learn how to make adjustments in your schedule. Eating part of your lunch as a small snack before the play begins, for example, may be enough to tide you over. There will be times when your family members feel that everything revolves around your meal schedule. But if you find creative ways to include flexibility in your plan, you can avoid some of the family stresses.

Your family members will also need to know how to handle emergencies. This means recognizing the warning signs, even if you downplay them or refuse help. They need to know when you are experiencing symptoms of hypoglycemia, for example, and when to call for help (see Chapter 2). They should also learn to recognize the signs of hyperglycemia, diabetic ketoacidosis, or hyperglycemic hyperosmolar state (see Chapter 3). Your family members should all know how to test your blood glucose levels, how to administer insulin, and how to give you a shot of glucagon. Have your family members come to some of your appointments with your diabetes educator. Your diabetes educator can help answer any questions your family may have about diabetes and also show them what to do should an emergency situation arise.

As much as you need your family's support, it is also important that you try not to place the bulk of responsibility for managing your diabetes on them. Don't make your wife nag you about eating too many helpings of mashed potatoes. Don't make your husband be the one who worries more about when you take your next insulin shot than you do. Take responsibility for your own situation, welcome your family's support, and try to meet your own goals, not someone else's.

During the period of adjusting to diabetes and for years to come, it will be important for both you and your family members to freely share your feelings about the condition. Don't try to hide how you are feeling from your family. If you feel overwhelmed, tell them. If they resent how diabetes affects them, encourage them to share those feelings so that together you can reach an understanding. Maybe a simple alteration in your routine will be enough to prevent those feelings from building up. The more you talk about diabetes and how it affects you as a family, the better you will be at making those changes that will help you balance both your diabetes care and family life.

Of course there may be some hidden benefits to diabetes, for both you and your family. Managing diabetes probably means changing your lifestyle as you start to eat better, exercise regularly, and develop habits that promote healthy living. This isn't something that only people with diabetes should do. These are habits that are good for everyone. As you pay attention to eating better, your family probably will begin eating the same way. As you start on your evening stroll after dinner, you may find that your whole family joins in. These sorts of activities can go a long way in promoting family togetherness. And as you struggle with the ups and downs of diabetes, and learn to communicate your feelings, you may find that you become closer to family members and develop strong emotional bonds you might not have created otherwise. The key is to try to work with your management plan to bring family members closer, not to drive them apart.

Developing Support Systems

One thing that can greatly help you on the road to living a healthier life with diabetes is developing a support system, a network of family, friends, health care professionals, and people with diabetes with whom you can share your feelings, concerns, and tips for healthy living.

■ WHAT TO DO

The first thing you can do to cultivate a support system is to reach out to those around you. Talk to your family and friends. Tell them about your diabetes and how you manage it. Discuss any specific concerns you have and let them know what they can do to help you. Make sure anyone who is close to you knows what to do in an emergency. More than anything, let them know you need their encouragement and support. Also, let them know that you are still the same person you always have been—just paying more attention to living a healthy lifestyle.

You may also want to enroll in some diabetes education classes. There you will meet other people facing the same day-to-day issues as you are. Many hospitals and community health organizations also offer diabetes support groups. Consider participating in one of these activities. You may also want to bring your family members or friends along so that they might understand some of the issues you are dealing with. Talking to other people who are going through the same thing as you will help you feel less alone, provide additional encouragement, and help you pick up tips for dealing with some of the more practical aspects of managing your diabetes.

Also, if you have access to a computer, you can tap in to a wealth of information and support on the internet. A good start is the American Diabetes Association's website, located at www.diabetes.org. For a directory and review of online resources related to diabetes, visit www.mendosa.com/diabetes.html. If you are interested in information and issues related to children with diabetes, visit www.castleweb.com/diabetes/. At these and many of the internet sites linked to these sites, you can meet people online, visit chat rooms, share in news groups, read message boards, and correspond by e-mail. There you can share your feelings and tips for survival with a community of people dealing with the same issues that you are dealing with.

Finally, don't forget your health care team. Not only are they there to see to your medical condition, but they can also help you deal with some of the practical aspects of dealing with diabetes, as well as some of the emotional issues.

Communicating with Your Health Care Team

Think of all the health care professionals that see to your medical health as members of your health care team. Your team should include your doctor, nurse educator, dietitian, eye doctor, podiatrist, exercise specialist, pharmacist, and mental health professional. Ideally, all these people should see themselves as a team that is committed to your welfare. The team is there to work together to make sure you have the knowledge to deal with your diabetes on a day-to-day basis, to provide the resources to help you make decisions that affect your health, to monitor your progress, and to help out if any medical needs arise.

■ WHAT TO DO

Make sure your doctor and other members of your team see themselves as a team and know about each other. Be sure that they have each other's phone numbers and addresses. If you are making any changes in your life—quitting smoking or taking up jogging, for example—make sure all your team members know about it. Also make sure everyone is fully informed if any problems should arise.

Don't forget that you are the captain of your team. You are ultimately responsible for your health, and you are the one who puts your diabetes care plan into action. It is important that you be able to communicate freely with the members of your team. You should not feel uncomfortable asking questions or telling them about any problems that may arise. But it is not always easy to feel comfortable when you feel nervous, are worried or stressed, or feel under pressure. Often just walking into a doctor's office can put you on edge. You may have specific things you want to discuss and then forget what you wanted to say. Here are a few tips to keeping the lines of communication open between you and the members of your health care team.

- Share the conversation. Your doctor should talk about 60 percent of the time and you should talk about 40 percent of the time. Make sure to speak up, ask questions, and share your concerns. But at the same time, don't forget to listen and hear what your health care professional has to say. If your doctor doesn't seem to have the time to listen to you, find a new doctor. Doctors have different strengths and weaknesses, so shop around, even within the same HMO.

- Write down everything you want to discuss with your team before your visit, and write down their answers as you go through each point.

- If your team member is saying something you don't understand, speak up. Sometimes health care professionals use jargon or technical terms that don't make sense to the nonprofessional. And sometimes the information is too complex to understand. If this happens, ask your team member to explain it to you in terms you will understand. Write down any information or instructions you are likely to forget when you leave. Don't worry about feeling "stupid" or asking something you think you ought to know already. It is important you understand everything your health care professional tells you before you leave the office.

- Don't be afraid to discuss sexual or personal topics. Your team members are professionals and prepared to deal with even the most sensitive topics. It's important for you to get all the help you need. Don't be embarrassed—many, many people have concerns just like yours.

- Don't be afraid to discuss money. Your team members realize that financial issues can be troubling and can contribute to your anxiety. If you don't think you can afford a treatment, or money concerns are keeping you from getting the care you need, talk to them. Many are willing to discuss payment options and may be able to direct you to the proper resources for additional assistance.

- Think about bringing a spouse or support person to sit in on the visit. Often, another party can help you to remember things you wanted to ask or can remember what the team member told you.

- If at any time you don't feel comfortable with any member of your health care team or feel that you are not communicating effectively, consider interviewing other professionals until you find someone with whom you feel at ease.

When You Travel

Whether you are camping in the backwoods of Maine or dining in the most elegant salons of Paris, traveling brings on its own set of challenges. It is difficult enough keeping your blood glucose levels under control when you are home with all its conveniences and following your regular routine. But when you travel, everything can be thrown out of whack. Not only do you have to plan for emergencies, worry about what to do if you run out of supplies, and deal with upsets in schedules, changing time zones, and altered exercise patterns, you also have to worry about eating right and keeping your blood glucose under control. The key to any successful trip, whether for business or pleasure, for a weekend or a month, is to plan ahead.

■ WHAT TO DO

Before You Go

Before leaving on any trip, talk to your doctor about any special precautions you might need to know about. If you are taking a short trip 50 miles away to visit your best friend, you may not get out of your routine all that much and may not need to take any special precautions. But if you are taking a long trip, especially if you are crossing time zones or visiting another country, you may have to prepare more carefully.

If you are going on an extended trip, traveling far from home, or visiting another country, make sure to schedule a visit with your doctor. Your doctor should examine you to make sure you are keeping your blood glucose levels under control. If you have any complications of diabetes, such as heart problems, these should also be assessed to make sure it is safe for you to travel. If possible, schedule this visit well in advance of your trip. This will give you time to get your diabetes under control, if necessary. If you will need any immunizations, you can take care of them at this time. Immunizations can sometimes leave you not feeling well and this can affect your blood glucose levels. If you take care of them in advance, you will have time to regain control of your blood glucose.

You will also need some papers from your doctor: a letter and your medical prescriptions. This is especially important if you are traveling far from home. The letter should explain how your diabetes is being treated. For example, it should state whether you are taking any oral agents, insulin shots, or using an insulin pump, and it should list all the supplies you currently use, such as insulin, lancets, test strips, and syringes. This letter can be useful should any questions arise through customs or if you need to seek treatment anywhere in your travels. The letter should also list any allergies you have or any foods or medications to which you are sensitive. It should also mention any complications or other medical conditions that affect you.

You should also have prescriptions for insulin or any oral agents you might be taking for diabetes. Don't rely on the prescriptions alone for obtaining supplies should you run out. Pack enough at the beginning to last you through your entire trip. But should you lose your bags, or some emergency occurs, you will have prescriptions available to get replacements.

The rules for getting prescriptions filled may vary from state to state and country to country. Make sure that you know the rules before you go. If you are traveling to another state within the United States, get a list of the ADA offices in the area or areas to which you are traveling. If you are traveling to one specific location, check with the local ADA office in advance to see if there will be any problem getting the prescription filled. If you are traveling to another country, get a list of International Diabetes Federation groups from the IDF, 40 Washington Street, B-1050 Brussels, Belgium. You may also want to get a list of English-speaking doctors in the country or countries you are visiting. This can be obtained from the International Association for Medical Assistance to Travelers, 417 Center Street, Lewiston, NY 14092. If you are traveling overseas and an emergency occurs or you need medical assistance, you can also seek help through the local American Consulate, American Express, or local medical schools.

Whether you are traveling around the block or around the world, wear a medical identification bracelet or necklace that identifies you as someone with diabetes. If you are traveling to a foreign country, ask your local ADA office for "Diabetes Identity Cards" written in the language of the country or countries you will be visiting. Also learn to say "I have diabetes" and "sugar or orange juice, please" in the language of the country you will be visiting.

What to Pack

If you are a seasoned traveler, you may be used to packing light. This is okay when it comes to clothes and accessories, but when packing your diabetes equipment, it's better to have and not need than need and not have. When packing your insulin, medications, and blood testing supplies, always pack at least twice as much as you think you'll need. Put half of your supplies in your carry-on bag and the rest in your regular suitcases. This way, if your bags are lost, you will still have an adequate supply to last you until you find your bags or replace your supplies. Keep your carry-on bag close by at all times, whether you are traveling by car, plane, train, boat, bike, foot, horse, or camel. Your carry-on bag should contain the following items:

- blood and urine testing supplies, including lancets, test strips, and meter

- extra batteries for your blood glucose meter

- all oral medications

- any other medications or medical supplies you may need, such as glucagon, antidiarrheal medicine, antibiotic ointment, antinausea drugs, or medication for any other conditions you have

- all the insulin, syringes, and/or infusion sets you will need for the trip (if you use a pump you may still want to pack some insulin syringes as an emergency backup)

- your diabetes identity card or other form of identification that indicates where you can be contacted while you are traveling, as well as your home address

- a snack of crackers and cheese or peanut butter, fruit, a juice box, and some form of fast-acting carbohydrate to treat hypoglycemia

When you pack insulin, pay special attention to how you store it. You don't want it to get too hot or too cold. If insulin freezes or is stored at temperatures below 36 °F, it may aggregate, or clump together, and become inactive. Also, keep insulin out of direct sunlight or in places that may get too hot. Insulin spoils if it is stored at temperatures greater than 86 °F. In general, if the temperature is comfortable for you, your insulin will be okay too. However, be careful about leaving it in the glove compartment or trunk of your car, or in a backpack or cycling packs that are exposed to direct sunlight. These can get quite hot. Instead, store your insulin in an insulated travel pack that will keep your insulin cool without freezing it. Also, make sure to keep all your insulin with you when traveling by plane, bus, or train, since the temperatures of luggage areas could harm your insulin.

When buying insulin overseas, be aware that insulins can come in different strengths in different countries. Nearly all insulin sold in the United States is of the same strength, U-100. This means there are 100 units of insulin in every cubic centimeter (cc) of fluid. When you use an insulin syringe, you are probably used to a U-100 syringe. This ensures that you deliver the right dose for your strength of insulin. In some countries, insulin may come as U-40 or U-80 solutions, which are more dilute than what you are used to. If you use one of these insulins, you also need to buy a matching U-40 or U-80 syringe. If you use a

U-100 syringe for U-40 insulin, you will end up injecting less insulin than you need. To avoid this, make sure your syringe matches your insulin strength. Ask your doctor how to make any adjustments in dose for any other insulin strength you may have to buy.

Eating on the Run

If you are flying or taking a train and eating en route, make sure to request a special meal in advance. You can request a special meal that is low in sugar, fat, or cholesterol. You should request your meal at least 2 days before you fly. A convenient time to do this is when you are making your seat reservations. Meal service is often slow on airlines, so make sure you see the cart coming down the aisle before you take your shot of insulin. Carry an extra snack with you in case your meal is delayed. Also make sure the flight attendant knows that you have diabetes. This could help expedite service if you are in need of a quick glass of orange juice or snack.

If you are flying in an airplane and need to inject insulin, be aware that the cabin is pressurized. Be careful not to inject air into the insulin bottle. In a pressurized cabin, this can make it difficult to move the plunger and you may end up injecting an inaccurate dose of insulin.

When traveling across time zones, be aware that some adjustments may be needed. If you are driving, this will probably only require a minor adjustment. But if you are flying across several time zones, it could make a difference. In general, remember that travel eastward shortens your day. If you use insulin, you will probably need less insulin. If you go west, your day is lengthened and you will need more insulin and perhaps an extra snack. Discuss your plans with your doctor or diabetes educator before your trip. Bring your travel plans and itinerary with you. Your doctor or diabetes educator can then help you make any required adjustments in your eating and insulin schedule. Don't forget to test your blood glucose level while you are traveling, especially if you are crossing time zones. If you are flying, test your blood glucose soon after you land and when you get settled into your lodgings. If you have jet lag and don't feel very well, it may be difficult to judge whether your glucose is too high or too low. Testing is the only way to know for sure.

Once you arrive at your destination, take it easy for a few days. Test your blood glucose levels more often than you usually do. Plan your activities around your insulin and meal schedules. Don't forget to take along snacks when hiking or sightseeing. Don't assume you can find food wherever you go. Try to experience the foods that will give you a sample of the local flavor, but avoid those foods you know will upset your stomach. When traveling in some foreign countries, you need to avoid the local tap water, even ice cubes. Rely instead on bottled water.

The most important thing to keep in mind is that diabetes need not interfere with your adventure. It just takes some advance planning and preparation. Once you integrate diabetes into your daily routine, whether at home or traveling, you are free to experience the world and all its pleasures.

Chapter 19
Solving Coping Problems

Adjusting to Diabetes

Maybe you were sailing along, enjoying life. Then, perhaps, things began to change and you didn't feel quite right. If you have type 1 diabetes, your symptoms may have appeared quite suddenly. If you have type 2 diabetes, you may have noticed that you felt worse over a period of time. Finally something happened that sent you to the doctor and you found out you had diabetes.

For some people, the diagnosis comes as a bit of a relief. "No wonder I have been feeling so awful!" you might remember saying. For others, the diagnosis hits like a ton of bricks. "My life will never be the same again," you might be thinking.

Being diagnosed with diabetes raises all sorts of conflicting emotions. It is often difficult to deal with these feelings as you also try to absorb all the medical information being thrown at you. It's difficult enough trying to stick to a diet and figure out how to give yourself insulin or work your blood glucose meter. It's easy to put these feelings aside. Or maybe you have decided to put off dealing with diabetes entirely. Maybe if you don't think about it, it will go away. Dealing with the reality of diabetes is not easy. And dealing with the conflicting emotions that come with it can be even harder. It doesn't help when you have bad feelings that go unresolved. You may feel edgy, anxious, nervous, depressed, or angry. And when you have these feelings, they can make your physical symptoms of diabetes even worse.

The best way to cope with diabetes, whether you are newly diagnosed or have been living with it for years, is to deal with both the physical symptoms and the emotional feelings. When you recognize and confront your feelings, you can resolve them. Once you resolve how you are feeling, you can move on with your life and begin to integrate your diabetes management into your day-to-day living.

Denial

When you were first diagnosed with diabetes, did you say to yourself, "Not me!" If so, you are not alone. Denial is a normal reaction when you are dealt troubling news. If your initial reaction to being diagnosed with diabetes is to deny that you have it, don't worry too much. Many doctors recognize denial as a normal stage you must pass through in order to accept your condition.

Denial can serve as a valuable coping mechanism. By denying bad news you can avoid slumping into a depression that can sometimes incapacitate you. The normal course of denial is to gradually come out of it, accepting little bits of information at a pace that you can handle. If you can come to terms with different aspects of diabetes at your own speed, then you may be able to make adjustments bit by bit. This is a way of dealing with the news in stages and may help you to avoid feeling so overwhelmed that you can't cope.

However, if you go on for months and months or sometimes even years denying that you have diabetes, you have a problem. Bad feelings don't go away just because you deny them. They are like a black cloud looming overhead, creeping in and affecting your outlook in ways you may not even realize. And the worst part is that by denying your condition, you put off taking care of yourself. Diabetes is a manageable disease, but only if you take charge and keep your blood glucose levels under control. If you deny you have it and don't take care of yourself, you make the condition worse and you face the risk of debilitating complications later.

■ SIGNS

Denial is normal during the first few weeks or even months following a diagnosis of diabetes. But if you were diagnosed with diabetes more than 6 months ago and you are still not changing your habits or giving it more than a fleeting thought, you may be in denial. Denial might be a problem for you if you still find yourself saying things like this:

- One bite of cheesecake won't hurt.

- This sore will heal by itself.

- I'll call the doctor next week.

- I don't have enough time to test my blood.

- I'm just taking pills so my diabetes isn't serious.

- They say I have diabetes, but what do they know?

- It's not really diabetes. I just have to take off a few pounds.

- I can't do anything about it, since my insurance won't cover it.

■ RISKS

The greatest risk of denial is neglecting your health. Diabetes won't go away if you don't take care of it, but it will get better if you do. When you deny diabetes, you may end up ignoring your meal plan, neglecting to test your blood glucose levels, or forgetting to take your medication. All these actions can cause your blood glucose levels to rise too high or fall too low. This can trigger an emergency situation that could send you to the hospital. And chronically high blood glucose levels over time can worsen the complications of diabetes. These include eye disease, nerve damage, cardiovascular disease, kidney disease, and infections. When you deny your diabetes, you may also neglect to do other things to ensure your health, such as taking care of your feet or quitting smoking.

■ WHAT TO DO

There is no single best way to break out of denial. Your spouse or health care professional can't do it for you. It may help you to realize that what you are going through is normal. It may also help you to talk to other people with diabetes and discuss how they got through it. You can meet other people with diabetes by joining a diabetes support group or signing up for a diabetes education class, often available at your local hospital or community center. You may also discover that the internet provides a wealth of information about diabetes, and you may link up with other people with diabetes through chat rooms, news groups, and message boards. To get started, check out the ADA website at www.diabetes.org.

Another way to break out of denial is to realize that you have two choices. Visualize yourself at a fork in the road. If you travel down one road, continuing to deny your diabetes, you will pass through periods of turmoil, marked by continued feelings of not feeling quite right, emergency episodes of hypoglycemia or hyperglycemia that may send you to the hospital, and along the way, dealing with the chronic conditions of a host of diabetes complications, including infections, skin problems, impotence, nerve damage, heart disease, stroke, kidney problems, leg pain, and foot ulcers. This road continues to climb uphill the further along you go. Or you can look down the other road. The other road has a few obstacles: watching what you eat, exercising, not smoking, monitoring your blood glucose levels, and taking your medication. Along the way you meet other people, say hello, and chat about how you are doing. There are a few bumps in the beginning and you may have to even slow down a few times, but as you go along, the path evens out and it is smooth going for a long, long way.

The point is, you have a choice. You can confront diabetes and take charge of your condition and get on the path to healthy living. Or you can continue to deny diabetes and face serious obstacles down the road. Taking the path to control may seem overwhelming. If this is your problem, slow down. Take a deep breath. And don't bite off more than you can chew, so to speak. Take it one step at a time. It may be too much to begin to change your eating patterns, start exercising, quit smoking, and start taking insulin all at once. Instead, realize that anything you do is better than nothing. Develop a long-term plan and a series of short-term plans. Tell yourself that this week, you are just going to focus on changing your eating. Or maybe you would rather start by getting used to monitoring your blood glucose levels. Think about getting an insulin pump or trying intensive therapy to give you the flexibility you need.

Where you should start depends on your exact condition. Talk to your doctor or diabetes educator. Tell her that you are overwhelmed, if that is the case, and you just want to start with one thing. Discuss what thing would be easiest for you to handle and the most beneficial to you. Then for a week or a few weeks, concentrate on just doing that one thing. Seek the help of your dietitian or exercise specialist or other health care professional, if necessary, to help with your goal. Once you have mastered that, you may feel better able to handle something else, such as beginning a walking program. If you take diabetes one step at a time, you may be better able to handle it emotionally, and that will put you down the right path physically.

Anger

Once you get over your feelings of denial, feelings of anger may begin to set in. Anger can also coexist alongside of feelings of denial or depression. Certain situations may trigger anger. And your anger may flare up in situations that on the surface have nothing to do with diabetes. Often people become angry about things they are really afraid of. Diabetes can be overwhelming and give rise to an array of fears. "How will I deal with hypoglycemia?" "Will I be able to have children?" "What will the other kids say when I have to give myself an insulin shot?" "Will I end up having my foot amputated?" These are all common reactions to scary thoughts. Once you voice those thoughts you may become angry. "Why did this have to happen to me?" "Why do I deserve this?" "Why don't you people just get out of my face?" Rest assured that these are normal feelings. It is normal to feel angry over something you feel you can't control, like diabetes. The trick to overcoming these feelings is to recognize them, realize they are normal, find ways to channel your energy, and ultimately realize that you can take charge of your diabetes.

■ SIGNS

The signs of anger are usually obvious. You flare up, turn red in the face, and clench your fists. Or you find yourself becoming agitated or easily annoyed. Something bothers you that shouldn't provoke a reaction. Someone says something and it ruffles your feathers. You can usually tell when you are feeling angry. But just what triggers the anger is not always obvious. You may find yourself getting angry when someone asks you about your diabetes. Or you may feel angry when you have to skip an activity to give yourself an insulin shot or test your blood glucose. But may also find yourself yelling at your kids for no apparent reason or becoming annoyed in traffic at a slight provocation. It may take some sorting out of your feelings to figure out why your behavior has changed. Diabetes can be a major factor in feelings of anger, especially if you are just coming to terms with the disorder.

■ WHAT TO DO

First, recognize that it is okay to feel angry. You have been dealt a bum deal and there is nothing wrong with feeling cheated. If you have been denying your feelings, it is perfectly normal to feel like lashing out. But uncontrolled anger on a regular basis can begin to eat away at you and alienate you from those who love you the most.

One way to begin to deal with your anger is to recognize it and take responsibility for it. Don't blame it on someone else if you get in an argument. Accept that you had an angry outburst. It may have been legitimately provoked, but it nevertheless made you lose your temper. At the same time, accept that it is okay to feel angry.

Next, begin to keep track of your angry episodes. Keep an anger journal. Write down all the things that make you angry during the course of a day. Write down the events that led up to the anger. Also record your general mood before you became angry. Do this for several days, or several weeks, if necessary.

Now sit down and review your notes. What makes you angry? When did it happen? Who was there? Do you notice any patterns? Maybe you get edgy when you are around other people in a social setting. Maybe your anger is triggered when you are asked about diabetes, or when people try to steer you away from the dessert table, or when you go out to eat with friends. Maybe you get angry when your mother or spouse asks you if you have tested your blood glucose level. By identifying those situations that trigger your anger, you can begin to come to terms with what makes you angry.

Once you have identified your anger triggers, think about what steps you can take to alleviate the situations that give rise to anger. You might even consider taking a day or even a week to let yourself be angry in the privacy of your own home, away from your family, before taking steps to control it. Get it out of your system. Then, begin a plan to control your anger.

You can start by learning to identify those situations you know will provoke anger. Become aware of the warning signs. You may start to tense up and feel your pulse quicken. Maybe you start talking louder or faster, or maybe you start to feel a little shaky. Whatever the sign, stop yourself. Close your eyes and count to 10. Talk slowly. Try to slow your breathing down. Get a drink of water. Sit down and lean back. Keep your hands at your side and zip your lips.

Controlling your anger doesn't mean you have to sweep it under the rug. Instead, think about how your anger is helping you to cope. Maybe if you don't like talking about diabetes, anger is helping you get around that. Instead of getting angry, think of other ways that will help you deal with the situation. For example, if you get angry every time your husband asks if you have tested your blood glucose level, tell him how you feel. And make a vow to head him off at the pass if he is making a reasonable request. For example, assure him that you will test your blood glucose at a certain time if he will lay off the nagging.

If you find yourself flaring up when asked about your diabetes, explain to your friends that you don't like to talk about it and ask them to refrain. At the same time you might examine why you are uncomfortable. You might find that you continue to be angry because you haven't fully accepted your condition. If this is the case, think about taking steps to help you accept it better. Think about joining a support group, educating yourself, and finding people to talk to.

Anger can work against you, but you can also think of anger as pent-up energy. Try to find ways to make your anger work for you. Your anger may be telling you that you need a change in your life. Perhaps you can channel your energy into becoming your own health advocate. Learn all you can about how to control your diabetes, develop a plan, and get to work at it.

Some people find that exercise is a good way to channel their anger. Going for a run or a brisk walk can do wonders when you are agitated. Many people find that this also helps them to settle down and think of a way to rechannel their energy. Exercise also has the added benefit of helping you control your blood glucose levels. Use your anger to educate yourself and put yourself in charge of your diabetes care. Anger can be a source of strength. It can give you the courage to speak up for yourself.

If you find it difficult to take steps to control your anger yourself, consider seeking help through counseling or expanding your support system. Often just talking about it can make you feel better.

Dealing with Stress

These days, we all live stressful lives, whether we have diabetes or not. Whether you are a student trying to cram for tomorrow's exam, a parent struggling with work and car pool arrangements, or a grandparent trying to adjust to the challenges of retirement, life can be stressful.

Throw in diabetes, and the stress level can be overwhelming. We feel stress when something happens that makes our bodies feel that they are under attack. Stress can be caused by physical things, such as injury or illness, or it can be caused by emotional problems, such as difficulties with a marriage, relationship, job, health, or money.

If you have diabetes, stress can be part of a vicious circle. Diabetes itself is stressful. And when you are overstressed, your body produces a cocktail of hormones. These hormones cause glucose and fat to be released into your bloodstream. It is nature's way of helping deal with the stress. For most people, that is good. But if you have diabetes, this response can throw your blood glucose levels out of whack. You do not always have enough insulin on hand to let glucose into cells. Your blood glucose level rises higher than it should. This can increase your stress level even further as you try to deal with the situation at hand.

It is important to find productive ways to deal with the stress in your life, especially if you have diabetes. Not only will this help prevent your blood glucose levels from going out of control as a direct reaction to the stress, but it will also help prevent the stress from triggering more serious psychological problems, such as depression and anxiety. When you are depressed or overly anxious about even minor concerns, you may let your diabetes care slide. When you feel miserable and have a sense of hopelessness, the last thing you want to do is check your blood glucose level. But neglecting your day-to-day diabetes care routine is the worst thing you can do in both the short and long term.

■ SIGNS

Stress can cause your blood glucose levels to rise unexpectedly. Any time you have unexplained hyperglycemia, ask yourself whether you have been under either physical or emotional stress. Stress can also give you an upset stomach, headaches, diarrhea, rashes, coughing, or feelings of nervousness, tiredness, or fatigue. It can make you feel sad or depressed or overanxious about things that are not normally a concern.

■ WHAT TO DO

If you frequently feel stressed out, overwhelmed, or unable to cope, there are several measures you can take to better handle the stress in your life. You may not be able to remove all the triggers of stress, but you may be able to handle how you react to them. If stress gets out of hand, you may experience periods of depression and/or anxiety. If this occurs, you may need to seek professional help.

The first thing to do is identify those times when you feel overwhelmed by stress. Make a list of all the things that contribute to your stress. Try to order them in terms of which things are most stressful. Look over the list. Ask yourself if there are triggers or situations on the list that you can do something about right away. For example, if you are constantly stressed out by a messy house, could you hire someone to help you clean once a month or even once a week? Can you enlist the help of family members? If you are having problems managing your workload at the office, can you talk to your boss about ways to decrease the workload? Can you afford to work part-time instead of full-time? If you are stressed out from driving the kids everywhere after school, can you carpool with your neighbors or get your spouse to pitch in? If traffic in general gets you riled up, can you find a new route to work or travel at a time when there is less congestion?

If your stress is related to more personal matters, such as marital problems or a particular family situation, enlist the help of your health care team. Maybe it would help to talk to a psychologist or social worker who can help you manage your emotional burdens and find ways to deal with your particular situation.

If you find that you are frequently caught in stressful situations and there is no way to prevent the situation from occurring, it may help to find better ways to control your reaction to the stress. Teach yourself some of the following ways to relax.

- Practice deep breathing exercises. To do this, sit or lie down with your arms and legs uncrossed. Try to make sure the room is quiet, with the lights turned down low. Take in a deep, deep breath, then push out as much air as possible. Breathe in and out again, relaxing your muscles as you breathe out. Do this for 5 to 20 minutes at a time at least once a day. If you find yourself in a stressful situation, try taking a few deep breaths until you feel relaxed.

- Exercise. Engaging in a daily physical activity can go a long way in relieving stress. When you feel stressed out, try going for a short jog, a walk, or a bike ride. You will be surprised at how soon you are feeling better. Regular physical exercise can prevent stress from getting out of hand.

- Memorize a prayer, poem, quote, or even a joke that makes you feel peaceful or even makes you laugh. When you begin to feel your stress level rising, think about these things that can make you smile.

- Learn how to control stress through relaxation therapy. This is a method of focusing on various muscle groups and learning to isolate and relax them. You can learn this through a class, a clinic, or an audiotape.

- Think of doing something new to reinvigorate or distract yourself from stress. Take a drawing class, get season tickets to the theater, join a sports team, or consider doing some volunteer work.

- Ask your doctor about seeking professional counseling if your problems have you too stressed out and you find them too difficult to deal with.

Some stresses will never go away. Diabetes is one of them. In those cases it may help to join a support group or talk to people in similar situations. Knowing how other people deal with the same stresses may help you cope better.

Depression

All people have periods when they feel a little blue every now and then. That's part of the ebb and flow of life. But if you have feelings of hopelessness or despair that last for weeks, you may be clinically depressed.

If you have diabetes, you may be even more susceptible to depression than someone without diabetes. Depression appears to be more common, last longer, and recur more frequently in people with diabetes than in the general population. Depression can occur when you are first diagnosed with diabetes, after you have gone through feelings of denial and anger, or later on, after you have been dealing with diabetes for years.

No one is really sure why people with diabetes are more prone to depression. It may be that the burden of diabetes management can wear on you and bring you down. It may arise out of feelings of isolation, feeling set apart from family and friends, and a sense that you are different than everyone else. Or it could be a physiological condition resulting from damage to the nerves that control your moods.

Whatever the reason, it is important to understand that if you are depressed, there is nothing wrong with you as a person. Depression can put you in a vicious cycle. You may feel depressed, have little energy for living, and neglect your diabetes care. This can make you feel worse physically, and even more depressed. Having high blood glucose levels for a period of time can make you feel sleepy and fatigued, for example. It can be difficult to break this cycle. The first step in dealing with depression is recognizing that you have it. Then you can take measures to break the cycle.

■ SYMPTOMS

One of the first signs of depression is a loss of pleasure. You no longer enjoy doing the things that once made you happy. You may also notice a change in sleep patterns. You may have trouble falling asleep at night, you wake up often during the night, or are restless during the night-time. You may wake up earlier than usual and find it difficult to get back to sleep. Alternatively, you may find that you want to sleep more than usual, even during the day.

You may also notice a change in appetite. Foods that once appealed to you no longer pique your interest. Or you may eat out of habit, without enjoyment. You may eat more or less than usual and may lose or gain weight quickly. You may have a hard time concentrating. Even watching a TV show or reading a magazine article may be difficult, because you are feeling restless. You may feel tired all the time and have no energy.

Some people with depression also feel nervous or anxious and have a difficult time just sitting still. You may have a hard time making decisions, even trivial or inconsequential decisions. You may also find yourself troubled by thoughts of guilt or self-deprecation. You feel like you can never do anything right. If you are depressed, you may feel worse in the morning than you do the rest of the day. When you are at your lowest point, you may even entertain suicidal thoughts. You may feel that you want to die or think about ways to hurt yourself.

■ WHAT TO DO

If you see yourself in three or more of these symptoms, you may have depression. Even if you only have one or two symptoms, but have been feeling bad for 2 weeks or more, it may be time to seek help.

The first thing to do is talk to your doctor. Tell her how you have been feeling. There may be an obvious physical reason for your depression and your doctor will want to examine you to see if anything else could be a factor. For example, some medications, alcohol or drug abuse, or poor blood glucose control can cause some of the same symptoms. Low blood glucose levels can make you feel hungry and cause you to overeat. They can also disturb your sleep at night. High blood glucose levels can make you get up during the night to urinate often. You may then feel tired all day. Thyroid problems can also cause symptoms of depression.

Once your doctor has ruled out any physical causes, you may be referred to a specialist. You may already be working with a mental health professional as part of your diabetes care team. If this is the case, it may be time to pay her a visit. If not, your doctor may recommend a psychiatrist, psychologist, psychiatric nurse, or licensed social worker. These professionals can help you get to the bottom of your feelings and suggest a course of treatment.

■ TREATMENT

There are two general types of treatment for depression: psychotherapy or counseling and antidepressant medication. Often, the best results come from a combination of the two.

Your psychotherapist can help you look at the problems that trigger your depression. Once you identify these triggers, you can then work on ways to resolve, or at least relieve, these problems. Sometimes all you need is a short-term course of therapy to help you get back on track. Other times, you may need to keep seeing your therapist for a longer period of time. It is critical that you feel comfortable with your therapist. You should feel at ease and be able to talk freely. If you are not comfortable with your counselor, shop around until you find someone you are able to connect with.

If your therapist feels that you would benefit from medication, you will need to see a psychiatrist. Psychiatrists are medical doctors and are the only mental health professionals who are allowed to prescribe medication. If you are referred to a psychiatrist, don't feel that something is wrong with you. Many people feel that if they need to see a psychiatrist, they must be crazy. Nothing could be further from the truth. Psychiatrists are trained professionals who are qualified to evaluate both the psychological and medical basis of any kind of emotional or mental problem. Many emotional disturbances are caused by physical problems, such as chemical imbalances in the nervous system or damage to the nerves. Your psychiatrist may be the best person to evaluate and treat such a situation.

Your psychiatrist may suggest an antidepressant medication. Most antidepressants work by increasing the amount of a chemical called serotonin in the synapses, or gaps, between the nerves. Too little serotonin can cause depression. Ask your psychiatrist and regular doctor how your antidepressant medication will affect blood glucose levels. Make sure your doctors are talking to each other about both your depression and your diabetes. If you do take an antidepressant, make sure to give it time to work. Usually a month or more is required before these medications work. If you don't see an improvement, tell your doctor. Often switching to another type of antidepressant will do the trick. You will probably benefit most by antidepressant medication if you also receive counseling at the same time.

If you have serious depression, the most important thing is to recognize the symptoms and seek help right away. It is usually a condition that can make you feel worse if left untreated and may be more than you alone can handle. If your doctor can't refer you to an appropriate mental health professional or you would like to switch mental health counselors, contact your local psychiatric society or psychiatry department of the closest medical school. Also contact the local branch of any organizations for psychiatric social workers, psychologists, or mental health counselors. Your local hospital may also have a referral service that can help you. Your local ADA office may also be able to help you find a counselor who is experienced in working with people with diabetes.

Anxiety

Anxiety can be a perfectly natural response to a stressful situation. It can serve as a valuable survival mechanism in a dangerous situation by making you more cautious. That is normal behavior and everyone experiences anxiety from time to time. When the boss invites you into her office, for example, or you are about to begin taking a test you didn't study for, you may feel worried. But anxiety can be a problem when it affects you at inappropriate times or when it is so intense and long lasting that it interferes with daily living. When this happens, you may have what is called an anxiety disorder. Anxiety disorders can be so distressing to some people that they lead to depression. Some people experience depression and anxiety at the same time. The signs and symptoms of anxiety and depression sometimes overlap, and they may also be caused by the same problems.

Life is stressful and can trigger anxiety in anyone at one time or another. But if you have diabetes, you face more stress than most people, day in and day out. Many people with diabetes learn to cope with this without too much of a problem. But for others, especially those with other stresses in their lives, diabetes can contribute to or even trigger anxiety. It's not enough that you have to face a deadline crunch, then come home to a house of screaming kids who need help with homework, but you also have to cook dinner and somewhere in there test your blood glucose and give yourself an insulin shot. That kind of stress can wear on you, and eventually, even little things make you feel anxious.

The key to dealing with anxiety, as is the case with most emotional problems, is to acknowledge the problem, identify the things that trigger undesirable behavior, try to alleviate the triggers, and find better ways to cope with the situation.

■ SYMPTOMS

Symptoms of anxiety include restlessness, feeling tired or easily fatigued all the time, difficulty concentrating, irritability, disturbed sleep, muscle tension, and a tendency to be overly worried or overly concerned. You may worry about work, school, money, your diabetes or general state of health, or relationships. You may also worry about more mundane things, such as getting the chores done or the car repaired. It is not a matter of these worries being unfounded, but usually the severity, duration, or frequency of these bouts of worrying is disproportionately greater than the situation calls for. The symptoms are the worst during times of greatest stress.

■ WHAT TO DO

If you think you worry too much or have been told you worry too much, and find that you have more than two of the symptoms above, you may have an anxiety disorder. This is especially true if you cannot see beyond your current concerns to enjoy things you once found pleasurable.

The first thing to do is talk to your doctor. Many medical conditions can trigger symptoms of anxiety and your doctor will first want to rule out any possible physical cause. Your doctor will also want to review your medications, because some medications can cause symptoms of anxiety. Your doctor will also want to check your records of your blood glucose levels over the past month, to see if extremes in your blood glucose levels might be triggering your feelings of anxiety. Anxiety itself, or the reaction to a stressful situation, can also alter blood glucose levels. As is the case with depression, this can lead to a cycle that needs to be broken.

Once any physical causes of anxiety are ruled out, your doctor will probably refer you to a mental health care professional. This could be a psychiatrist, psychologist, psychiatric nurse, or licensed social worker. You may already have one of these professionals on your health care team. Your mental health counselor will help you work through your problem. This can be accomplished through counseling or psychotherapy, medication, or a combination of counseling and drug therapy.

■ TREATMENT

The exact course of treatment for any anxiety disorder depends on the nature of the problems and what sorts of things trigger anxiety. This may be related to the physical stress or emotional burden of dealing with diabetes, or it could be completely unrelated. In some cases, underlying insecurities and inner conflicts may be a major factor in anxiety. Getting to the bottom of those feelings through counseling and psychotherapy may be of help. Trying to identify and understand those situations that provoke anxiety may also help.

However, frequently there is no clear-cut reason why a person experiences inappropriate anxiety. In these situations, drug therapy may help relieve the symptoms. Antianxiety drugs must be prescribed by a psychiatrist or other medical doctor and should be given with great care. Make sure your regular doctor and your psychiatrist are in contact with each other. Ask whether any medication will affect your blood glucose control. Some antianxiety drugs, such as benzodiazepines, can lead to physical dependence. If you discontinue such a drug, it must be done gradually. As with many drugs used to treat emotional disorders, they are usually more effective if used in conjunction with counseling. Talk to your doctor about what will work best for you.

Motivation

One of the most difficult aspects of diabetes is the fact that it is a chronic condition. It never goes away. You may be able to manage it well and feel no ill effects. But in order for that to occur, you have to work at it. Sometimes you don't mind. It can almost be like a second career for some people as they learn the ins and outs and ups and downs of controlling blood glucose levels. Maybe you initially attack your diabetes care plan with gusto, carefully adhering to the prescribed meal plan, dutifully checking blood glucose and injecting insulin on schedule. But at some point, you may very well just get tired of it. You want to take a break, take a day off perhaps. It's just too hard keeping on top of things, never getting a chance to rest—or feeling guilty if you do. Just how do you stay motivated to keep up the good work day in and day out, 24 hours a day, 365 days a year?

There are no easy answers. Everyone is motivated by different things. For some people it helps to have a partner, supporting and encouraging them. Other people prefer to go it alone, do it their own way. Whatever your style, it is important to figure out what works for you. You may not be able to keep up with a plan developed with someone else in mind. You may need meals that take your likes and dislikes into account and a schedule that fits in with your lifestyle. It will be easier to be motivated if your plan lets you live life the way you like to live.

■ WHAT TO DO

First, evaluate where you are. If you have already written down a list of goals, dig them out and look them over. If you have never written out your goals, this may be a good time to do it. Next, evaluate where you are. Are your blood glucose levels where you want them to be? Are you at your ideal weight? Do you feel good about your progress? If so, you are probably right on track and have been able to motivate yourself. It is not unusual to have a day every now and then when you just don't feel like doing everything you should. That is probably okay just as long as you don't slack off entirely and let your blood glucose levels get too high or too low.

If, however, you are not anywhere near reaching your goals, it is time to take a closer look and figure out why. Where are you falling short? Not sticking to your meal plan? Not always taking your insulin or monitoring blood glucose? Do you exercise? If there are one or more aspects of your diabetes care plan that you tend to neglect, ask yourself why. Chances are, if you are not doing what you want to be doing or feel you should be doing, you may have a motivation problem.

If you are having a difficult time motivating yourself to follow your plan, it may be because your plan does not suit you. Do your meals take into account your likes and dislikes? Does your insulin schedule allow you enough flexibility? Are you trying to do exercises that you don't like to do? If your diabetes care plan does not take into account your needs, it is time to talk to your doctor or diabetes educator about your diabetes care plan. You may due for an overhaul. Make sure your health care providers know what your schedule is like, whether you follow the same pattern every day, or if your hours and activities change all the time. Do you like to cook or eat out? Which foods do you like? Which foods do you hate? What kinds of activities do you like to do? Ask your doctor or diabetes educator to help you design a plan that suits your living style. Once you have something that you can live with, you might find that you are more motivated.

You may find it easier to become motivated by talking to other people with diabetes. Join a diabetes support group. By talking to others about what helps them to feel motivated, you may feel more like making an extra effort yourself and may get some good tips. Investigate the internet and join in a chat session with other people with diabetes.

Another way to get motivated might be to team up with a buddy. This could be someone with diabetes or someone without diabetes who just wants support in reaching his or her goals. Maybe you have a friend who wants to start exercising or lose weight. Try meeting for workouts or sharing recipes. Set goals that are realistic, not something you can never hope to attain. Track your progress and reward yourself when you succeed.

Alcohol Abuse

If you have good control of your diabetes, it probably won't hurt you to have a drink every now and then with your meals. But if you drink too much alcohol, are unable to stop drinking or abstain even when you want to, or drink even when it interferes with your family, friends, job, or social standing, then you may have an alcohol abuse problem.

■ SYMPTOMS

The first step in dealing with alcoholism is to admit you have a problem. This is probably the most difficult step. It can sometimes seem like a fine line between social drinking or having a drink or two after work to unwind to considering yourself an alcoholic. In the early stages, alcohol abuse may be difficult to recognize, even by relatives or close friends. If you have an alcohol abuse problem, you may also be reluctant to admit it. If you have more than two of the following symptoms listed below, then it is very likely that you have a serious alcohol abuse problem. Even if only one or two symptoms apply to you, you may be at risk of becoming dependent on alcohol.

- You tend to want to drink more or longer than the rest of the crowd. At a party you may look for a refill right away when you finish a drink instead of waiting to be offered one. Or you might pour yourself a little more than others seem to be drinking.

- You become preoccupied with drinking. You might often drink two or more alcoholic drinks when alone, either at home or in a bar, or feel a need to have a drink at a certain time each day, such as right after work. You feel a need to have at least one alcoholic drink each day and feel physically deprived if you don't. You look for a drink when you are feeling pressured or stressed. You may even crave a drink in the morning.

- Your drinking may trigger family arguments or your arguments may occur mostly when you have been drinking.

- You begin to hide alcohol or sneak drinks. When questioned about your drinking, you may tend to be less than honest or try to stretch the truth.

- You sometimes miss appointments and work, or are late for work, because of your drinking.

- You sometimes have blackouts, in which you forget what happened while you were drinking the night before.

- You notice an increasing tolerance to alcohol. You can "hold your liquor."

- You deny that you have a problem, even if you show many of the signs listed above.

■ RISKS

Drinking too much alcohol can be a problem for anyone. It can interfere with work, family life, and day-to-day living. Some people who are alcoholics are frequently intoxicated and often have a problem controlling their behavior. Others may manage to function in one area of their lives, but other areas suffer. In addition, alcohol abuse can also damage the body. It can lead to inflammation of the esophagus, which sometimes progresses to cancer, can cause anemia and birth defects when it occurs in pregnant women, can cause stomach problems, liver disease, heart problems, high blood pressure, atherosclerosis, stroke, inflammation of the pancreas, nerve damage, and brain damage.

If you have diabetes, alcohol abuse can be even more dangerous. It can worsen many of the complications of diabetes, especially nerve damage, eye disease, high blood pressure, kidney disease, and cardiovascular disease. It can also damage the liver, which is where your body stores glucose. When your liver is damaged, your blood glucose levels can be difficult to control. Also, if you have an alcohol abuse problem, you are much less likely to be able to give your diabetes care the attention you need to. If you are intoxicated, you may be unable or unwilling to test your blood glucose level and take the steps to treat high or low blood glucose levels.

Hypoglycemia is much more common among people with diabetes who have alcohol abuse problems. When your blood glucose levels drop too low, the liver releases glucose, which is stored there as glycogen. But if you have too much alcohol in your body the liver is too busy trying to get rid of the alcohol, which it sees as a toxin, and does not release glucose efficiently. As a result, your blood glucose levels can drop dangerously low. You could risk coma or even death.

■ WHAT TO DO

The first step, of course, is to recognize there is a problem. Unfortunately, this is also the most difficult step. This is one situation where you can't expect anyone to do it for you or nag you into better behavior. You have to want to stop drinking to excess and you yourself have to take the steps to recovery. Even if your drinking problem is in its early stages, you have to be the motivating force behind curtailing your alcohol intake.

The first thing to do if you show any of the symptoms listed above or feel that you are drinking too much is to try to cut down on the amount of alcohol you drink. If you have a drink or two every night, cut back to drinking every other night or only on weekends. If you only drink on weekends, but tend to drink to excess, stop after one drink. If you cannot do this, because you feel either a psychological or physical need to drink, then you need professional help right away. Talk to your doctor or call your local chapter of Alcoholics Anonymous (AA).

If you have been drinking for a long time, you may experience symptoms of withdrawal if you try to quit cold turkey. If you have decided to end your alcohol abuse, you should do so under a doctor's supervision. If you quit abruptly, within 12 to 48 hours you may experience symptoms of withdrawal, such as tremor, weakness, sweating, or nausea. Heavier drinkers may also hallucinate and hear voices. This stage can last for days, but it can be controlled with antipsychotic drugs. If untreated, alcohol withdrawal may progress to delirium tremens, a more serious condition that usually appears 2 to 10 days after you stop drinking. Initial anxiety may give way to confusion, sleeplessness, nightmares, excessive sweating, and deep depression. Your pulse may quicken and you may have a fever. You may also experience hallucinations, restlessness, and terror. If untreated, delirium tremens can be fatal.

If you have a serious alcohol abuse problem, your best bet is to be treated in an inpatient detoxification program at a clinic or hospital. There, your symptoms of withdrawal will be monitored and treated with medications such as benzodiazepines or antipsychotic drugs. You may even need intravenous fluids, sedatives, and antifever drugs. You should be closely supervised at all times.

Once you are through the symptoms of withdrawal and detoxification, you can begin a program of rehabilitation. Without help, most alcoholics relapse within a few weeks. Treatment in a group setting seems to be the most successful. You may want to seriously consider a long-term inpatient rehabilitation program at your local hospital. Ask your doctor how to go about arranging this. Usually this is coordinated along with detoxification.

The AA program has helped more people in this country than any other program. When you are ready to begin your rehabilitation program, have your doctor put you in touch with your local AA chapter. You may also want to join AA even if you have been through a long-term detoxification and rehabilitation program in a clinical setting. If AA is not your style, check into other local support groups for alcoholics or any programs run by your local hospital or community health center. Once you leave the hospital, make sure you seek counseling or support in one setting or another to continue your sobriety.

Even with detoxification and rehabilitation, some recovering alcoholics may still have trouble staying sober. If this happens to you, you may want to ask your doctor about drug therapy. One drug called disulfram (Antabuse) is taken on a regular basis. If you drink alcohol while on disulfram, acetaldehyde, a by-product of alcohol metabolism, will build up in your bloodstream and cause a violent reaction. Acetaldehyde is a toxin to your body and causes facial flushing, throbbing headache, rapid heart beat, rapid breathing, and sweating within 5 to 15 minutes of drinking alcohol. This adverse reaction is usually enough to keep you from drinking alcohol again. You should only take this route if you really and truly want to stop drinking. It should not be given within 7 days of your last drink and should not be taken if you have another serious illness or are pregnant. People with diabetes should not take disulfram without a doctor's supervision.

Another drug therapy, naltrexone, can help people refrain from alcohol. It should only be used as part of a comprehensive treatment program that includes counseling or some sort of group therapy. Naltrexone alters the effect of alcohol on the brain. Its big advantage is that it will not make you sick and may be safer for people with diabetes. However, because it doesn't make you sick, you may continue to drink. If you have liver disease or hepatitis, you should not take naltrexone.

Ending alcohol abuse can be tricky for anyone, but even more so for someone with diabetes. If you suspect you have a problem, talk to your doctor and carefully review your options. Your doctor and other members of your health care team can help guide you on your road to recovery.

Eating Disorders

If you have diabetes, it is not unusual to be preoccupied with what you eat and worry about whether you are eating too much or gaining too much weight. This shows that you are doing your part to keep your diabetes under control. Even people who don't have diabetes often fuss over their weight and diet. However, if you are excessively concerned over your weight to a point that threatens your health, you may have an eating disorder. You may also have an eating disorder if you seek psychological comfort in food and are unable to control what you eat.

There are three major types of eating disorders, all of which can seriously affect people with diabetes. Anorexia nervosa often affects teens and young women. If you have anorexia nervosa, you eat very little food and probably exercise to excess. Bulimia nervosa is also common in young women. If you have bulimia nervosa, you tend to binge eat and then purge. Purging is usually accomplished by vomiting, taking laxatives, or overexercising. A binge eating disorder usually affects older people who are obese. If you have this condition, you are prone to binge eating without purging. Because all of these conditions involve uncontrolled patterns of eating, they can make diabetes extremely difficult to manage.

Anorexia Nervosa

Anorexia affects mostly young women. In fact, 95 percent of those who have anorexia are women. It seems to be more common among people from middle and upper socioeconomic classes. It can be a mild, transient phenomenon that some women go through and outgrow. Or it can be part of a lifelong pattern that is severe and life-threatening. There are multiple causes of anorexia, but it is important to remember all eating disorder behaviors are symptoms of other psychological problems. Treat those problems, and the food-related symptoms will improve. Half of all people with anorexia also have bulimia.

■ SYMPTOMS

If you are anorexic, you probably weigh less than 85 percent of normal body weight. You have an intense fear of gaining weight even though you are thin and probably consider yourself too fat. You may exercise to excess and may even resort to bingeing and purging. You are probably preoccupied with food, even though you tend to eat far less than you should. You may hoard, conceal, or even waste food. You may cook elaborate meals for others, but refuse to eat anything yourself. It is likely that you frequently miss at least three consecutive menstrual cycles. When confronted by others, you probably deny that you have an eating problem.

If you have diabetes and are anorexic, you may frequently take part in a very dangerous practice. You may deliberately take less insulin than you know you should. The intent here is to keep from gaining weight by passing excess glucose into the urine. By excreting glucose you thus absorb less calories. This practice is extremely dangerous. It can lead to emergency situations requiring hospitalization and can even lead to coma and death. It can also worsen the complications of diabetes.

■ WHAT TO DO

As with any psychiatric disorder, you cannot be successfully treated until you recognize the problem and agree to seek treatment. Treatment of anorexia usually focuses first on restoring normal body weight and second on psychotherapy. Sometimes antidepressant medication is needed.

If weight loss is severe, it can be life-threatening. If you have lost more than 25 percent of your ideal body weight, you will most likely be treated in a hospital setting. Usually you will be encouraged to eat solid food. Only rarely will you be fed intravenously. Once you have gained enough weight, psychotherapy—in an individual, group, or family setting—can begin.

Your doctor may also suggest that you meet with your dietitian and diabetes educator. Your dietitian can work with you to develop an eating plan that encourages you to eat sensibly and nutritiously. You can learn to eat the right foods without gaining excessive amounts of weight. If you are taking insulin, talk to your educator about finding out how to devise a schedule that fits in with your eating plan.

Bulimia Nervosa

Bulimia also affects mostly young women. In fact, if you are bulimic, you may also be anorexic. Like people with anorexia, bulimics are also of upper socioeconomic classes and are excessively preoccupied with weight. This preoccupation is only a symptom of a deeper problem.

You may have bulimia if you binge eat and then purge to eliminate the food or overexercise to rid yourself of the calories. This means you eat very large amounts of food in a single setting at least twice a week. Usually this behavior has gone on for 3 months or more. You may feel that you can't stop eating or have a hard time controlling how much or what you eat. If food is there, you eat it, whether you are hungry or not. Once you binge, you will try to get rid of the food you have eaten by vomiting, using laxatives, or taking other medications to lose weight or prevent weight gain. You may also resort to using less insulin than you need to get rid of excess calories as glucose in the urine. If you are bulimic, you are less likely to deny your eating problem than someone with anorexia, and you are more likely to feel guilty about it.

■ WHAT TO DO

If you have bulimia or suspect you have bulimia, talk to your doctor right away. You will be referred to a psychotherapist for counseling in a group or individual setting. You should try to find someone who specializes in eating disorders. Often antidepressant drugs are helpful in treating bulimia, even if you are not diagnosed with depression. However, the symptoms can recur when the drug is discontinued.

You should also meet with your dietitian and diabetes educator. Your dietitian can work with you to develop an eating plan that encourages you to eat sensibly and nutritiously. Your eating plan should incorporate foods you like and should help you maintain a healthy weight. If you are taking insulin, talk to your educator about devising a schedule that fits in with your eating plan.

Binge Eating Disorder

Unlike anorexia and bulimia, binge eating disorders affect both men and women. Almost half of all binge eaters are male. Binge eaters tend to be older than those with anorexia and are frequently obese. Binge eating involves consuming excessive amounts of food without purging. As with other eating disorders, binge eating can make diabetes difficult to control. Excessive amounts of food can send blood glucose levels skyrocketing. Also, the eating pattern is often erratic and unpredictable, and it is difficult to maintain any regular diabetes care schedule. Binge eaters usually continue to gain weight as the bingeing continues, which makes insulin resistance even worse.

■ SYMPTOMS

If you are a binge eater, you eat large amounts of food and feel that you have no control over what you eat. You are probably distressed about your pattern of eating. Often binge eaters try to lose weight, but cannot control their behavior. About half of all binge eaters also suffer from depression.

■ WHAT TO DO

If you suspect that you are a binge eater, talk to your doctor right away. You may be referred to a psychotherapist and may benefit from group or individual counseling. You may also find relief with antidepressant or appetite suppressant therapy. Drug therapy will be more successful if prescribed along with counseling.

Chapter 20
Solving Discrimination and Insurance Problems

When you were first diagnosed with diabetes, you were probably overwhelmed with information. And if you were like most people, you probably spent a lot of time educating yourself, learning how to manage your diabetes, and getting your life on track. Once you learned to keep your diabetes under control and maintain a style of healthy living, you probably realized that living with diabetes is not all that different from living without diabetes. You could do all of the same things as someone without diabetes, and do them well. Then at some point, just when you thought things were starting to settle down, you hit a roadblock: the rest of the world.

Before you were diagnosed, you probably didn't know much about diabetes. One of the problems you may confront is the fact that most people don't know all that much about it either. And when people don't understand something, they often have misconceptions. These misconceptions can lead to discrimination in the workplace, in schools, in the military, and in seeking health insurance. Years ago, people with diabetes were denied fair treatment in many aspects of life. It was not unusual to be denied a job outright because of diabetes. The Americans with Disabilities Act of 1990 has done a lot to level the playing field for people with diabetes. However, discrimination can be more subtle today, and people with diabetes still face hurdles. Your task in seeking fair treatment as a person with diabetes is to know your rights, to educate those who might be in a position to deny you your fair shake, and to take action, if necessary.

Discrimination in the Workplace

In the past, it was not uncommon to face outright discrimination in the workplace. You might have been told point-blank that you weren't being hired because of your diabetes. Or you might have been faced with being fired or being denied a promotion in your present job when you were diagnosed with diabetes. The Americans with Disabilities Act changed all that in 1990. This law protects all civilian employees who work for companies that employ more than 15 people from discrimination. In much the same way that companies cannot discriminate against people on the basis of sex, race, or religion, the act also ensures that people with disabilities are also protected in the workplace. People with disabilities who work for the federal government or companies receiving federal funding have been protected from discrimination under the Rehabilitation Act of 1973. Under these laws, if you are qualified for the job and are able to carry out the work with reasonable accommodation, a company cannot discriminate against you. That means they are not allowed to carry out unfair practices in hiring, firing, promoting, training, and paying you. Employers must also avoid unfairness in recruiting, advertising, tenure, or layoffs.

But is diabetes really a disability? You have been working hard to keep your diabetes under control and live a normal life. You may have a hard time thinking of yourself as disabled. If so, this is good and it is likely that those around you will not consider you disabled and will not discriminate against you. But under the law, you are protected in the event your employer or potential employer thinks of you as disabled and treats you unfairly. The law defines a disabled person as anyone who has a physical or mental impairment that substantially limits one or more major life activities, has a record of such impairment, or is regarded as having such impairment.

Major life activities include seeing, hearing, speaking, walking, breathing, doing manual tasks, learning, caring for oneself, and working. If your diabetes has ever caused you any of these impairments, then you are covered under the first two definitions of disability. But even if you have never been disabled or impaired by diabetes, if your employer sees you as impaired, and discriminates against you just because he knows you have diabetes, you are also covered under the third definition of being disabled.

But how do you know whether you are being discriminated against? Were you not hired because you told them you had diabetes, or because the person hired had more experience? Were you passed over for a promotion because your coworker is really a better worker than you, or was it because you have diabetes? Sometimes it is difficult to tell and you may never know for sure.

■ INDICATIONS

It is hard to tell if you are being discriminated against if you have diabetes. Before these laws were passed, a company was allowed to ask you questions or require a physical before you were hired. If you then were not hired, it was not always easy to know why. Today, you are not required to take a physical before being offered a job. If you are hired for a job and then the offer is retracted after you tell them you have diabetes, or after you have a physical, then it might seem that you are being discriminated against.

If you are passed over for hiring, promotion, or a pay raise, and someone with lesser qualifications or less productivity is hired, promoted, or given a raise, then you might have been discriminated against.

Under the law, your employer is supposed to provide a "reasonable accommodation" to allow you to do your job. But the company does not have to make accommodations that will cause "undue hardship" to the company. Just what constitutes reasonable accommodation and undue hardship is not always clear. Often it is up to the courts to decide. If your company does not allow you time to test your blood glucose or give yourself an insulin injection, they may be discriminating against you. If they don't allow you work breaks to go to the bathroom more often or don't let you keep snacks or diabetes supplies near by, they may be discriminating against you. If your company forces you to work a swing shift instead of a standard shift, you may be a victim of discrimination. If they restrict your job opportunities or responsibilities because of your diabetes, you may have a case for discrimination. If your company refuses to give you flexibility in your working hours that you may need to accommodate your diabetes care schedule, it is possible that they are discriminating against you. However, this is only the case if accommodating you would not cause them undue hardship.

An employer is allowed to discriminate against you if it would be too hard or cost too much to meet your needs. If they would have to hire another person to cover you while you take time off, for example, they may not be discriminating against you. But if you have the kind of job in which you could get the job done just as well by working different hours and they won't let you, then it is possible that discrimination has occurred.

A company does not have to give you more sick leave than someone else. But it can't give you less. It does not need to find you health insurance without a preexisting condition clause. It can hold you to the same standards of performance or production as other workers. But it cannot hold you to a higher standard than other workers. A company does not have to give you a job or promotion just because you are disabled. And it does not have to give you preference over other qualified people who apply for the job. But neither can it give others preference over you if the others are not qualified.

Since it is not always clear when you are being discriminated against, sometimes misunderstandings can be cleared up by talking things over with your boss. Other times, more drastic action is needed.

■ WHAT TO DO

First of all, you need to decide whether or not to tell your employer that you have diabetes. There are reasons both to tell and not to tell. Here are some reasons you might want to tell:

- If you take insulin or oral diabetes medications, you may experience hypoglycemia. If you have a severe reaction, you may need the help of others. Those around you should be aware you have diabetes and should know what to do should an emergency occur.

- If you are open about your diabetes, people will understand it better and may be less likely to treat you unfairly. If you tell, you can show your coworkers that people with diabetes are just like anyone else.

- If you tell everyone, you don't have to hide a major part of your life. You avoid sending the message that you have something to hide. You don't have to keep track of who knows and who doesn't know.

- When you talk about your diabetes, other people can become aware of the symptoms and treatment. This may alert them to any warning signs and help them seek treatment if they also develop diabetes.

Of course there are also legitimate reasons not to tell:

- You may want to keep your privacy. You may not feel comfortable telling everyone about your condition, just as some people feel uncomfortable talking about money or religion.

- If you don't tell, you are less likely to be discriminated against because of your diabetes. Sometimes, people change their attitudes when they know someone has a disability. Discrimination may be very subtle and difficult to prove.

If you think you have been discriminated against, either while seeking a job or while presently employed, there are some steps you can take to resolve the situation. The first step is to talk to your employer directly. Often you can clear up any misunderstandings through open communication. Your employer may not know that much about diabetes, and you may be providing a valuable service by educating him. Sometimes information about how you manage your diabetes may be enough to convince your employer that a person with diabetes can be easily accommodated in that job. Also, don't forget to listen to your employer's concerns. If there are reasons your employer is discriminating against you or refusing to accommodate you, propose solutions to arrive at a mutually satisfactory agreement. Make sure to document any conversations, communication, or proposals you have had in attempts to remedy your situation.

If open communication and education doesn't work, you may want to seek the help of a union or employee group. You should also consult with a lawyer. Your lawyer may be able to resolve the situation with a simple telephone call or letter. You and your lawyer may want to remind your employer of his responsibility and provide information about the Americans with Disabilities Act.

If your employer refuses to negotiate or listen to your concerns, you may have no choice but to take legal action. Your first step may be to file charges with the Equal Employment Opportunity Commission (EEOC). This should be done within 180 days of the act of discrimination. You should know, however, that there is only a 1 in 665 chance that the EEOC will file a lawsuit on your behalf. The average wait for a complaint to be processed is 297 days. Filing an EEOC complaint is, however, a requirement for a later lawsuit if you need a "right to sue" letter. This is a letter the EEOC gives you if they don't take your case. The EEOC will give free information for both the public and employers.

If you do file a lawsuit, be aware that it is your job to prove you have been discriminated against. Just because you have diabetes and were passed up for promotion is not enough. You need to provide evidence, either direct or strongly circumstantial. The best evidence is a written statement from your employer stating why you weren't hired, were passed over, or were let go. If you are not hired, are not promoted, or refused a raise, ask for a written statement outlining the reasons. There may be other reasons for your employer's decision of which you should be aware.

The problem here is that your employer may not admit in writing to his reasons for discriminating against you. In that case you may have to work a little harder to gather circumstantial evidence. Gather together materials such as the employer's job application form, policy manuals, or statements regarding the employer's position on equal employment opportunity and any rules or regulations cited by the employer as the reason you were discriminated against. Save copies of job advertisements, the job description, and any job performance criteria. Record the date, time, place, and context of any offhand comments that may lead you to think you are a victim of discrimination.

You should also compile a list of potential witnesses, including their work titles and how to contact them. Include some information about their duties at work and how they would know about your situation.

Also, compile a diary or "paper trail" of events in chronological order. Keep copies of all documents related to your case. Create a list of the dates, places, and people you have talked to in the process of seeking a job, promotion, raise, or reasonable accommodation. Even your own notes or a memo following any conversation may be helpful.

To bolster your case, don't quit your job. If you must leave, look for other work. The courts are more likely to rule in your favor if you show that you are willing and able to work. Keep records of your blood glucose levels throughout your ordeal to show that you keep good blood glucose control and can do the job. Also see your doctor regularly. You may need your doctor's word that you are in good health and are doing a good job of controlling your diabetes.

You may also be able to get help dealing with your diabetes in the workplace under another federal law. The Family Medical Leave Act was passed in 1993 and allows you to take up to 12 weeks of unpaid leave each year to care for your own serious illness or to help ill family members. You can take leave under the act as a single 12-week stretch or in shorter intervals, such as 1 day off per week. If your company normally pays your health insurance, it must continue to do so while you are on leave.

In order to take advantage of this leave, you must work for a company that employs at least 50 people within 75 miles of the workplace. You must have been working with your employer for at least 1 year and put in at least 1,250 hours. In most cases, workers must request leave 30 days in advance. Some top-level executives may be ineligible for leave. This act allows you to take care of yourself, your spouse, parents, step- and foster parents, minor children, minor step- and foster children, and adult children who cannot take care of themselves. It will not cover leave to take care of unmarried partners, in-laws, siblings, grandchildren, or grandparents.

Discrimination in Schools and Day Care

It is not always easy to tell when an adult is being discriminated against. And if you have a child with diabetes who attends school or day care, it may be even more difficult. You are not there all day and you may not be aware of everything that goes on. Maybe your child is denied permission to go to the bathroom or isn't allowed to eat a morning snack. Maybe she isn't allowed to test her blood in the classroom or isn't allowed on a field trip. If you find that your child's needs are not being met, there may be a problem. Often schools and day care centers don't understand the needs of a child with diabetes. They are doing what seems to them to be appropriate and they don't even realize they are being discriminatory. It may be your job as a parent to first educate them about diabetes and your own child's needs. And you might inform them that some of their practices may, in fact, be illegal.

Two federal laws guarantee all students with disabilities a free and appropriate public education without discrimination. Section 504 of the Rehabilitation Act of 1973 prohibits discrimination against individuals with disabilities in any federally funded program. This includes the public school system. The Education for All Handicapped Children Act was passed in 1975. This law was amended in 1990 and given a new name:

the Individuals with Disability Education Act. This law guarantees "free appropriate public education, including special education and related service programming for all children with disabilities."

You probably don't think of your child as "handicapped" or "disabled." After all, you have probably been struggling to give your child a normal life and ensure that she fits in. However, any child with diabetes has special needs. Meeting those special needs—making sure your child eats on schedule, receives insulin when needed, and is able to test blood glucose levels regularly—is essential to leading a healthy and normal life. As long as your child can keep blood glucose levels in control, she can go about life just like any other kid. These laws ensure that your child is able to do this.

■ INDICATIONS

Your child's school should be taking steps to provide a learning environment that accommodates her needs. If your child's school is not accommodating these needs, then she might be being treated unfairly. For example, you might expect that your child should be able to:

- Eat whenever and wherever necessary. This could include keeping snacks or glucose tablets close at hand.

- Go to the bathroom or water fountain when necessary.

- Participate fully in all extracurricular activities, including sports or field trips.

- Refrain from physical activity when blood glucose levels are too high or too low.

- Eat lunch on schedule with enough time allotted to finish eating.

- Be absent more than the traditional limit.

- Be excused for tardiness in case of blood glucose problems.

- Ask for assistance with blood glucose monitoring or insulin injections, if needed.

If your school is neglecting to accommodate these or any other of your child's needs, then you may have a legitimate complaint. Also, if a school or day care refuses to admit your child and you suspect that it is because of diabetes, you may have a basis for complaint.

■ WHAT TO DO

The best way to deal with your child's diabetes in a school or day care setting is to head off any problems before they arise. The first step is to educate school personnel. If your child with diabetes is entering school or day care for the first time, starting at a new school, starting a new school year, or is newly diagnosed with diabetes during the current school year, you should first meet with school staff members who will affect your child's care.

Meet first with the school principal and ask him to explain how the school's policies would affect your child's need to test blood glucose, administer insulin or glucagon, or have a carbohydrate snack on hand for low blood glucose emergencies. Also find out what time your child would be eating meals, whether there is a designated snack time, whether there is a nurse on duty to handle any emergencies that may arise, whether the meals served at the school are suitable for a child with diabetes, whether there are any restrictions on your child's participation in school events or physical activities, and any other concerns you might have. If there are any problems with the school policies that might interfere with your child's well-being, raise them at this time and ask whether any accommodations can be made.

Also, ask to meet with your child's teachers. You should talk not only to your child's main classroom teacher, but also to any special activity teachers. It's especially important to meet with the physical education teacher. During your meetings with your child's teachers, make sure to tell them that your child has diabetes and explain how your child cares for it. Describe the basics of diabetes and what it means to live with it. You may even want to get a hold of pamphlets from the ADA to give your child's teachers. There is one called "Children with Diabetes: Information for Teachers and Child-Care Providers" on the ADA internet website you can print out. Use the search function to find the pamphlet. The ADA internet address is www.diabetes.org.

Make sure to tell your child's teacher that your child must eat mid-morning and mid-afternoon snacks, and tell the teacher what time those snacks need to be eaten. Make sure the teacher understands that these snacks are not optional. This could mean bringing snacks to assemblies or on field trips.

Find out what time your child will be eating lunch, so you can help figure out her insulin schedule. Whether your child has lunch at 11 a.m. or 1 p.m. could make a big difference. Also ask to be notified if there is any change in the scheduled lunchtime.

Talk to your child's teacher about what happens during an episode of hypoglycemia. Tell her what to look for in your own child. Ask her to ensure that your child be able to test her blood glucose level, whether your child does this independently or needs the assistance of a nurse or teacher. Find out whether your child will test for blood glucose in the classroom or nurse's office and make sure this is acceptable to you. Your child's teacher should understand what blood glucose levels are too low for your child and how hypoglycemia should be treated. Give the teacher a supply of fast-acting carbohydrate snacks to keep on hand for your child. You might also give the school nurse a similar supply. Make sure the teacher understands that if your child has an episode of hypoglycemia, under no circumstances should she be left alone. Even if your child is sent to the nurse's office, someone must go with your child. There is an instruction sheet called "Diabetes Care Guide" you can print out from the ADA internet website. Fill out the sheet for your child and give it to your child's teachers. The ADA internet address is www.diabetes.org.

Your child's teacher should also know what hyperglycemia is and how to be alert for signs of diabetic ketoacidosis. Make sure that your child's gym teacher understands that your child should not exercise with a blood glucose level of 240 mg/dl or higher. Your child may need more insulin with a blood glucose level in this range. Talk to your doctor about how to deal with this situation and make sure your child's teacher and gym teacher understand what to do. If your child has high blood glucose due to insufficient insulin and she exercises, her blood glucose level could rise even higher. Any time your child's blood glucose is this high, your child also needs to be tested for ketones and be alert for signs of diabetic ketoacidosis.

If possible, get yourself a pager. Make sure your child's teacher and the school nurse and/or administrator have your pager number. Have them send a page with your child's blood glucose level whenever it is out of the range of what you and your child's doctor think are acceptable. Also make sure that the school has your child's doctor's phone number and pager number.

Once you meet your child's teachers and school administrators and convey your child's needs, it is likely that the school will make an effort to accommodate your child. If the school receives federal funding as any public school and some private schools do, the next step is to document how the school will meet the needs of your child. The accommodation must be documented in either a Section 504 plan under the Rehabilitation Act of 1973 or in an Individualized Education Program (IEP) under the Individuals with Disabilities Education Act. If you develop an IEP, your child's school is eligible for federal funds to defray the cost of implementing the plan. If you develop a 504 plan, your school will not qualify for federal funds.

Make sure to talk to the members of your child's health care team in developing your child's school accommodation plan. This could include making sure that the school lunch program meets your child's nutritional needs, that your child be allowed to keep snacks close at hand, that your child be allowed to test blood glucose levels during the day, that your child be given adequate time to eat meals, and that your child not be excluded from activities. Make sure to think through what things are important to your child's well-being and include those in the plan. In developing this accommodation plan, you have the right to expect that reasonable accommodations be made. You will probably get more cooperation from the school officials if you show a willingness to understand their concerns and to negotiate an agreement both parties are happy with. Try to encourage the attitude that you are all members of the same team, not adversaries.

If, however, you do not feel that your child's needs are being met, you may be forced to take stronger action. Contact an attorney for help in deciding the best course of action. You can start by filing an administrative complaint with the Department of Education in your state. Do not delay in getting legal help. Administrative appeals and other actions need to be initiated right away or you lose the ability to use them. You may need to be prepared to take your case to court.

Discrimination in the Military

If you think dealing with problems in the workplace and schools is bad, try taking on the U.S. military. A few years ago, you couldn't enlist in the military if you had diabetes. You weren't even allowed to serve if your parents had diabetes. And if you developed diabetes while serving, you were immediately discharged.

Much of this has changed, although you are still not allowed to enlist in the military if you have diabetes. If you develop diabetes while serving, your fate is not so clear. The military will make a decision of whether to let you continue serving depending on whether you have type 1 or type 2 diabetes, whether you require insulin or other medications, and the nature of your service duties.

■ WHAT TO DO

The military reviews all medical conditions on a case-by-case basis. If you are diagnosed with diabetes while serving, your case will first be reviewed by a medical board. This board could consist of just one person—the doctor who diagnosed you. The board summarizes your condition and general state of health and assesses how well you control your diabetes and whether you have any complications. The board's findings are then referred to the Physical Evaluation Board (PEB). The PEB consists of a physician and two nonmedical officers. This board decides whether you can continue service based on what you do. This review can take weeks or even months. The PEB will declare you either fit or unfit to serve. If you are declared fit, you could return to your present duties or you could be reassigned. Either way, you will be given a profile that states you have diabetes and lists any restrictions you might have. For example, your profile might state that you cannot be assigned to areas that lack medical facilities. Your profile will also state that you need three meals each day. If you are declared unfit, you will be discharged. This decision can be appealed.

If you have type 2 diabetes and you are able to control your blood glucose levels through diet and exercise alone, the chances are quite high that you will be allowed to return to your unit as though nothing happened. If you require insulin or oral agents, your fate rests in the hands of the PEB. If you are diagnosed with type 1 diabetes, you could remain in the military, but you will probably be restricted from worldwide deployment or combat. If you have a duty that does not require you to be deployable, then you have a chance of remaining in that position. But if your job requires deployment, you could be discharged or face reassignment.

Problems with Health Insurance

If you have diabetes, you need health insurance. Medical costs are high for anyone these days, but if you have diabetes, the costs can be staggering. Getting good coverage is important not only for your family's pocketbook, but also for your health. Having adequate coverage will ensure that you receive the routine care you need now and will help prevent complications from crippling you and your pocketbook later. You also need insurance to help pay for any emergencies that may arise.

Unfortunately, health insurers also know that care for someone with diabetes can be expensive. If your insurance is covered by your employer or your spouse's employer, consider yourself lucky. If you have to pay for your own health care, you probably already know that it can expensive and difficult to obtain.

If you have diabetes, you have to give a lot of thought to switching jobs or retiring because of it. You have what insurers call a "preexisting condition." If you sign up for a new health plan, you may have to pay premiums for 6 months to years before receiving benefits because of your preexisting condition, or you may have to pay higher premiums. Some insurance companies may even refuse to insure you. So when making any life changes, be certain that your insurance needs are covered.

■ WHAT TO DO

In choosing a health care plan, you have several options.

Types of Policies

Your best bet if employed is to enroll in a group policy if offered by your employer. Group policies are usually offered to all employees regardless of their health. Under the Americans with Disabilities Act, employers who grant insurance to one employee must grant it to all employees. If your company employs less than 15 people, you may need to undergo a health screening and a medical history.

Some employers will pay the entire insurance premium. But most likely, you will have to pay a portion of that premium. Health care premiums are considered nontaxable. You can probably have your health insurance premiums deducted from your paycheck before taxes are withheld.

If you are changing jobs or leaving your parents' policy for the first time, you may need insurance to cover the period of transition, especially if your new employer has a preexisting condition clause. There is a federal law that can help you. Under the Consolidated Omnibus Budget Reconciliation Act (COBRA), your employer must allow you to keep your existing health insurance policy with equal coverage for up to 18 months after you leave your job. You will have to pay the entire premium and you may be charged up to 2 percent more than the rate the company charges your employer. Even still, this is almost always less expensive than paying for coverage on your own. If you are disabled, COBRA coverage can be extended to 29 months. Dependents can continue their coverage for up to 36 months. COBRA also covers spouses who become widowed or divorced. If you are a recent high school or college graduate and have not yet secured a job with your own insurance policy, you may be covered under this law. While searching for a new job, you will also be covered during any exclusion period imposed by your new insurance company if you have a preexisting condition. This could mean that you are paying double for a period of time, but it is still better than getting insurance on your own.

If you are laid off or leave a company, you have 60 days to accept COBRA benefits. During that time, employers must pay the insurance bills. However, if your company has less than 20 employees, or if you work for the federal government or some churches, you will not be covered under COBRA.

If your COBRA runs out, or if you don't qualify for COBRA, then you still have other options. Many states require employers to offer conversion insurance during the interim, regardless of your health or physical condition. However, 15 states and the District of Columbia do not require this. In most states, if an insurance company terminates a company's group plan, it is required to offer you a conversion policy as well. When you convert your policy, you remain with the same insurer, but begin paying for your own insurance. Conversion coverage is almost always less expensive than paying for insurance on your own. However, it can cost more than what you were paying while employed and may offer fewer benefits. Once your COBRA insurance runs out or you leave your job, you have 31 days to accept or reject this type of insurance. So make sure to explore all insurance options in advance, if possible.

Another option is to purchase temporary short-term health care coverage on your own. This is called a stop-gap policy and usually lasts for 1 year. It is designed to accommodate people in between jobs. Shop around to get the best coverage at the lowest price possible.

Alternatively, you can seek help through any professional or trade organizations you might belong to. Check with your professional organization to see what kinds of insurance they may offer.

Still another possibility is something called "pooled risk" health insurance. This kind of plan is offered by certain states to people who have lived in the state for 6 to 12 months and have been rejected for group or individual coverage. The coverage is usually good, but the costs can vary widely from state to state. Some states have waiting lists to buy into the pool. Contact your state's insurance commissioner or health department for information on your own state's policies.

As a last resort, you can seek individual coverage with Blue Cross and Blue Shield. They are known to insure anyone, regardless of health problems, especially people who live in states without pooled risk insurance. However, only a portion of these companies now hold open enrollment periods during which anyone may apply for coverage and many now exclude preexisting conditions, such as diabetes, for a year or more, just as other insurance companies do.

Types of Health Care

The two major types of health care plans offered by insurance companies today are fee-for-service and managed care. The difference in plans depends on what arrangements are made between the insurer and the doctors and hospitals as to how services will be provided. Many agreements limit your choice of doctors in exchange for more affordable premiums.

In the past, fee-for-service plans were the most common type of plan. They are set up so that you or your employer pays a set premium each year. You are then allowed to choose your own doctors and hospitals. The insurance company usually pays for some or all of your care. You must usually pay a small amount for your care as an out-of-pocket deductible. Once you have met your yearly deductible, your insurance kicks in to pay for your remaining expenses during the year, according to the particulars of your contract. You might also be required to pay a portion of the cost of each visit to your doctor. Most plans have a maximum out-of-pocket expense limit. Once you have paid that minimum, they will pay 100 percent of the additional expenses. When comparing plans, pay special attention to the cost of premiums, deductibles, co-payments, and out-of-pocket limits. Less expensive plans usually have higher deductibles and out-of-pocket limits.

The great advantages of fee-for-service plans are that you get to choose your own doctors and have greater leverage in choosing the course of your care. The main disadvantages are that these plans are more costly and do not always cover preventive health care such as mammograms, pap smears, or well-child visits.

Under managed care plans, you or your employer usually pays a fixed premium and you receive a comprehensive care package. This package includes routine visits, preventive care, and hospitalization. Often you are assigned a primary care practitioner you must see first. Your primary care practitioner will refer you to other professionals as required. You usually do not pay a deductible or any large out-of-pocket expenses.

The big disadvantage to managed care programs is that your choice of doctors and hospitals is often limited. Any tests or procedures must be approved by your insurer. If you need to see a specialist, this must also be approved, and you usually must see your primary care doctor first. This can make it more difficult to seek a second opinion.

Health Maintenance Organizations (HMOs) are the most common type of managed health care service. HMOs usually create a full-service health center by hiring or contracting with health care professionals. You must see someone under contract or employed by the HMO to receive prepaid health care. The HMO makes arrangements for coverage of sickness or accidents when you travel outside the area.

A preferred provider organization (PPO) is another type of managed care plan. With this type of service doctors make an arrangement with an insurer, such as Blue Cross and Blue Shield, to discount their fees. The doctors are then paid by the insurer. Under a PPO you will receive full coverage if you choose a doctor who is a preferred provider of the plan. You will usually visit doctors in their own private offices. If you choose someone outside of the plan, however, you may end up paying for most of the bill.

In choosing your insurance, you want to take into account the kinds of services you might need and the amount of coverage you expect your provider to cover. Here are some questions to ask when choosing an insurer or insurance plan:

- Are visits to my primary care physician covered?

- Is there a limit on how many visits are allowed?

- How much will I have to pay for each visit to my doctor?

- Does the plan cover visits to my diabetes educator?

- Does the plan cover visits to my dietitian?

- What mental health benefits are covered?

- What medications are covered?

- Is there a prescription plan to reduce costs? Is a co-payment required for each prescription?

- How often can prescriptions be refilled?

- Does the plan cover my diabetes supplies? Will it pay for my insulin and insulin supplies? An insulin pump? How about my monitor and test strips?

- Does the plan cover the other members of my health care team? My podiatrist? Eye doctor? Dentist?

- Can I make an appointment with my podiatrist, eye doctor, dentist, or other team member without first seeing my regular doctor?

- Which hospitals can I use?

- What kind of home health care coverage is included? Are there limitations?

- What happens if I am away from home and something happens?

In seeking out the answers to these questions, be persistent. Find out exactly which supplies are covered. Make a list of everything you typically need, including all supplies, medications, and equipment, and which doctors you visit or think you will need to visit. When you talk to your insurance representative, go down the list and get an answer for each specific question. Be a pest, if necessary, until you get all the answers you need.

Medicare and Medicaid

If you are over the age of 65, are disabled and unable to work, or have a very low income, you may have other insurance options. Medicare, a federal insurance program, covers part of the hospital bills, doctor fees, and other expenses for people over the age of 65 and for some people with disabilities who cannot work. However, if you are eligible for Medicare, you may still have to pay for a large portion of your medical bills. Many people buy policies called Medigap plans to pay for expenses not covered by Medicare. If you are considering one of these plans, be sure to read the policy carefully and compare prices before buying anything.

You can sign up for Medicare 3 months before the month of your 65th birthday. For more information on Medicare, call your local Social Security Administration office, listed under the U.S. Government listings in your telephone book. When you apply, you will need your birth certificate. Not everyone over the age of 65 is eligible for Medicare. For example, some people who have worked at state or local government jobs may not be eligible for Medicare. If you are not sure about your coverage, contact your local Social Security Administration office.

Here are some of the things that Medicare covers.

- Medicare pays 80 percent of the cost of blood glucose meters for people who are prescribed insulin. It also pays the same amount toward lancets, strips, and other supplies used with the meter. It will only pay for test strips if you are using a meter. You must have a written prescription for all of these items, even if they are purchased over the counter, in order to get reimbursed. You will also need a written statement from your doctor that details your diagnosis, fluctuations in your blood glucose levels, and your recommended self-monitoring schedule. Make copies of these written statements. Give a copy to your pharmacist to be submitted with your Medicare claim each time you buy supplies.

- In some states, Medicare pays for diabetes outpatient education. Certain criteria are usually required. For example, the program may need to be conducted in a hospital, the curriculum approved by Medicare, and the education considered to be a medical necessity. Your doctor may have to write a "prescription" for your education.

- Medicare will not pay for routine foot care.

- Medicare will help pay for laser treatment for retinopathy and for cataract surgery and for kidney dialysis and transplants.

- Medicare does not cover the cost of diabetes pills, insulin, syringes, or insulin pumps.

- Medicare may pay for outpatient nutrition counseling or dietitian services.

- Medicare does not pay for regular eye exams or for prescription eyeglasses or contact lenses.

If you have a very low income, you might be eligible for Medicaid. This is a federal and state assistance program. Requirements of Medicaid eligibility can vary from state to state. Contact the Medicaid office in your state to find out whether you qualify. Also ask about what health expenses will be covered. If you have questions, a social worker can help you with this.

Chapter 21
Solving Other
Medical Problems

Managing your diabetes can be a challenge in itself. Sometimes it may seem that your whole life revolves around your diabetes care plan. Even if you have gotten things well under control, other problems completely unrelated to diabetes are likely to come up. When you are dealing with diabetes day in and day out, you may forget that you can still catch a cold or the flu, require hospitalization or surgery, or deal with other conditions such as allergies, asthma, or arthritis, just like anyone else. But as a person with diabetes, other conditions may affect you differently. It's bad enough that you can barely breathe or get out of bed because of the flu. But being sick can also throw your blood glucose levels out of whack. The important thing is to be prepared and know in advance how to handle these adversities when they arise.

Handling Sick Days

Any kind of illness or infection stresses your body. This includes the sort of respiratory infection that gives you a cold and the viruses that cause the flu. When you are sick, whether it is a head cold, the flu, or a stomach virus, your body is stressed. Your body reacts to stress by releasing a cocktail of hormones that helps you fight disease. These so-called stress hormones, such as cortisol and glucagon, cause the liver to release glucose and inhibit the effect of insulin. The net result is that blood glucose levels rise. If not taken care of, these high blood glucose levels can lead to life-threatening situations, such as diabetic ketoacidosis and hyperglycemic hyperosmolar state. An important aspect of handling sick days is to plan ahead and keep a close watch on your blood glucose levels.

■ SYMPTOMS

If you have a common cold caused by a respiratory virus, it usually runs its course in 4 to 10 days, but sometimes a bacterial infection can set in. The flu is a different illness than the common cold and is caused by a different virus. However, some of the symptoms are similar, and sometimes one infection can follow another. The flu usually lasts 2 or 3 days, although bronchitis can develop and persist for weeks. A viral infection of the stomach that causes the stomach flu usually lasts 24 to 48 hours.

■ WHAT TO DO

If you are feeling under the weather because of a cold, flu, or stomach virus, make sure to keep close tabs on your blood glucose levels. Monitor your blood glucose levels at least every 3 to 4 hours. Also test your urine for ketones at the same time. (See Chapter 1 for more information on monitoring blood glucose and ketones.) If your levels are too high or if you are pregnant, you should monitor more often. You may need to take an extra dose of insulin if your blood glucose level climbs too high. You should talk to your doctor in advance about what levels are too high for you and how much extra insulin you should take. In general, anything over 250 mg/dl or any sign of moderate to high levels of ketones in your urine needs to be treated.

If you are sick, never skip an insulin dose. Always take your normal dose of insulin, even if you can't eat. If you take oral agents to control your blood glucose, take your medication. Your doctor may even suggest taking an extra dose of insulin when you are sick, whether you normally take insulin or an oral diabetes medication. Talk to your doctor in advance about whether you need to take extra insulin when you are sick, and how much you should take.

If you are feeling nauseous and are vomiting, or even if you just don't feel like eating, you may have to replace your normal meal plan with a sick-day plan. Talk to your doctor or dietitian about what foods you should eat when you are sick, and when you should eat them. Rice, soup, crackers, or frozen fruit juice bars are good choices. Try to keep these on hand when the cold and flu season starts. Also drink plenty of fluids, but try to avoid caffeine. If you are vomiting or have a fever or diarrhea, you could be losing fluid and are at risk of dehydration. If this is the case, you may need to drink nondiet soft drinks or sports drinks that contain sugar and carbohydrate. This can help prevent the hypo-glycemia that can occur when you are not eating enough or if you are taking extra insulin. If your vomiting is severe, try drinking 3 to 6 ounces every hour in small sips. This will help to keep your blood glucose levels stable.

Keep a fever thermometer on hand and keep tabs on your tempera-ture. Call your doctor if your fever rises above 103 °F. Ask your doctor in advance what cold medicines are safe to take. Many over-the-counter medicines should not be taken if you have diabetes. For example, decongestants contain ingredients that raise blood glucose levels, inter-act with oral agents, and raise blood pressure. Pseudoephedrine, phenylpropanolamine, and phenylephrine are examples of deconges-tants that can affect blood glucose levels. Ask your doctor for other drugs to watch out for. Don't take any over-the-counter or prescription medication without first talking to your diabetes care doctor.

In addition to the medicines or "active ingredients" found in many cold remedies, you also have to look out for the "inactive ingredients." These are additives that affect the color, taste, or consistency. Read the label and be on the lookout for added sugar or alcohol. A small amount of sugar is probably okay, as long as you are aware you are taking it. However, if you are taking many doses or large doses of a particular medication with sugar, you might be better off looking for a sugar-free version. Alcohol is also added to many medicines, especially nighttime cold remedies, such as Nyquil. Alcohol can lower blood glucose levels. So if you do take medicine that contains alcohol, make sure to also eat something first.

Pain medications such as aspirin and acetaminophen (Tylenol) are also usually safe in small doses. Many doctors, in fact, prescribe low doses of aspirin on a daily basis to guard against cardiovascular disease. This is safe if you have diabetes. However, ibuprofen is not safe for any-one with kidney disease. It can cause acute renal failure for anyone with kidney problems. If you have diabetes, do not take ibuprofen without first talking it over with your doctor.

If you are sick, you probably feel awful. It is hard to know when you are feeling bad because of your cold, or whether there is a problem with your diabetes or blood glucose control. You should call your doctor if you experience any of the following conditions:

- You have been sick for 1 or 2 days without any improvement.

- You have had vomiting or diarrhea for more than 6 hours.

- You have moderate to large amounts of ketones in your urine.

- You are taking insulin and your blood glucose levels continue to be above 250 mg/dl, even though you have taken two or three supplemental doses of regular insulin. Discuss in advance with your doctor just how much extra insulin you need to take on sick days.

- You are taking insulin and your blood glucose level is under 60 mg/dl.

- You are controlling your type 2 diabetes with oral agents and your blood glucose levels are above 250 mg/dl for more than 24 hours.

- You have any signs of severe hyperglycemia (very dry mouth, fruity odor on your breath, dehydration, confusion, or disorientation).

- You are sleepier than usual.

- You have any stomach pain, chest pain, or difficulty breathing.

- You have any doubts or questions about what you should be doing for your illness.

When you call, your doctor will need some information. As difficult as it may be to take records when you are feeling sick, any notes you might take can make it easier for her to figure out whether there is a serious problem. Your doctor will want to know when you first started feeling ill and what your symptoms have been. Share any records of blood glucose tests or ketone testing. Also make note of any insulin doses or diabetes medications you have taken and when you took them, as well as any other medications you have taken. Your doctor will also want to know what your temperature is, whether you can take fluids and foods, and whether you have lost weight. Make sure to have your pharmacist's phone number on hand, if possible.

Hospitalization

Let's face it. Almost no one looks forward to a stay in a hospital. But there may come a time, whether you have scheduled minor elective surgery or are in the throes of an emergency, when you need to check into a hospital. You may be nervous about this and not like the feeling that you have no control. You are out of your normal routine and may worry about how long you will be there, how quickly you will recover, and whether or not your diabetes will be adequately cared for.

Even though you are not sick now and don't plan to be anytime soon, anything could happen at any time. The best time to plan your hospital stay is before you even have the need. Taking the time now to think about your hospital stay will go a long way in making sure you get the best care possible.

■ WHAT TO DO

The first thing to do is to choose a hospital. You can't always choose a hospital in an emergency situation. It is best to do the legwork now, not when you have other things on your mind. Start by finding out where your doctor has privileges. Ask your doctor if she has a preference or would recommend one hospital over the other. One hospital may be more experienced in dealing with people with diabetes, for example, or may be better equipped to handle emergencies. Ask your doctor where she would send a family member.

Depending on where you live, your choices may be restricted. You may live in an urban area with dozens of hospitals nearby, or there could only be one hospital within an hour's drive. If you do have a choice, consider what kind of hospitals are available. In general, three kinds of hospitals are available: city or county hospitals, private community hospitals, and hospitals that serve as teaching centers, often affiliated with a medical school. Sometimes there is overlap. A county or city hospital could be affiliated with a medical school.

If your doctor strongly recommends a particular hospital, that may be enough to help you decide. But you can also seek other opinions. Ask your friends, neighbors, or relatives who have had recent hospitalizations about their experiences. Check with your local ADA office or diabetes support group to find out more about your local hospital's reputation. Also ask your health insurance provider which hospital services they will cover and whether there is any restriction on the choice of hospital. Many insurance companies require that you let them know in advance of any scheduled inpatient or outpatient hospital visit. Often, you must be precertified in order to have the services covered, unless there is an emergency situation.

When choosing a hospital, find out if there are any endocrinologists on staff. Endocrinologists specialize in hormonal disorders and are experienced with treating diabetes. Find out whether the hospital has diabetes educators or dietitians on staff who have experience working with people with diabetes and whether they are available to both inpatients and outpatients. Also find out whether the hospital sponsors any diabetes education programs, support groups, or other types of support services.

Once you are in the hospital, it is important to communicate your needs as a person with diabetes to both admitting personnel and clinical staff. If you are not in any condition to communicate directly, make sure that a family member or friend can speak up for you. Make sure that the doctors and nurses taking care of you know that you have diabetes. Tell them what medications you are currently taking. Write a list ahead of time that includes all your medications, how often you take them, and in what doses. If you have any other conditions, such as allergies or complications of diabetes, be sure to tell your attending staff. If you have high blood pressure, you may require special treatment before surgery, for example. If you take any heart medications, these may need to be adjusted. If you are prone to hypoglycemia, make sure to let them know. If possible, bring your blood glucose monitoring records with you. Also tell them about your meal plan. Ask to meet with the hospital dietitian and discuss your particular dietary needs.

With enough advance planning that allows you to investigate your hospital and provide them with enough information about you and your diabetes care plan, you can ensure that your hospital stay goes as smoothly as possible.

Surgery and Anesthesia

The thought of surgery can make you nervous. Even the most routine outpatient surgical procedures are not without their risks. If you have diabetes, you can expect to recover as well as anyone without diabetes. However, you may find that maintaining blood glucose control during and immediately after surgery can be tricky. That's because surgery imposes a major stress on your body. And the way your body reacts to stress is to secrete hormones that trigger the release of glucose into the bloodstream and inhibit the effects of insulin. The net result is that blood glucose levels can rise. It is important that your medical staff takes steps to keep your blood glucose levels under control to avoid any complications. You can help the process by maintaining good blood glucose control before your surgery.

Unless you are having emergency surgery, the first question to ask is whether you really need it. If you doctor recommends surgery, make sure to take the time to discuss your options with her. Ask your doctor whether there are any alternatives and what will happen if you elect not to be operated on. Also discuss the risks involved. No surgical procedure is without risk. Ask what tests and other procedures you might be expected to go through in conjunction with the surgery. Also find out whether you will be under the care of your primary care physician in the hospital or whether you will be seen by a doctor on staff at the hospital. If you will see other doctors, do they specialize in diabetes? Make sure to get all your questions answered before agreeing to any elective surgery.

Of course, if after discussing your surgery with your doctor, you are still unsure or have reservations, feel free to seek a second opinion. Anytime a doctor recommends surgery, a long-term medication, or other treatments that may affect your lifestyle, it is a good idea to think about getting a second opinion. You may also want a second opinion if your doctor tells you that your condition is incurable or there is no therapy that can help you.

If you are considering surgery, ask your insurance company if they will pay for the procedure that is being recommended. Also ask if they will pay for a second opinion. Some insurance companies will require a second opinion before they will fully cover any surgery. And some insurers will reimburse you for the expense of seeking a second opinion. Also ask the insurance company if they will only pay for a second opinion if you see one of the doctors they recommend.

It is not always easy to figure out who to ask for a second opinion. Don't ask your doctor whether you need a second opinion. But if you have reservations, tell your doctor you would like a second opinion. Ask your doctor or another doctor you trust to recommend someone with whom you can consult. Look for a doctor who is board-certified in the field in which you are seeking information. For example, if you are considering heart surgery, find someone who is board-certified in cardiology or surgery. The person answering the phone will be able to tell you if the doctor is board-certified. Make sure that the physician with whom you are consulting knows that you have diabetes.

If your problem is related to diabetes, call your local ADA office for the names of specialists in your area. The ADA may also be able to recommend doctors for problems unrelated to diabetes. Or you can try calling the appropriate department of a nearby major medical center or teaching hospital. Ask for the names of specialists in the field. Also ask your friends and neighbors for recommendations.

When you seek a second opinion, here are some things you might want to ask.

- What is the diagnosis and how was it determined?

- Which treatments are available? Which treatments are most common? Most successful?

- Do you recommend this particular treatment for me? Why?

- What are the potential risks, side effects, and complications of the treatment and how likely are they?

- Is the treatment reversible?

- How will the treatment affect my diabetes control?

- How long will I have to be in the hospital? When can I expect a complete recovery?

- Will I need follow-up care?

- Are there hidden costs? Will I have to undergo repeated blood tests, physical therapy, or nursing care?

- Is this treatment experimental? Will I be participating in research?

- Would you recommend this treatment for a member of your family?

Once you decide on surgery or a particular treatment, and if time allows, try to work with members of your health care team to achieve good blood glucose control. The better your general state of health, the better your chances of withstanding the stress of surgery. This will help reduce the chance of developing infection and will help speed your recovery.

However, if you are brought into the hospital for emergency surgery, or if your blood glucose levels are not well controlled, don't panic. The medical staff will take great care in keeping your blood glucose levels within an acceptable range for surgery. This may be done through intravenous insulin and a glucose drip that will be monitored throughout surgery.

If you routinely keep your blood glucose levels under good control, your doctor will probably not recommend any changes in your diabetes care routine before you enter the hospital. However, you can expect that once you enter the hospital, the staff will keep close tabs on it. Don't be surprised if your blood glucose levels swing once you have been admitted. This can occur as a result of the stress or anxiety in anticipation of surgery, your medical condition that is making the surgery necessary, and the changes in your eating and exercise routine that occur when you check into the hospital. Don't be surprised if you are put on insulin, even if you are used to controlling your diabetes through diet and exercise alone or with the help of oral agents. It is usually a temporary measure and once you recover, you will probably resume your normal routine.

If you are given insulin, you may be prescribed several injectable doses each day. If you are already using insulin, don't be surprised if your dose is increased. Some doctors may prefer to give you a continuous infusion of insulin intravenously. You will probably also be given glucose intravenously. This allows your medical staff to keep your blood glucose levels stable by checking them frequently and making adjustments in insulin and glucose infusion rates.

Don't panic if your blood glucose levels are kept higher than what you are used to. This may be done deliberately to avoid the risk of hypoglycemia. Most doctors think that keeping them a little higher than normal is preferable, as long as they don't go over 200 mg/dl. However, if you feel any symptoms of hyperglycemia or hypoglycemia, make sure to tell your nurse or doctor right away.

Before any scheduled surgery, you should expect to meet with your surgeon at least once before your operation. The surgeon should explain the surgery and what you should expect afterwards. If possible, keep a list of questions to ask the surgeon beforehand. Nurses will also be on hand to answer questions you may have.

The anesthesiologist will also visit you to tell you what you should expect. During any kind of surgery, you will be given anesthesia, or a pain killer, so that you don't feel the pain. Your anesthesiologist is a doctor who specializes in administering anesthesia. Under certain circumstances, you may have choices in anesthesia, and these should be explained to you. For most major operations, and many minor ones, you will be given a general anesthesia. This means you will be asleep during the entire procedure. Many general anesthetics, however, can cause blood glucose levels to rise. You will be given an anesthetic that will be less likely to disrupt your metabolism and blood glucose control. Many physicians prefer a local anesthetic for surgery, but this depends on the type of surgery you are having done. Epidurals, spinal taps, and other locally administered anesthetics are less likely to cause hyperglycemia. Many doctors also prefer dealing with a patient who is awake, because there is a greater chance that you will notice any symptoms of hyperglycemia or hypoglycemia should they occur. Don't be afraid to ask your anesthesiologist questions about what to expect during surgery and about how the anesthesia will affect your blood glucose levels.

After surgery, you may be switched from intravenous insulin to subcutaneous insulin. Depending on the operation, you may be able to eat right away. In some cases, you may not be able to eat for several days. You may require intravenous feeding and will be given a continuous infusion of glucose. Your blood glucose levels should be monitored frequently. It is important to keep tight control of your blood glucose levels during this period to avoid the possibility of infection and other complications.

Accidents and Emergencies

If you are faced with a medical emergency or are a victim of an accident, you don't have the luxury of advance preparation. Depending on the extent of your injuries, you may require major surgery or a relatively noninvasive hospital stay to ensure that you are stable.

■ WHAT TO DO

If you are involved in an accident or other emergency situation, you will probably not have any choice in hospitals. You will be taken to the nearest hospital that can provide the care you need. If you are conscious, make sure to tell the attending medical personnel that you have diabetes. That may influence their decision about where to take you. Make sure to always wear some sort of jewelry that identifies you as a person with diabetes, in case you are not conscious. If you do have a preference of hospitals, tell those in attendance in the event that they can take you there. Also make sure that those close to you know to tell anyone about your diabetes, should an emergency situation arise.

If you have been in an accident, it is very likely that your blood glucose levels will swing widely. Even a relatively minor accident can stress the body. As long as your medical personnel are aware that you have diabetes, they will make every attempt to bring your blood glucose levels under control.

The combination of trauma and any other emergency procedures will most likely cause your blood glucose levels to rise. Don't panic. You will probably be given intravenous insulin and glucose and your blood glucose levels will be monitored frequently. If you are able, any information that you can give your medical personnel about your diabetes care, insulin or medication schedule, or how you control your blood glucose will help them better attend to your situation. Also tell them if you have any diabetes complications, such as heart disease, kidney disease, or neuropathy. Once in a hospital setting, the staff can keep close tabs on your blood glucose levels as they tend to your injuries.

Of course, the better your general state of health and the better your blood glucose control, the better your chances of surviving any accident or medical emergency. In addition to wearing a medical ID tag, consider keeping information on your diabetes care and important aspects of your medical history, including any medications you currently take, on hand at all times. Any information you can provide in an emergency setting will help the medical staff attend to your needs.

Arthritis

There are several types of arthritis. If you have arthritis, it won't directly affect your diabetes. However, many of the medications you may take for arthritis can affect blood glucose control. And arthritis can make it more difficult to do the things you need to do to give yourself good diabetes care.

The three most common types of arthritis are degenerative joint disease, rheumatoid arthritis, and gout. Degenerative joint disease is the most common type of arthritis. It results from wear and tear on your joints. This can lead to stiffness and pain. Rheumatoid arthritis is an autoimmune disease thought to be caused by an immune system attack on the tissues of the joints. It is marked by red, swollen, and extremely painful joints. Gout is a somewhat rare, painful condition that occurs more often in people with diabetes than in the general population. It is caused by crystals of uric acid that collect in the joints. High blood pressure medications and eating animal organs such as kidney and liver can also contribute to gout. Avoiding these and other foods can diminish the symptoms of gout.

■ WHAT TO DO

If you have arthritis, ask your doctor about what medications can affect your blood glucose control. Large doses of aspirin (12 tablets daily), which are frequently taken to relieve symptoms of arthritis, lower blood glucose levels and make you more prone to hypoglycemia. Phenacetin and nonsteroidal anti-inflammatory drugs can harm the kidneys. If you have a history of kidney disease, do not take any arthritis medication without first checking with your doctor. Make sure you tell any arthritis specialist you see that you have diabetes. And make sure any arthritis medication you take has the approval of your diabetes care doctor.

If you have arthritis, you may also have mobility problems. You have probably been told to exercise to control your diabetes, but this can be hard if you have arthritis. Depending on the extent to which you are affected, you may be able to find some exercises to do that will not damage your joints. Swimming, for example, is an excellent choice. Many health clubs or the YMCA offer aquatics classes or water therapy sessions specifically designed for people with arthritis or mobility problems. Consider becoming involved with something like this. It could go a long way toward controlling your diabetes and also providing therapy to relieve the symptoms of arthritis.

Arthritis can also make it more difficult to take care of your diabetes. If your joints are severely affected, even testing your blood glucose or injecting insulin can become a major challenge. If this is the case, try to solicit help from a family member or friend. Talk to your doctor or diabetes educator about particular products that may be easier to use for a person with arthritis. For example, you may find it more convenient to use an insulin pump than to deal with insulin syringes. An automatic lancing device can make blood testing easier than pricking your finger manually. Make sure your doctor and other members of your health care team understand your limitations so they can help you make the adjustments you need.

Taking Non-Diabetes Medications

Other medical conditions, such as asthma and allergies, do not necessarily affect diabetes directly. However, whenever you suffer from any other disease or condition, and take medication either on an occasional or regular basis, check with your doctor to see how it might affect your blood glucose control. For example, corticosteroids used to treat asthma, allergies, and some joint disorders can raise blood glucose levels. However, do not under any circumstances discontinue any medication out of concern for your blood glucose level without first checking with your doctor. In some cases, discontinuing certain medications can be life-threatening. Do not start or stop taking any drug without your doctor's approval. You may need to consult with both your diabetes care doctor and the doctor who is treating your other conditions. Also, check with your doctor before taking any over-the-counter medications.

Glossary

autoimmunity . . . . a condition in which the body's own immune system attacks cells of the body. This is the basis of type 1 diabetes, in which the immune system attacks the beta-cells of the pancreas, and insulin is no longer produced.

basal insulin . . . . intermediate- or long-acting insulin that is absorbed slowly and gives the body a steady low level of insulin. This mimics the body's natural low-level steady background release of insulin. Also used to describe the low-level steady background release of fast-acting insulin by an insulin pump.

beta-cells . . . . cells that make insulin. These cells are found in the islets of Langerhans in the pancreas.

blood glucose meter . . . . a hand-held instrument that tests the level of glucose in the blood. A drop of blood (obtained by pricking a finger) is placed on a small strip that is inserted in the meter. The meter calculates and displays the blood glucose level.

bolus insulin . . . . fast-acting insulin injected before meals that gives the body a quick rise in insulin levels. This mimics the body's natural after-meal release of insulin that stops the rise in blood glucose. Also used to describe the before-meal insulin dose given with an insulin pump.

calories . . . . units that represent the amount of energy provided by food. Carbohydrate, protein, and fat are the primary sources of calories in the diet, but alcohol also contains calories. If all calories consumed aren't used as energy, they may be stored as fat.

carbohydrate . . . . one of three major sources of calories in the diet. Carbohydrate comes primarily from sugar (simple carbohydrate) and starch (complex carbohydrate, found in bread, pasta, and beans). Carbohydrate is broken down into glucose during digestion and is the main nutrient that raises blood glucose levels.

cholesterol . . . . a waxy, fat-like substance used by the body to build cell walls and make certain vitamins and hormones. The liver produces enough cholesterol for the body, but we also get cholesterol when we eat animal products. Eating too much cholesterol and saturated fat can cause the blood cholesterol to rise and accumulate along the inside walls of blood vessels. This is a risk factor for heart attack and stroke.

DCCT . . . . the Diabetes Control and Complications Trial. This was a 10-year study sponsored by the National Institutes of Health. More than 1,400 people with type 1 diabetes were divided into two groups: those who aimed for near-normal blood glucose levels and those with standard goals. The study showed that tight blood glucose control reduces the risk of diabetic complications.

diabetes . . . . a disease in which the body cannot produce insulin or cannot use insulin properly. It is characterized by high blood glucose levels.

endocrinology . . . . the study of hormones at work in the body. Because insulin is a hormone, diabetes is a disease of the endocrine system. Many "diabetes doctors" are endocrinologists.

exchanges . . . . the food lists used in the American Diabetes Association, the American Dietetic Association *Exchange Lists for Meal Planning*. There are seven basic food groups: Starch, Other Carbohydrates, Meat and Meat Substitutes, Vegetables, Fruits, Milk, and Fat. Any food in a given list can be exchanged for any other food in that list in the appropriate amount.

fats . . . . the most concentrated source of calories in the diet. Saturated fats are found primarily in animal products. Unsaturated fats mainly come from plants and can be monounsaturated (olive or canola oil) or polyunsaturated (corn or other oils). Excess intake of fat, especially saturated fat, can cause elevated blood cholesterol, increasing the risk of heart disease and stroke.

fiber . . . . the parts of plants that the body can't digest, such as fruit and vegetable skins. Fiber aids in the normal functioning of the digestive system, specifically the intestinal tract.

gestational diabetes . . . . diabetes that develops during pregnancy. The mother's blood glucose rises in response to hormones secreted during pregnancy, and the mother cannot produce enough insulin to handle the higher blood glucose levels. Although gestational diabetes usually goes away after pregnancy, about 60 percent of women who have had gestational diabetes eventually develop type 2 diabetes.

glucagon . . . . a hormone produced by the pancreas that raises blood glucose levels. An injectable preparation is available by prescription for use in treating severe insulin reactions.

glucose . . . . a simple form of sugar that serves as the body's fuel. It is produced when foods are broken down in the digestive system. Glucose is carried by the blood to cells. The amount of glucose in the blood is known as the blood glucose level.

**glycohemoglobin or
glycated hemoglobin** . . . . describes the attachment of glucose to red blood cells. When blood glucose levels are high, the percentage of glucose attached to red blood cells increases. Doctors take blood samples to evaluate average blood glucose control over the past 3 to 4 months. One such test measures HbA_{1c}.

health care team . . . . the group of health care professionals who help patients manage diabetes. This team may include a physician, registered dietitian, and certified diabetes educator. (A certified diabetes educator can also be a physician, registered nurse, or registered dietitian.) Ophthalmologists, podiatrists, exercise physiologists, mental health professionals, and other specialists can also be part of the team and may also be certified diabetes educators.

heart disease . . . . a condition in which the heart cannot efficiently pump blood. Coronary artery disease is the most common form of heart disease. It occurs when the arteries that nourish the heart muscle narrow or become blocked. People with diabetes have a higher risk than the general population for developing heart disease.

hyperglycemia . . . . a condition in which blood glucose levels are too high (generally, 200 mg/dl or above). Symptoms include frequent urination, increased thirst, and weight loss.

hypoglycemia . . . . (or insulin reaction) a condition in which blood glucose levels drop too low (generally, below 60 mg/dl). Symptoms include moodiness, numbness in the arms and hands, confusion, and shakiness or dizziness. When left untreated, this condition can become severe and lead to unconsciousness.

immunosuppression . . . . suppression of the immune system. People who receive kidney and pancreas transplants take immunosuppressive drugs to prevent the immune system from attacking the new organ.

impaired glucose tolerance . . . . a condition diagnosed when oral glucose tolerance test results show that a person's blood glucose level falls between normal and diabetic levels. It isn't considered a form of diabetes, but people with this condition are at an increased risk for developing diabetes.

insulin . . . . a hormone produced by the pancreas that helps the body use glucose. It is the "key" that unlocks the "doors" to cells and allows glucose to enter. The glucose then fuels the cells.

insulin resistance . . . . a condition in which the body does not respond to insulin properly. This is the most common cause of type 2 diabetes.

intensive diabetes management . . . . a way of treating a person with diabetes who has the goal of achieving near-normal blood glucose levels. The approach involves using all available resources, including multiple daily injections of insulin, frequent blood glucose monitoring, exercise, and diet.

**ketoacidosis or
diabetic coma** . . . . a severe condition caused by a lack of insulin or an elevation in stress hormones. It is marked by high blood glucose levels and ketones in the urine, and it occurs almost exclusively in those with type 1 diabetes.

ketones . . . . acids produced when the body breaks down fat for fuel. This occurs when there is not enough insulin to permit glucose to enter the cells and fuel them or when there are too many stress hormones.

metabolism . . . . describes the body's capture and use of energy to sustain life. Diabetes is a metabolic disease because it affects the body's ability to capture glucose from food for use by the cells.

mg/dl . . . . milligrams per deciliter. This is the unit of measure used when referring to blood glucose levels.

nephropathy . . . . kidney damage. This condition can be life-threatening. When kidneys fail to function, dialysis (filtering blood through a machine) or kidney transplantation becomes necessary.

neuropathy . . . . damage to the nerves. Peripheral neuropathy, which affects the nerves outside the brain and spinal cord, is the most common form of neuropathy. Peripheral neuropathy can damage motor nerves (which affect voluntary movement, such as walking) sensory nerves (which affect touch and feeling), and autonomic nerves (which affect bodily functions such as digestion).

obesity . . . . an abnormal and excessive amount of body fat. Obesity is a chronic illness. It is on the rise and is a risk factor for type 2 diabetes.

oral diabetes medications or oral hypoglycemic medications . . . . medications taken orally that are designed to lower blood glucose levels. They are used by some people with type 2 diabetes and are not to be confused with insulin.

pancreas . . . . a comma-shaped gland located just behind the stomach. It produces enzymes for digesting food and hormones that regulate the use of fuel in the body, including insulin and glucagon. In a fully functioning pancreas, insulin is released through special cells located in clusters called islets of Langerhans.

protein . . . . one of three major sources of calories in the diet. Protein provides the body with material for building blood cells, body tissue, hormones, muscle, and other important substances. It is found in meats, eggs, milk, and certain vegetables and starches.

retinopathy . . . . damage to small blood vessels in the eye that can lead to vision problems. In nonproliferative retinopathy, the blood vessels bulge and leak fluids into the retina and may cause blurred vision. Proliferative retinopathy is more serious and can cause vision loss. In this condition, new blood vessels form in the retina and branch out to other areas of the eye. This can cause blood to leak into the clear fluid inside the eye and can also cause the retina to detach.

receptors . . . . molecules that often sit on cell surfaces and play a role in chemical "communication." For example, insulin cannot allow glucose to enter cells unless it first binds to the receptors on the cells and they respond properly.

stress hormones or
counterregulatory
hormones . . . . hormones released during stressful situations. These hormones include glucagon, epinephrine (adrenaline), norepinephrine, cortisol, and growth hormone. They cause the liver to release glucose and the cells to release fatty acids for extra energy. If there's not enough insulin present in the body, these extra fuels can lead to hyperglycemia and ketoacidosis.

sugar . . . . a simple carbohydrate that provides calories and raises blood glucose levels. There are a variety of sugars, such as white, brown, confectioner's invert, and raw. Fructose, lactose, sucrose, maltose, dextrose, glucose, honey, corn syrup, molasses, and sorghum are also sugars.

sugar substitutes . . . . sweeteners used in place of sugar. Note that some sugar substitutes have calories and will affect blood glucose levels, such as fructose (a sugar, but often used in "sugar-free" products), and sugar alcohols, such as sorbitol and mannitol. Others have very few calories and will not affect blood glucose levels, such as saccharin, acesulfame K, and aspartame (NutraSweet).

triglycerides . . . . simple fatty acids found in both plants and animals. Vegetable oils contain triglycerides with unsaturated fatty acids and tend to be liquid at room temperature, whereas animal sources of triglycerides contain mostly saturated fatty acids and tend to be solid at room temperature.

type 1 diabetes . . . . (or immune-mediated diabetes). A form of diabetes that tends to develop before age 30 but may occur at any age. It's usually caused when the immune system attacks the beta-cells of the pancreas and the pancreas can no longer produce insulin. People who have type 1 diabetes must take insulin to survive.

type 2 diabetes . . . . (or insulin-resistant diabetes). This form of diabetes usually occurs in people over the age of 40, but may develop in younger people, especially minorities. Almost all people who develop type 2 diabetes are insulin resistant, and most have a problem with insulin secretion. Some simply cannot produce enough insulin to meet their bodies' needs, and others have a combination of these problems. Many people with type 2 diabetes control the disease through diet and exercise, but some must also take oral medications or insulin.

urine tests . . . . tests that measure substances in the urine. Urine tests for blood glucose levels do not provide the timely information that is important in blood glucose control. Urine tests for ketones are very useful for monitoring diabetes control and are important in preventing or detecting ketoacidosis.

Resources

For the Visually Challenged

American Council of the Blind
1155 15th Street, NW, Suite 720
Washington, DC 20005
(202) 467-5081
(800) 424-8666
(202) 331-1058
e-mail: ncrabb@acb.org
website: http://www.acb.org
National information clearing-house and legislative advocate that publishes a monthly magazine in Braille, large print, cassette versions, and computer disk.

American Foundation for the Blind
11 Penn Plaza, Suite 300
New York, NY 10001
(212) 502-7600
(800) 232-5463
e-mail: asbinfo@asb.org
internet: gopher.asb.org_5005
Works to establish, develop, and provide services and programs that assist visually challenged people in achieving independence.

American Printing House for the Blind
1839 Frankfort Avenue
PO Box 6085
Louisville, KY 40206
(502) 895-2405
(800) 223-1839
(502) 899-2274 (fax)
Concerned with the publication of literature in all media (Braille, large type, recorded) and manufacture of educational aids. Newsletter provides information on new products.

Division for the Blind and Visually Impaired
Rehabilitation Service Administration
U.S. Department of Education
Room 3229, Mary Switzer Building
330 C Street, SW
Washington, DC 20202
(202) 205-9309
Provides rehabilitation services, through agencies in each state, to

those who have become visually impaired who wish to maintain their employment or train for new employment.

National Association for Visually Handicapped (NAVH)
22 West 21st Street
New York, NY 10010
(212) 889-3141

or

NAVH San Francisco regional office (for states west of the Mississippi)
3201 Balboa Street
San Francisco, CA 94121
(415) 221-3201
A list of low-vision facilities is available by state. Visual aid counseling and visual aids, peer support groups, and more intensive counseling are offered at both offices. Some counseling is done by mail or phone. Maintains a large-print loan library.

National Federation of the Blind
1800 Johnson Street
Baltimore, MD 21230
(410) 659-9314 (for general information)
(800) 638-7518 (for job opportunities for the blind)
website: http://www.nfb.org
Membership organization providing information, networking, and

resources through 52 affiliates in all states, DC, and Puerto Rico. Some aids and appliances available through national headquarters. The Diabetics Division publishes a free quarterly newsletter, *Voice of the Diabetic*, in print or on cassette.

National Library Service (NLS) for the Blind and Physically Handicapped
Library of Congress
1291 Taylor Street, NW
Washington, DC 20542
(202) 707-5100
(202) 707-0744 (TDD)
(800) 424-8567 (to speak with a reference person)
(800) 424-9100 (to leave a message)
Encore, a monthly magazine on flexible disk (record), includes articles from *Diabetes Forecast*. It is available on request through the NLS program to individuals registered with talking book program.

Recordings for the Blind and Dyslexic (RFBD)
20 Roszel Road
Princeton, NJ 08540
(609) 452-0606 (voice)
(609) 987-8116 (fax)
(800) 221-4792 (weekdays 8:30–4:45 EST)
website: http://www.rfbd.org

Audiotape library for the print-handicapped registered with RFB. Free loan of cassettes for up to a year; 80,000 titles on cassette.

The Seeing Eye, Inc.
PO Box 375
Morristown, NJ 07963-0375
(201) 539-4425 (voice)
(201) 539-0922 (fax)
e-mail: semaster@seeingeye.org
Guide dog training and instruction on working with a guide dog.

For Amputees

American Amputee Foundation
PO Box 250218
Little Rock, AR 72225
(501) 666-2523 (voice)
(501) 666-8367 (fax)
Peer counseling to new amputees and their families. Information and referral. Has local chapters. Maintains list of support groups throughout U.S. Publishes newsletter.

National Amputation Foundation
73 Church Street
Malverne, NY 11565
(516) 887-3600 (voice)
(516) 887-3667 (fax)
Sponsor of Amp-to-Amp program in which new amputee is visited by amputee who has resumed normal life. A list of support groups throughout the country is available.

For Those Needing Long-Term or Home Care

National Association for Home Care (NHAC)
228 7th Street SE
Washington, DC 20003
(202) 547-7424
(202) 547-3540 (fax)
website: http://www.nahc.org
Free information for consumers about how to choose a home care agency. Send self-addressed stamped envelope.

Nursing Home Information Service
c/o National Council of Senior Citizens
8403 Colesville Road, Suite 1200
Silver Spring, MD 20910
(301) 578-8800, ext. 8839
(301) 578-8999 (fax)
Information on selecting and paying for a nursing home and choosing other long-term care alternatives.

For Finding Quality Health Care

American Medical Association
515 North State Street
Chicago, IL 60610
(312) 464-4818
website: http://www.ama–assn.org
Will tell you how to contact your county or state medical society, which will provide you with a referral to a local physician.

American Board of Medical Specialties
47 Perimeter Center East, Suite 500
Atlanta, GA 30346
(800) 776-2378
Record of physicians certified by 24 medical specialty boards. Certification status of physician available to callers. Directories of certified physicians organized by city of medical practice and alphabetically by physician names available in many libraries.

American Association for Marriage and Family Therapy
1133 15th Street NW, Suite 300
Washington, DC 20005-2710
(202) 452-0109
(800) 374-2638
(202) 223-2329
Referral to local professional marriage and family therapist.

National Association of Social Workers
750 First Street, NE, Suite 700
Washington, DC 20002-4247
(202) 408-8600
(800) 638-8799
Referral to local professional social worker.

American Association of Sex Educators, Counselors, and Therapists
PO Box 238
Mount Vernon, IA 52314-0238
For a list of certified sex therapists, send a self-addressed stamped business-size envelope.

American Association of Diabetes Educators
444 North Michigan Avenue, Suite 1240
Chicago, IL 60611
(312) 644-2233
(800) 832-6874
(312) 644-4411 (fax)
Referral to local professional diabetes educator.

The American Dietetic Association
216 West Jackson Boulevard, Suite 800
Chicago, IL 60606
(312) 899-0040
(800) 366-1655 consumer hotline; 9–4 CST, M–F only
(312) 899-1979 (fax)
Information, guidance, and referral to local professional dietitian plus Consumer Nutrition Hotline.

American Optometric Association
243 N. Lindbergh Boulevard
St. Louis, MO 63141
(314) 991-4100

Referral to state optometric association for local referral to professional optometrists.

American Board of Podiatric Surgery
1601 Dolores Street
San Francisco, CA 94110
(415) 826-3200
(415) 826-4640 (fax)
Referral to board-certified local podiatrist.

For Miscellaneous Health Information

American Academy of Ophthalmology
655 Beach Street
San Francisco, CA 94109-1336
(415) 561-8500
website: http://www.eyenet.org
For brochures on eye care and eye diseases, send a self-addressed, stamped envelope.

American Heart Association
7272 Greenville Avenue
Dallas TX 75231
(800) 242-8721
website: http://www.amhrt.org
For referral to local affiliate's Heartline, which provides information on cardiovascular health and disease prevention.

Impotence World Association
10400 Little Patuxent Parkway, Suite 485
Columbia, MD 21044
(800) 669-1603
(410) 715-9609
For information, guidance, and physician referral in each state on impotence.

Medic Alert Foundation
PO Box 1009
Turlock, CA 95381-1009
(800) 432-5378
(209) 668-3331
(209) 669-2495 (fax)
website: http://medicalert.org
To order a medical ID bracelet.

National Kidney Foundation
30 E. 33rd Street
New York, NY 10016
(800) 622-9010
(212) 889-2210
(212) 689-9261 (fax)
website: http://www.mcw.edu/nkf
For donor cards and information about transplants.

National AIDS Hotline
Centers for Disease Control and Prevention
(800) 342-2437 (24-hour)
(800) 344-7432 (Spanish)
(800) 243-7889 (TTY)
Information, counseling, and referral on issues of HIV and

AIDS, pamphlets and brochures available on request.

National Chronic Pain Outreach Association
P.O. Box 274
Millboro, VA 24460
(540) 997-5004
(540) 997-1305 (fax)
e-mail: ncpoa1@aol.com
To learn more about chronic pain and how to deal with it.

Pedorthic Footwear Association
9861 Broken Land Parkway, Suite 255
Columbia, MD 21046-1151
(800) 673-8447
Provides referrals to local certified pedorthists (people trained in fitting prescription footwear).

For Travelers

Centers for Disease Control, U.S. Government Printing Office
Superintendent of Documents
PO Box 371954
Pittsburgh, PA 15250-7954
(202) 512-1800
(202) 512-2250 (fax)
Order the brochure, *Health Information for International Travelers* (stock # 017-023-00195-7), by credit card by phone or send a check or money order for $14.

International Association for Medical Assistance to Travelers
417 Center Street
Lewiston, NY 14092
(716) 754-4883
(519) 836-3412 (fax)
A list of doctors in foreign countries who speak English and who received postgraduate training in North America or Great Britain.

International Diabetes Federation
40 Washington Street
B-1050 Brussels, Belgium
A list of International Diabetes Federation groups that can offer assistance when you're traveling.

For Exercisers

International Diabetic Athletes Association
1647 W. Bethany Home Road, #B
Phoenix, AZ 85015
(800) 898-IDAA
email: idaa@getnet.com
website: http://www.getnet.com/~idaa/
For people with diabetes interested in sports at all levels, as well as health care professionals. Newsletter available.

President's Council on Physical Fitness and Sports
701 Pennsylvania Avenue, NW, Suite 250
Washington, DC 20004
(202) 272-3421

(202) 504-2064 (fax)
For information about physical activity and fitness.

American College of Sports Medicine
PO Box 1440
Indianapolis, IN 46206-1440
(317) 637-9200
(317) 634-7817 (fax)
website: http://www.acsm.org/sportsmed
For information about health and fitness.

For People Over 50

American Association for Retired Persons (AARP)
601 E Street, NW
Washington, DC 20049
(202) 434-2277
(800) 456-2277 (pharmacy)
(202) 434-2558 (fax)
(800) 424-3410 (membership)
website: http://www.aarp.org
Prescriptions mailed to your door. Prices the same for members and nonmembers. $1 postage and shipping per order. Possible savings over drugstore prices on generic drugs, but no prices are guaranteed.

National Council on the Aging
409 3rd Street, 2nd Floor
Washington, DC 20024
(800) 424-9047
(202) 479-1200

(202) 479-0735 (fax)
Advocacy group concerned with developing and implementing high standards of care for the elderly. Referral to local agencies concerned with the elderly.

For Equal Employment Information

Equal Employment Opportunity Commission
1801 L Street NW
Washington, DC 20507
For technical assistance and filing a charge:
(800) 669-4000 (connects to nearest local EEOC office)
(202) 663-4900
(202) 663-4912 (fax)
For publications on the Americans With Disabilities Act:
(800) 669-3362
(800) 800-3302 (TDD)

American Bar Association
Commission on Mental and Physical Disability Law
740 15th Street, NW
Washington, DC 20005-1009
(202) 662-1570
(202) 662-1032 (fax)
(202) 662-1012 (TTY)
website: http://www.abanet.org
Provides information and technical assistance on all aspects of disability law.

**Disability Rights Education
and Defense Fund, Inc.**
2212 6th Street
Berkeley, CA 94710
(800) 466-4232 (voice/TDD)
(510) 644-2555 (voice/TDD)
(510) 841-8645 (fax)
e-mail: dredfca@aol.com
Provides technical assistance and
information to employers and
individuals with disabilities on disability rights legislation and policies. Assists with legal
representation.

**National Information Center for
Children and Youth With
Disabilities**
PO Box 1492
Washington, DC 20013-1492
(800) 695-0285 (voice)
(202) 884-8200 (voice and TDD)
(202) 884-8441 (fax)
website: http://www.aed.org/
nichcy
Maintains database containing up-
to-date information on disability
topics.

Health Insurance Information

Social Security Administration
(800) 772-1213

Medicare Hotline
(800) 638-6833

The booklet, *Guide to Health
Insurance for People With Medicare,*
written by the National
Association of Insurance
Commissioners and the Health
Care Financing Administration of
the Department of Health and
Human Services, is updated every
year and is available through any
insurance company. Ask for it. It
contains the federal standards for
Medigap policies and general
information about Medicare. For
a more detailed explanation of
Medicare, ask for *The Medicare
Handbook,* available from any
Social Security Administration
office. It is also available from:

Medicare Publications
Health Care Financing
Administration
6325 Security Boulevard
Baltimore, MD 21207

**Health insurance through the
AARP:**
(800) 523-5800
The AARP administers 10 health
insurance plans. For some plans,
individuals with diabetes or other
chronic illnesses are eligible within
6 months after enrolling in
Medicare Part B. For other plans, a
3-month waiting period is required
for those with conditions preexis-
tent in the 6 months preceding the

effective date of the insurance, if not replacing previous coverage.

State Insurance Departments
You may need to contact your state's insurance department, insurance commission, or health department if you have questions about insurance policy options within your state. If you want to report a complaint because your insurer has denied a claim, you should also contact the insurance department. Also, you may want to ask whether your state has an insurance risk pool. Some states have formed insurance risk pools to make it possible for individuals to obtain health insurance regardless of their state of health.

Index

Pruritus, 303
    symptoms, 303
    what to do, 303
Psychological counseling, 315, 328, 424,
        426
Psychological trauma, 112
Psychotherapy, 426–427, 437
Pubococcygeal muscles, exercising, 331
Pyelonephritis, 267–268
    prevention, 268
    symptoms, 267
    treatment, 267–268
    what to do, 267

Racial factors, 188–189
Radial nerve entrapment, 202
    symptoms, 202
    what to do, 202
Radiculopathy, 200, 262
    symptoms, 200
    what to do, 200
Reactions to diabetes medications,
        310–311
    to insulin, 310–311
    to sulfonylureas, 311
Rebound hyperglycemia, 115–117
Record keeping, 87
Rehabilitation Act of 1973, 442, 447, 451
Relationship problems, 315, 327
Relaxation therapy, 424
Renal disease, end-stage, 226–229
    symptoms, 226
    treatment, 227–229
    what to do, 227
Renal insufficiency, 224–226
    symptoms, 224
    treatment, 225–226
    what to do, 224–225
Repaglinide, 153–154
Retinal hemorrhaging, 235
Retinopathy, 232–240
    cryotreatment, 239
    laser treatment, 237–239
    nonproliferative, 233–236

prevention, 235–236
    proliferative, 236–240
    symptoms, 223, 233, 236
    treatment, 186, 234–235, 237–240
    vitrectomy, 239–240
    what to do, 233–234, 236–237
Rheumatoid arthritis, 471–472
Rhinocerebral mucormycosis, 271

Sample insulin plans, 132–137
"Saturday Night Palsy," 202
School discrimination problems, 366,
        447–451
    indications, 448
    what to do, 449–451
Sciatica, 203
Scleredema, 300
    symptoms, 300
    what to do, 300
Secondary failure, 157
Seizures flowchart, 21
Self-responsibility, 404
Sensorimotor neuropathy, 279
Severe hypoglycemia, 93–96
Sex. *See* Gender
Sexual activity, 326–332
    and blood glucose control, 323–324,
        332–333
    and hypoglycemia, 98
Sexual problems in men flowchart, 66–67
Sexual problems in women flowchart,
        70–71
Sick days, 461–464
Sick leave, 444
Side effects
    with alcohol, 153
    allergic reactions, 153
    in hypoglycemia, 153
    of oral medication, 151–154
    prevention, 154
    symptoms, 154
    what to do, 154
Signs
    of anger, 419

About the American Diabetes Association

The American Diabetes Association is the nation's leading voluntary health organization supporting diabetes research, information, and advocacy. Founded in 1940, the Association provides services to communities across the country. Its mission is to prevent and cure diabetes and to improve the lives of all people affected by diabetes.

For more than 50 years, the American Diabetes Association has been the leading publisher of comprehensive diabetes information for people with diabetes and the health care professionals who treat them. Its huge library of practical and authoritative books for people with diabetes covers every aspect of self-care—cooking and nutrition, fitness, weight control, medications, complications, emotional issues, and general self-care. The Association also publishes books and medical treatment guides for physicians and other health care professionals.

Membership in the Association is available to health care professionals and people with diabetes and includes subscriptions to one or more of the Association's periodicals. People with diabetes receive *Diabetes Forecast*, the nation's leading health and wellness magazine for people with diabetes. Health care professionals receive one or more of the Association's five scientific and medical journals.

For more information, please call toll-free:

Questions about diabetes: 1-800-DIABETES

Membership, people with diabetes: 1-800-806-7801

Membership, health professionals: 1-800-232-3472

To order ADA books or receive a free catalog: 1-800-232-6733

Visit us on the Web: www.diabetes.org

Visit us at our Web bookstore: merchant.diabetes.org